Diversified Health Occupations 4TH EDITION
ESSENTIALS

Diversified Health Occupations 4TH EDITION
ESSENTIALS

LOUISE SIMMERS, M.Ed., R.N.

◆

Madison Comprehensive High School
Mansfield, Ohio

Delmar Publishers

an *International Thomson Publishing company* I**T**P®

Albany • Bonn • Boston • Cincinnati • Detroit • London • Madrid
Melbourne • Mexico City • New York • Pacific Grove • Paris • San Francisco
Singapore • Tokyo • Toronto • Washington

Notice to the Reader

Publisher does not warrant or guarantee any of the products described herein or perform any independent analysis in connection with any of the product information contained herein. Publisher does not assume, and expressly disclaims, any obligation to obtain and include information other than that provided to it by the manufacturer.

The reader is expressly warned to consider and adopt all safety precautions that might be indicated by the activities described herein and to avoid all potential hazards. By following the instructions contained herein, the reader willingly assumes all risks in connection with such instructions.

The publisher makes no representations or warranties of any kind, including but not limited to the warranties of fitness for particular purpose or merchantability, nor are any such representations implied with respect to the material set forth herein, and the publisher takes no responsibility with respect to such material. The publisher shall not be liable for any special, consequential, or exemplary damages resulting, in whole or in part, from the readers' use of, or reliance upon, this material.

Dedication

This text is dedicated to my husband, Floyd Simmers, and our children, Joe, Karen, and Sharon, who tolerated so many things with patience and who provided encouragement, support, and assistance during its development and revision.

COVER: Design by Spiral Design Studio
Cover paintings by Alex Piejko

DELMAR STAFF

Publisher: Tim O'Leary
Acquisitions Editor: Sandy Clark
Senior Project Editor: Andrea Edwards Myers

Production Manager: Wendy A. Troeger
Production Editor: Carolyn Miller
Marketing Manager: Maura Theriault

COPYRIGHT © 1998
By Delmar Publishers
a division of International Thomson Publishing Inc.
The ITP logo is a trademark under license

Printed in the United States of America

For more information, contact:

Delmar Publishers
3 Columbia Circle Box 15015
Albany, New York 12212-5015

International Thomson
   Publishing Europe
Berkshire House 168-173
High Holburn
London WC1V7AA
England

Thomas Nelson Australia
102 Dodds Street
South Melbourne, 3205
Victoria, Australia

Nelson Canada
1120 Birchmount Road
Scarborough, Ontario
Canada M1K 5G4

International Thomson Editores
Campos Eliseos 385, Piso 7
Col Polanco
11560 Mexico D F Mexico

International Thomson Publishing Gmbh
Königswinterer Strasse 418
53227 Bonn
Germany

International Thomson Publishing Asia
221 Henderson Road #05-10
Henderson Building
Singapore 0315

International Thompson
   Publishing—Japan
Hirakawacho Kyowa Building, 3F
2-2-1 Hirakawacho
Chiyoda-ku, 102 Tokyo
Japan

6 7 8 9 10   XXX 02 01

ISBN: 0-8273-7817-3

Library of Congress Catalog Card Number: 96–13882
CIP

CONTENTS

Diversified Health Occupations, 4th Edition, Essentials was written to provide the beginning student in health occupations with the basic entry-level knowledge and skills required for a variety of health occupations. Although each specific health occupation requires specialized knowledge and skills, some knowledge and skills are applicable to many different health occupations. In short, this book was developed to provide some of the core knowledge and skills that can be used in different fields.

Diversified Health Occupations, 4th Edition, Essentials provides the student with the basic knowledge and skills required for many different health occupations. Each unit has a list of objectives, a list of key terms (with pronunciations for more-difficult words), and a list of suggested references from which the student can obtain additional information.

For each skill included in the text, both the knowledge necessary for the skill and the procedure to perform the skill are provided. By understanding the principles and the procedure, the student will develop a deeper understanding of why certain things are done and will be able to perform more competently. Procedures may vary slightly depending on the type of agency and on the kind of equipment and supplies used. By understanding the principles of the procedure, however, the student can adapt the procedure as necessary and still observe correct technique. A glossary and metric conversion chart are also provided as references for the student.

Because regulations vary from state to state regarding which procedures can be performed by a student in health occupations, it is important to check the specific regulations for your state. A health occupation worker should never perform any procedure without checking legal responsibilities. In addition, no procedure should be performed by a student unless the student has been properly taught the procedure and has been authorized to perform the procedure.

The author, Louise Simmers, received a B.S. in Nursing from the University of Maryland and an M.Ed. in Vocational Education from Kent State University. She has worked as a public health nurse, medical-surgical nurse, charge nurse in a coronary-intensive care unit, and instructor of practical nursing. She currently teaches Health Occupations at Madison Comprehensive High School in Mansfield, Ohio. She is a member of the University of Maryland Nursing Alumni Association, Sigma Theta Tau, Phi Kappa Phi, National Education Association, and American Vocational Association, and is a volunteer worker for the Richland County Red Cross. As an active member of the Health Occupations Division of the Ohio Vocational Association, Ms. Simmers has served on numerous committees and was elected to serve as president of this organization for 1982–1983. In 1980, she received the Vocational Educator of the Year Award for Health Occupations in the State of Ohio; and in 1990, she received the Diversified Health Occupations Instructor of the Year Award for the State of Ohio.

ABOUT THIS BOOK

Diversified Health Occupations, 4th Edition, Essentials was created to provide a concise, "core" foundation of learning that will enable the student to move into any health occupations career. Whether used for a tech-prep program, school-to-work program, or introductory "core" course, this text is an essential guide that meets the changing needs of health occupations education and the workplace. For best results, you may want to become familiar with the features incorporated into this text as well as the accompanying learning tools.

ADDED FEATURES

◆ Full-color design and photos enhance learning and clarify technical content.
◆ Icons denote the *integration of academics* such as math, science, and communication; *occupational safety issues* such as universal precautions, safety, OBRA requirements, and instructor's check; and *workplace-readiness* issues such as career, legal responsibility, and technology information.
◆ The text material covers the *National Health Care Skill Standards*, helping teachers implement the curriculum elements of this important document.
◆ Design ensures easy-to-read Information and Procedure sections.

CONTENT HIGHLIGHTS

◆ Basic information and skills every health occupations student needs for any variety of careers.

◆ Information on managed care to help students better understand the changing work environments they will encounter.

◆ The latest information on universal precautions, OBRA requirements, and isolation techniques.

◆ Information on the National Health Care Plan and how changing economic and workplace conditions may affect health care workers.

◆ Information on workplace-readiness skills to help prepare students for the workplace and to meet the needs of school-to-work programs.

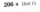

◆ Information on workplace technology to help prepare students for the modern workplace.

◆ Information on cultural diversity to prepare students for encountering people and patients of differing cultures, thus helping to foster sensitivity when dealing with others' cultural practices and beliefs.

◆ Information on legal directives to make students aware of the options of a living will and Power of Attorney so that they are knowledgable about the 1991 Patient Self-Determination Act.

EXTENSIVE TEACHING AND LEARNING PACKAGE

Diversified Health Occupations, 4th Edition, Essentials has a complete and specially designed supplement package to enhance student learning and workplace preparation. It also is designed to assist instructors in planning and implementing their instructional programs for the most efficient use of time and resources. The package contains:

Teacher's Resource Kit

Order # 0-8273-7824-6
A complete guide to implementing a diversified health occupations course! The kit explains how to apply content to applied academics and the National Health Care Skill Standards. It also provides classroom-management ideas, lesson plans, various testing materials, classroom activities, leadership-development activities, and various resource materials such as transparency masters. The kit also contains a **Computerized Testbank** of over 1,000 questions that can be used to create quizzes and tests.

Computerized Testbank

Order # 0-8273-7825-4
Contains over 1,000 questions and answers in both MAC and 3.5" Windows® format.

Student Workbook

Order # 0-8273-7820-3
Contains perforated, performance-based assignment and evaluation sheets. The assignment sheets are designed to help students review learning. The evaluation sheets are designed to provide criteria or standards for judging student performance for each procedure in the text.

Instructor's Guide

Order # 0-8273-7818-1
Provides easy-to-find answers to questions in the *student workbook.*

Anatomy and Physiology Transparencies

Over 100 Anatomy and Physiology transparencies—in full color—reinforce learning in a visual format.

Diversified Health Occupations Activity Software (3.5" Windows™)

Order # 0-8273-7954-4
A great way to assess and reinforce your understanding of skills and knowledge required for success. Each activity draws from over 900 random questions, so you never play the same game twice!

Diversified Health Occupations Videos

A set of four videos that directly correlate to the text. The videos present career- and workplace-readiness issues.

Complete Video Package
Order # 0-8273-7982-X

Video Series Instructor's Manual

Video 1: Is a Career in Health Care for You?,
Order # 0-8273-8276-6 • Video 2: A Day in the Life of Health Care Services, **Order # 0-8273-8277-4** • Video 3: Professional and Personal Standards for Health Care Careers, **Order # 0-8273-8278-2** • Video 4: How to Succeed in Your Health Care Career, **Order # 0-8273-8279-0**

ACKNOWLEDGMENTS

The author would like to thank everyone who participated in the development of this text, including

Nancy L. Raynor, Chief Consultant, Health Occupations Education, State of North Carolina, who served as a consultant

Dr. Charles Nichols, Department Head, and Ray Jacobs, Teacher Educator, Kent State University

Nancy Webber, R.N., Diversified Health Occupations Instructor

Each person who consented to be a subject in the photographs

Administrative staff at Madison Comprehensive High School

Carolynn Townsend, Lisa Shearer Cooper, Donna Story, and Dorothy Fishman, who contributed unit information

The author and Delmar Publishers would like to thank those individuals who reviewed the manuscript and offered suggestions, feedback, and assistance. The text has been improved as a result of the reviewers' helpful, insightful, and creative suggestions. Their work is greatly appreciated.

Lauretta Atkinson
Mays Landing, New Jersey

Janet Bailey
Plano, Texas

Jeannette Bice
Talladega, Alabama

Diana Bontempo
Orlando, Florida

Marge Connelly
Rochester, Minnesota

Marla Keeth
Sunland, California

Caroly Kellam
Bryan, Texas

Barbara Lenta
Syracuse, New York

Meri-Kathryn Peed
Charlotte, North Carolina

Vickie Poole
South Boston, Virginia

Cheryl Volkmer
Toledo, Ohio

The author also wishes to thank the following companies for information and/or illustrations.

A-dec, Inc.
Belmont Equipment Corporation
Burdick Corporation
Computer Identics
Control-o-fax Office Systems
Food and Agriculture Organization of the United Nations
Harbor UCLA Diagnostic Imaging Center
Health Occupations Students of America
J. T. Posey Company
Physician's Record Company
UNISYS Corporation
Vocational Industrial Clubs of America, Inc.

Basic Health Care
CONCEPTS and SKILLS

A LETTER TO THE STUDENT

Welcome to the world of health occupations. You have chosen a career in a field that offers endless opportunities. If you learn and master the knowledge and skills required, you can find employment in any number of rewarding occupations.

There will always be a need for workers in health occupations because such workers provide services that cannot be performed by automation or a machine. Thus, although the future will bring changes, you will always be an important part of providing care or services needed.

The material that follows will provide you with a good start toward your career goal. As you learn to use the information presented in the pages that follow, I encourage you to always continue to learn and to grow. All material is presented in a manner to make learning as easy as possible. However, you must still make the effort to achieve the standards set and to perform to the best of your ability.

I expect that you will find this book different from previous books that you have used. If you read the introductory material that follows, you will understand how to use this book. I think you will enjoy working with it, because it will allow you to constantly see how much progress you are making. In addition, it is probably the only book you will have used that allows you to practice tests or evaluations before you actually take them.

One final word. You are entering a field that provides one of the greatest rewards: that of working to assist others. Although the work is hard at times, you will always have the satisfaction of knowing that you are helping other people. So, be proud of yourself. When you learn the concepts and skills well, you will provide services that are appreciated by all.

INTRODUCTION

This text is divided into fifteen units. Each unit covers several topics. The topics presented are designed to provide you with the basic knowledge and skills required for many different health careers. Before starting a unit, read the unit objectives so you will know exactly what is expected of you. The objectives identify the competencies you should have mastered upon completing the unit.

Diversified Health Occupations, 4th Edition, Essentials has a textbook and a workbook. Each unit in the textbook is subdivided into Information sections. At the end of most of these sections you will find a statement telling you to go to the workbook to complete an assignment sheet on the information covered. Some units also include Procedure sections, each of which refers you to an evaluation sheet in the workbook. Following are brief explanations of these main components.

1. *Information Sections (Textbook)*: The Information sections are designed to provide the basic knowledge you must acquire. These sections explain why the knowledge is important, the basic facts regarding the particular topic, and how this information is applied in various health careers. Most Information sections refer you to specific assignment sheets in the workbook.

   Some Information sections are designed to provide the basic knowledge you must have to perform a given procedure. These sections explain why things are done, give necessary facts, stress key points that should be observed, and, again, refer you to specific assignment sheets in the workbook.

2. *Assignment Sheets (Workbook)*: The assignment sheets provide review of the main facts and information presented in the textbook. After you have read an Information section in the text, try to answer the questions on the assignment sheet. Refer back to the Information section to see whether your answers are correct. Let your instructor grade your completed assignment sheets. Note and learn from any changes or corrections. Be sure you understand the information before going on to another Information section or performing the corresponding procedure.

3. *Procedure Sections (Textbook)*: The Procedure sections provide step-by-step instructions on how to perform the procedures. Follow the steps while you practice the procedures. Each procedure begins with a list of the necessary equipment and supplies. On occasion, you will see any or all of three words within the procedure sections: Note, Caution, and Checkpoint. Note means to carefully read the comments following. These comments usually stress points of knowledge or explain why certain techniques are used. Caution means that a safety factor is involved and that you should proceed carefully while doing the step in order to avoid injuring yourself or the patient. Checkpoint means to ask your instructor to check you at that point in the procedure. Checkpoints are usually located at critical points in the procedures. Each procedure section refers you to a specific evaluation sheet in the workbook.

4. *Evaluation Sheets (Workbook)*: Each evaluation sheet contains a list of criteria on which you will be tested when you have mastered a particular procedure. Make sure that your performance meets the standards set. When you feel you have mastered a particular procedure, sign the evaluation sheet and give it to your instructor. Your instructor will grade you by using the listed criteria and checking each step against your performance.

In addition to these components, you will also find a list of Suggested References at the end of each unit in the textbook. If you want additional information about the topics discussed, refer to these references.

Finally, you will notice various icons throughout the textbook. The purpose of these icons is to accentuate particular factors or denote specific types of knowledge. The icons and their meanings are as follows:

 Observe Universal Precautions   Instructors Check—Call Instructor at This Point

 Safety—Proceed with Caution   OBRA Requirement— Based on Federal Law

 Math Skill   Legal Responsibility

 Science Skill   Career Information

 Communications Skill   Technology

UNIT 1

Health Care Systems

After completing this unit of study, you should be able to:

◆ Describe at least eight types of health care facilities
◆ Analyze at least two government agencies and the services offered by each
◆ Describe at least three services offered by nonprofit agencies
◆ Compare the basic principles of at least four different health insurance plans
◆ Explain the purpose of organizational structures in health care facilities
◆ Identify at least three current trends or changes in health care
◆ Define, pronounce, and spell all of the key terms

KEY TERMS

Centers for Disease Control (CDC)
clinics
cost containment
dental offices
diagnostic related groups (DRGs)
emergency care services
Food and Drug Administration (FDA)
geriatric care
health departments
health insurance plans
health maintenance organizations (HMOs)
home health care
hospice

hospitals
industrial health care centers
laboratories
long-term care facilities (LTCs or LTCFs)
managed care
Medicaid
medical offices
Medicare
mental health
National Institutes of Health (NIH)
nonprofit agencies
Occupational Safety and Health Administration (OSHA)

Omnibus Budget Reconciliation Act (OBRA)
organizational structure
preferred provider organization (PPOs)
rehabilitation
school health services
U.S. Department of Health and Human Services (DHHS)
voluntary agencies
wellness
Worker's Compensation
World Health Organization (WHO)

Note: *To further emphasize the Key Terms, they appear in color in the unit copy.*
You will notice beginning in Unit 2 on page 16 that pronunciations have been provided for the more difficult key terms.
The single accent mark, _'_, shows where the main stress is placed when saying the word. The double accent, _"_, shows secondary stress (if present in the word).

INTRODUCTION

Health care systems include the many agencies, facilities, and personnel involved in the delivery of health care. According to U.S. government statistics, health care is one of the largest and fastest-growing industries in the United States. This industry employs over 9.8 million workers in over 200 different health careers. By the year 2005, employment is expected to increase to over 13.8 million workers. Health care has become a 2-billion-dollar-per-day business.

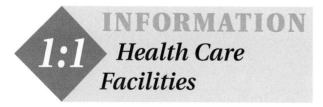

INFORMATION
1:1 Health Care Facilities

Many different health care facilities provide services that are a part of the industry called *health care,* figure 1-1. A basic description of the various facilities will help provide an understanding of the many different types of services included under the umbrella of the health care industry.

Hospitals are one of the major types of health care facilities. They vary in size and types of service provided. Some hospitals are small and serve the basic needs of a community; others are large, complex centers offering a wide range of services including treatment, education, and research. Hospitals are also classified as private, religious, nonprofit, and government, depending on the sources of income received by the hospital. Some hospitals are general hospitals treating a wide range of conditions, but others are speciality hospitals caring for only special conditions or age groups. Examples of speciality hospitals include burn hospitals, cancer hospitals, pediatric (or children's) hospitals, psychiatric hospitals (dealing with mental diseases and disorders), orthopedic hospitals (dealing with bone, joint, or muscle disease), and rehabilitative hospitals (offering services such as physical and occupational therapy). Government hospitals include the many facilities located throughout the world that provide care for government service personnel and their dependents.

Figure 1-1 Different health care facilities *(Top photo by Michael Dzaman; Middle photo courtesy of Metro Life Flight, Cleveland, OH)*

Other examples of government hospitals include Veterans Administration hospitals (which provide care for veterans), state psychiatric hospitals, and state rehabilitation centers. University or college medical centers provide hospital services along with research and education. They can be funded by private and/or governmental sources. In any type of hospital facility, a wide range of trained health workers is needed at all levels.

Long-term care facilities (LTCs or LTCFs) mainly provide assistance and care for elderly patients, usually called *residents.* However, they also provide care for individuals with disabilities or handicaps and individuals with chronic or long-term illness. Some facilities are called *nursing homes* or *geriatric homes.* These are designed to provide basic physical care to individuals who can no longer care for themselves. Others are called *extended care facilities.* These are designed to provide skilled nursing care and rehabilitative care to prepare patients or residents for return to home environments or other long-term care facilities. Many of these facilities also offer special services such as the delivery of meals to the homes of the elderly, chronically ill, or people with disabilities. Some facilities offer senior citizen or adult day care centers, which provide social activities and other services for the elderly. The need for long-term care facilities has increased dramatically due to the large increase in the number of elderly people. Therefore, many health career opportunities are available in this field.

Medical offices vary from offices that are privately owned by one doctor to large complexes that operate as corporations and employ many doctors and other health care professionals. Medical services obtained in these facilities can include diagnosis (determining the nature of an illness), treatment, examination, basic laboratory testing, minor surgery, and other similar care. Some medical doctors treat a wide variety of illnesses and age groups, but others specialize in and handle only certain age groups or conditions. Examples of specialities include pediatrics (infants and children), cardiology (diseases and disorders of the heart), and obstetrics (care of the pregnant female).

Dental offices vary in size from offices that are privately owned by one or more dentists to dental clinics that employ a number of dentists. In some areas, major retail or department stores operate dental clinics. Dental services can include general care provided to all age groups or specialized care offered to certain age groups or for certain dental conditions.

Clinics are health care facilities found in many types of health care. Some clinics are composed of a group of medical or dental doctors who share a facility and other personnel. Other clinics are operated by private groups who provide special care. Examples include surgical clinics that perform minor surgical procedures; emergency care clinics; rehabilitation clinics that offer physical, occupational, speech, and other similar therapies; and specialty clinics such as diabetic or oncology (cancer) clinics. Many hospitals operate clinics for outpatients (patients who are not admitted to the hospital). Health departments offer clinics for pediatric health care; treatment of sexually transmitted diseases and respiratory disease; immunizations; and other special services. Medical centers at colleges or universities offer clinics for various health conditions. These clinics often offer free care and treatment to provide learning experiences for medical students.

Emergency care services provide special care for victims of accidents or sudden illness. Facilities providing these services include ambulance services, both private and governmental; rescue squads, frequently operated by fire departments; emergency care clinics and centers; emergency rooms operated by hospitals; and helicopter or airplane emergency services that rapidly transport patients to medical facilities for special care.

Laboratories are often a part of other facilities but can operate as separate health care services. Medical laboratories can perform special diagnostic tests such as blood or urine tests. Dental laboratories can prepare dentures (false teeth) and many other devices used to repair or replace teeth. Medical and dental offices, small hospitals, clinics, and many other health care facilities frequently use the services provided by laboratories.

Home health care agencies are designed to provide care in a patient's home. The services of these agencies are frequently used by the elderly and disabled. Examples of such services include nursing care, personal care, therapy (physical, occupational, speech, respiratory, etc.), and homemaking (food preparation, cleaning, etc.). Health departments, hospitals, private agencies, government agencies, and nonprofit or volunteer groups can offer home care services.

Hospice agencies provide care for terminally ill persons with life expectancies of 6 months or less. Care can be provided in the person's home or in a hospice facility. Care is directed toward allowing the person to die with dignity and in comfort. Psychological, social, spiritual, and financial counseling are provided for both the patient and the family.

Mental health facilities treat patients with mental disorders and diseases. Examples of these facilities include guidance and counseling centers, psychiatric clinics and hospitals, chemical abuse treatment centers (dealing with alcohol and drug abuse), and physical abuse treatment centers (dealing with child abuse, spousal abuse, etc.).

Rehabilitation facilities are located in hospitals, clinics, and/or private centers. They provide care to help patients with physical or mental disabilities obtain maximum self-care and function. Services may include physical, occupational, recreational, speech, and hearing therapy.

Health maintenance organizations (HMOs) provide total health care directed toward preventative health care. Services include examinations, basic medical services, health education, and hospitalization or rehabilitation services as needed. Some HMOs are operated by large industries or corporations; others are operated by private agencies. They often use the services of other health care facilities including medical and dental offices, hospitals, rehabilitative centers, home health care agencies, clinics, and laboratories.

Industrial health care centers are found in large companies or industries. Such centers provide health care for employees of the industry or business by performing basic examinations; teaching accident prevention and safety; and providing emergency care.

School health services are found in schools and colleges. These services provide emergency care for victims of accidents and sudden illness; perform tests to check for health conditions such as speech, vision, and hearing problems; promote health education; and maintain a safe and sanitary school environment. Many school health services also provide counseling.

All health care facilities require many different health care workers at all levels of training.

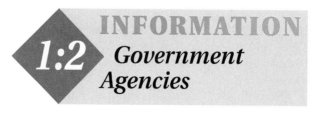

1:2 INFORMATION
Government Agencies

In addition to the government health care facilities mentioned previously, other health services are offered at international, national, state, and local levels.

The World Health Organization (WHO) is an international agency sponsored by the United Nations. It compiles statistics and information on disease, publishes health information, and investigates and addresses serious health problems throughout the world.

The U. S. Department of Health and Human Services (DHHS) is a national agency that deals with the health problems in the United States. One division of the DHHS is the National Institutes of Health (NIH), which is involved in research on disease. Another division is the Centers for Disease Control (CDC), which is concerned with causes, spread, and control of diseases in populations. The Food and Drug Administration (FDA) is a federal agency responsible for regulating food and drug products sold to the public. Another important federal agency is the Occupational Safety and Health Administration (OSHA). It establishes and enforces standards that protect workers from job-related injuries and illnesses.

State and local (county and city) health departments provide health services as directed by the Department of Health and Human Services (DHHS) and also provide specific services needed by the state or local community. Examples of services include immunization for disease control; inspections for environmental health and sanitation; collection of statistics and records related to health, health education, and clinics; and other services needed in a community.

Government services are tax supported. To provide all necessary services, many health care workers are needed at all levels.

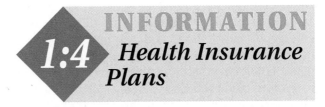

INFORMATION
1:3 Nonprofit Agencies

Nonprofit agencies, frequently called voluntary agencies, are supported by contributions. They provide health services at national, state, and local levels.

Examples of nonprofit agencies include the American Cancer Society, the American Heart Association, the American Respiratory Disease Association, the Diabetic Association, the National Association of Mental Health, the National Foundation of the March of Dimes, and the American Red Cross. Many of these organizations have national offices as well as branch offices in states and/or local communities.

As indicated by their names, many such organizations focus on one specific disease or group of diseases. Each organization typically studies the disease, provides funding to encourage research directed at curing or treating the disease, and promotes public education regarding information obtained through research. These organizations also provide special services to victims of disease, such as purchasing medical equipment and supplies, providing treatment centers, and supplying information regarding other community agencies that offer assistance.

Nonprofit agencies employ many health care workers in addition to using volunteer workers to provide services.

INFORMATION
1:4 Health Insurance Plans

In order to pay for the costs of health care, most people rely on health insurance plans. Without insurance, the cost of an illness can mean financial disaster for an individual or family.

Hospital and other health insurance plans are offered by several thousand insurance agencies. A common example is Blue Cross-Blue Shield. In this type of plan, a premium (or payment) is made to the insurance company. When the insured individual incurs health care expenses covered by the insurance plan, the insurance company pays for the services. The amount of payment and the type of services covered vary from plan to plan. Most insurance plans have limits on payments and deductibles. *Deductibles* are amounts that must be paid by the patient. Another term for deductibles is *co-insurance*, where expenses are shared by the patient and insurance company. For example, in an 80%—20% co-insurance, the company pays 80% of covered expenses, and the patient pays the remaining 20%. Many individuals have insurance coverage through their places of employment (called group insurance), where the premiums are paid by the employer and/or individual. Private policies are also available for purchase by individuals.

A health maintenance organization is another type of health insurance plan. A monthly fee or premium is paid for membership, and the fee stays the same regardless of the amount of health care used. The premium can be paid by an employer and/or an individual. Total care provided is directed toward preventative type health care. An individual insured under this type of plan has ready access to health examinations and early treatment and detection of disease. Because most other types of insurance plans do not cover routine examinations and preventative care, the individual insured by an HMO can therefore theoretically maintain a better state of health. The disadvantage of an HMO is that the insured is required to use only HMO-affiliated health care providers (doctors, labs, hospitals) for health care. If a non-affiliated health care provider is used instead, the insured usually must pay for the care.

A preferred provider organization (PPO) is another type of health insurance plan usually provided by large industries or companies to their employees. The industry or company forms a contract with certain health care agencies, such as a large hospital and/or specific doctors and dentists, to provide certain types of health care at reduced rates. Employees are restricted to using the specific hospital and/or doctors, but the industry or company can provide health care at lower rates.

The government also provides health insurance plans for certain groups of people. Two of the main plans are Medicare and Medicaid.

Medicare provides hospital care for almost all individuals over the age of 65 and for any person with a disability who has received Social Security benefits for at least 2 years. Medicare consists of two kinds of coverage: type A for hospital insurance, and type B for medical insurance. Type A covers hospital care and care provided by an extended care facility or home-health care agency after hospitalization. Type B offers additional coverage for doctor's services, outpatient treatments, therapy, and other health care. The individual does pay a premium for type B coverage and also must pay an initial deductible for services. In addition, Medicare pays for only 80% of the services; the individual must either pay the balance or have another insurance policy to cover the expenses.

Medicaid is a medical assistance program operated by individual states. The individuals covered under this program vary slightly from state to state. This health insurance plan usually pays for the health care of welfare recipients, individuals who are physically disabled or blind, and needy people over age 65.

Worker's Compensation is a health insurance plan providing treatment for workers injured on the job. It is administered by the state, and payments are made by employers and the state. In addition to providing payment for needed health care, this plan also reimburses the worker for wages lost because of on-the-job injury.

The United States government also provides health care for all military personnel. In addition, a health insurance plan called CHAMPUS (the Civilian Health and Medical Programs for the Uniform Services) provides care for military dependents and retired members of the Armed Forces. The Veterans Administration provides for military veterans.

Managed care is an approach that has developed in response to rising health care costs. Employers as well as insurance companies who pay large medical bills want to ensure that such money is spent efficiently rather than wastefully. The principle behind managed care is that all health care provided to a patient must have a purpose. A second opinion or verification of need is frequently required before care can be provided. Every effort is made to provide preventative care and early diagnosis of disease in order to avoid the high cost of treating disease. Employers and insurance companies create a network of doctors, specialists, therapists, and health care facilities that provide care at the most reasonable cost. Health maintenance organizations and preferred provider organizations are the main providers of managed care, but many private insurance companies are establishing health care networks to provide care to their subscribers. As these health care networks compete for the consumer dollar, they are required to provide quality care at the lowest possible cost. The health care consumer who is enrolled in a managed care plan receives quality care at the most reasonable cost, but is restricted in choice of health care providers.

Health insurance plans do not solve all health care problems, but they do help many people, paying for all or part of the cost of health services.

All health care facilities must have some type of **organizational structure.** The structure may be complex, as in larger facilities, or simple, as in smaller facilities. Organizational structure always, however, encompasses a line of authority or chain of command. The organizational structure should indicate areas of responsibility and lead to the most efficient operation of the facility.

A sample organizational chart for a large general hospital is shown in figure 1-2. This chart shows organization by department. Each department, in turn, can have an organizational chart similar to the one shown for the nursing department in figure 1-2. A simple organizational chart for a small medical office is shown in figure 1-3. The organizational structure will vary with the size of the office and the number of people employed.

In both organizational charts illustrated, the lines of authority are clearly indicated. It is important for health care workers to identify and understand their respective positions in a given facility's organizational structure. By doing this, they will know their lines of authority and understand who are the immediate supervisors in charge of their work. It is also important for health care workers to understand the functions and goals of the organization.

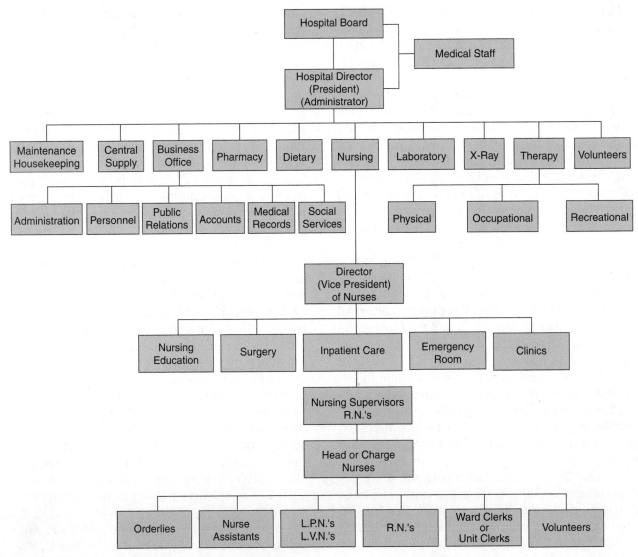

Figure 1-2 A sample hospital organizational chart

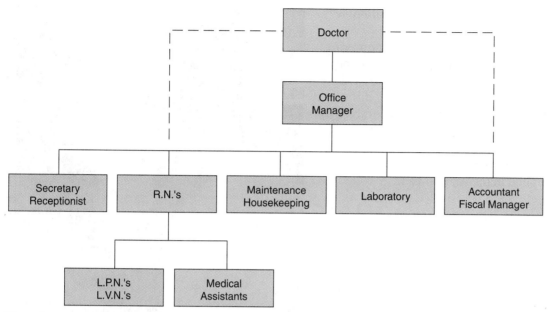

Figure 1-3 A sample medical office organizational chart

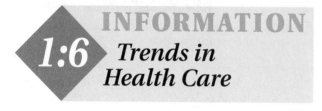

INFORMATION
1:6 *Trends in Health Care*

Health care has seen many changes during the past several decades, and many additional changes will occur in the years to come. An awareness of such changes and trends is important for any health care worker.

COST CONTAINMENT

Cost containment, a term heard frequently in health care circles, means trying to control the rising cost of health care. Highly technical and specialized procedures such as heart, lung, liver, or kidney transplants can cost hundreds of thousands of dollars. Even so, many of these procedures are performed daily throughout the United States. Artificial hearts are another new technology being used. Computers that can be used to examine internal body parts are valuable diagnostic tools. These devices can cost thousands and even millions of dollars. Since the expenses must be paid, health care costs could rise to levels that could prohibit the use of new technology. All aspects of health care are therefore directed toward cost containment. Although there is no firm answer to controlling health costs, most agencies that deliver health care are trying to provide care at the lowest possible price.

Diagnostic related groups (DRGs) are one way Congress is trying to control costs for government insurance plans such as Medicare and Medicaid. Under this plan, patients with certain diagnoses who are admitted to hospitals are classified in one payment group. A limit is placed on the cost of care, and the agency providing care receives this set amount. This encourages the agency to make every effort to provide care within the expense limit allowed. If the cost of care is less than the amount paid, the agency keeps the extra money. If the cost of care is more than the amount paid, the agency must accept the loss.

Many agencies are combining services to eliminate duplication of services. Clinics, laboratories shared by different agencies, health maintenance organizations, and other similar agencies all represent attempts to control the rising cost of health care.

Outpatient services, where patients receive care without being admitted to hospitals or other care facilities, have increased greatly. Surgery, X-rays, diagnostic tests, and many other procedures that once required admission to a hospital are now done on an outpatient basis.

Mass or bulk purchasing—buying equipment and supplies in larger quantities at reduced prices—is another means of controlling costs. This can be done by combining the purchases of different departments in a single agency, or by combining the purchases of several different agencies.

The preceding are just a few examples of cost containment, and many other methods will undoubtedly be applied in the years ahead.

HOME HEALTH CARE

Home health care is a rapidly growing field. Diagnostic related groups and shorter hospital stays have created a need for providing care in the home. Years ago, home care was the usual method of treatment. Doctors made house calls, private duty nurses cared for patients in the patients' homes, babies were delivered at home, and patients died at home. Current trends show a return to some of these practices. Home care is also another form of cost containment because it is usually less expensive to provide this type of care. All aspects of health care can be involved. Nursing care; physical and occupational therapy; respiratory therapy; social services; nutritional and food services; and many other types of care can be provided in the home environment.

GERIATRIC CARE

Geriatric care, or care for the elderly, is another field that will continue to experience rapid growth in the future (figure 1-4). This is due in part to the large number of individuals who are experiencing longer life spans thanks to advances in health care. Many people now enjoy life spans of eighty years or more. Years ago, very few people lived to be 100 years old. This is becoming more and more common. Also, the "baby boom" generation—the large number of people born after World War II—will reach the geriatric age classification in the near future. Many different facilities will be involved in providing care and resources for this age group. Adult day care centers, retirement commu-

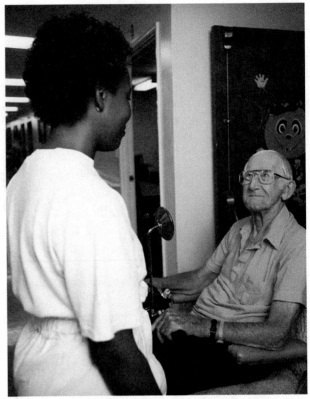

Figure 1-4 Geriatric care is a field that will continue to experience rapid growth.

nities, long-term care facilities, and other organizations will all see increased demand for the services they provide.

OBRA The Omnibus Budget Reconciliation Act (OBRA) of 1987 has led to the development of many regulations regarding long-term care and home health care. This act requires states to establish training and competency evaluation programs for nursing and geriatric assistants. Each assistant working in a long-term care facility is now required under federal law to complete a mandatory, state-approved training program and pass a written and/or competency examination to obtain certification or registration. Each state then maintains a registry of qualified individuals. The Omnibus Budget Reconciliation Act also requires compliance with patients'/residents' rights, and forces states to establish guidelines to ensure that such rights are observed and enforced. These regulations serve to ensure certain standards of care. As the need for geriatric care increases, additional regulations may be created. It is important that every health care worker be informed about all OBRA regulations in order to comply with these regulations.

WELLNESS

Wellness, or the state of being in optimum health, is another major trend in health care. People are more aware of the need to maintain health and prevent disease. More individuals are recognizing the importance of exercise, good nutrition, weight control, healthy living habits, and other similar factors. This has led to the establishment of wellness centers, weight control facilities, health food stores, nutrition services, and other organizations.

ALTERNATIVE METHODS OF HEALTH CARE

Many alternative forms of health care are receiving recognition. Individuals disenchanted with regular medical or surgical care are seeking other types of treatments for a variety of conditions. Three main examples of such alternative methods are acupuncture, positive thought, and therapeutic touch. Acupuncture involves the insertion of needles at specific points in the skin to restore the internal energy balance the body requires to heal itself. It is an ancient art that modern practitioners are using to treat chronic pain, obesity, and nicotine addiction. Positive thought involves developing self-awareness, self-esteem, and love for oneself to allow the body to heal itself and eliminate disease. In the positive thought approach, disease is viewed as a negative process that can be reversed by an individual's mental processes. Relaxation techniques, yoga, meditation, and other similar therapies are also used to decrease the effects of disease and/or eliminate pain. Therapeutic touch practitioners believe in a life energy that permeates every body cell and creates a bioelectric field that extends beyond the body surface. Therapeutic touch practitioners use their hands to locate areas of weakness in this field and direct energy into the field to correct such weakness. Studies have shown that touch can induce physical relaxation and reduce anxiety, which, in turn, can decrease pain and stimulate healing. Other examples of alternative methods include hydrotherapy (water therapy); herbal medicine; massage; Shiatsu and acupressure (finger pressure

similar to acupuncture without needles); ionization therapy (wherein air ionizers produce negatively charged air particles or ions to treat common respiratory disorders); tissue salts therapy (to replace inorganic minerals missing in the body); t'ai chi (a series of flowing movements and meditation to tone both the mind and body); Gestalt therapy (self-discovery leading to self-liberation); and hypnosis. As greater numbers of individuals choose to use one or more of these forms of treatment, it will be important for health care providers to become aware of these methods in order to provide total patient care.

NATIONAL HEALTH CARE PLAN

The high cost of health care and large number of uninsured individuals have created a demand for a national health care plan. Many different types of plans have been proposed. One plan involves nationalized medicine, where the federal government would pay for all health services and levy taxes to pay for those services. Another plan involves the creation of health care cooperatives, which would allow consumers to purchase health care at lower costs. A third plan is based on managed care and requires employers to provide coverage and the federal government to subsidize insurance for the poor. Still another plan would allow each state to establish its own health care plan paid for by employers, individuals, and/or government subsidies.

The main goal in health care reform is to ensure that all Americans can get health coverage. Related problems include the cost of creating such a system, the fact that those with insurance may pay more to cover uninsured individuals, the lack of freedom in choosing health care providers, and the regulations that will have to be created to establish a national health care system.

Although the preceding are just several of the trends in health care, they do illustrate how health care has changed and how it will continue to change. Every health care worker must stay abreast of such changes and make every attempt to learn about them.

STUDENT *Go to the workbook and complete the assignment sheet for Unit 1, Health Care Systems.*

Unit 1 Summary

Health care, the largest and fastest growing industry in the United States, encompasses many different types of facilities that provide health-related services. These include hospitals; long-term care facilities; medical and dental offices; clinics; laboratories; industrial and school health services; and many others. Government and nonprofit or voluntary agencies also provide health care services. All health care facilities require different health care workers at all levels of training.

Many types of health insurance plans are available to help pay the costs of health care. Insurance does not usually cover the entire cost of care, however. It is important for consumers to be aware of the types of coverage provided by their respective insurance plans.

Organizational structure is important in all health care facilities. The structure can be complex or simple, but it should show a line of authority or chain of command within the facility and indicate areas of responsibility.

As health care continues to grow as an industry, changes and trends will occur. Issues of primary importance are cost containment to control the high cost of health care, home health care, care for the elderly, wellness to prevent the need for health care, alternative methods of health care, and a national health care plan.

Unit 1 Suggested References

Castro, Janice. *The American Way of Health.* Boston, MA: Little, Brown, and Co., 1994.

Feltman, John (Ed.). *Health Remedies and Techniques.* Emmaus, PA: Rodale Press, 1992.

Hegner, Barbara, and Esther Caldwell. *Nursing Assistant: A Nursing Process Approach.* 7th ed. Albany, NY: Delmar Publishers, 1995.

Inglis, Brian, and Ruth West. *The Alternative Health Guide.* New York, NY: Alfred Knopf, 1993.

Locke, Steven, and Douglas Colligan. *The Healer Within.* New York, NY: E.P. Dutton, 1986.

Raffel, Marshall W., and Norma K. Raffel. *The U. S. Health System: Origins and Functions.* 4th ed. Albany, NY: Delmar Publishers , 1994.

Siegel, Bernie. *Love, Medicine, and Miracles.* New York, NY: Harper and Row, 1986.

U. S. Department of Labor. *Occupational Outlook Handbook.* 1996–1997 ed. Washington, D.C.: U. S. Government Printing Office, 1996.

Williams, Catherine, and Jim Zukowski. *Basic Allied Health Education Core.* Austin, TX: EIMC, University of Texas at Austin, 1992.

Williams, Stephen. *Essentials of Health Services.* Albany, NY: Delmar Publishers, 1995.

UNIT 2

Careers in Health Care

UNIT OBJECTIVES

After completing this unit of study, you should be able to:

♦ Compare the educational requirements for associate's, bachelor's, and master's degrees

♦ Contrast certification, registration, and licensure

♦ Describe at least ten different health careers by including a definition of the career, three duties, educational requirements, and employment opportunities

♦ Investigate at least one health career by writing to listed sources to request additional information on the career

♦ Interpret at least ten abbreviations used to identify health occupations workers

♦ Define, pronounce, and spell all of the key terms (see page 5 for explanation of accent mark use)

KEY TERMS

admitting officers/clerks

animal health technicians

art, music, dance therapists

associate's degree

athletic trainers

audiologists

bachelor's degree

biomedical equipment
  technicians

central/sterile supply workers

certification

dental assistants

dental hygienists
  (den´-tall hi-geen´-ists)

dental laboratory technicians

dentists

dialysis technicians
  (die-ahl´-ih-sis tek-nish´ins)

dietetic assistants

dietetic technicians

dietitians

Doctor of Chiropractic (D.C.)
  (Ky-row-prak´-tik)

Doctor of Medicine (M.D.)

Doctor of Osteopathy (D.O.)
  (Oss-tee-ohp´-ath-ee)

Doctor of Podiatric Medicine
  (D.P.M.)
  (Poh″-dee´-ah-trik)

doctorate/doctor's degree

electrocardiograph (ECG or
  EKG) technicians
  *(ee-lek″-trow-car´-dee-oh-graf
  tek-nish´-ins)*

electroencephalographic (EEG)
  technologist
  *(ee-lek″-troh-en-sef-ahl-oh-
  graf´-ik tek-nahl´-oh-jist)*

emergency medical technician
  (EMT)

endodontics
  (en´-doe-don´-tiks)

entrepreneur
  (on″trah-peh-nor´)

geriatric aides/assistants
  (jerry-at´-rik)

health care administrators

health occupations education
  (HOE)

home health care assistants

housekeeping workers/sanitary
  managers

licensed practical/vocational
  nurses (LPNs/LVNs)

licensure
  (ly´-sehn-shur)

master's degree

medical assistants

medical laboratory assistants

medical laboratory technicians

medical records administrators

medical records technicians

medical technologists

nurse assistants

occupational therapists (OTs)

occupational therapy assistants

ophthalmic laboratory
  technicians

ophthalmologists

opticians
  (ahp-tish´-ins)

optometric
  technicians/assistants
  *(ahp-tow-meh´-trik tek-nih´-
  shins)*

optometrists (ODs)
  (ahp-tom´-eh-trists)

oral surgery

orthodontics
  (or″-thow-don´-tiks)

paramedic (EMT-P)

pedodontics
  (peh″-doe-don´-tiks)

perfusionists
  (purr-few´-shun-ists)

periodontics
  (peh″-ree-oh-don´-tiks)

pharmacists
  (far´-mah-sists)

pharmacy technicians

phlebotomists

physical therapists (PTs)

physical therapy assistants

physicians

physician assistants

prosthodontics
  (pross″-thow-don´-tiks)

psychiatric/mental health
  technicians

psychiatrists

psychologists
  (sy-koll″-oh-jists)

radiologic technologists
  *(ray″-dee-oh-loge´-ik
  tek-nahl´-oh-jists)*

recreational therapists

recreational therapy assistants

registered nurses (RNs)

registration

respiratory therapists (RTs)

respiratory therapy technicians

social workers

speech-language therapists

surgical technicians/
  technologists

unit secretaries/unit
  coordinators

veterinarians (DVM or VMD)
  (vet″-eh-ran-air´-e-ans)

veterinary assistants

ward clerks

INFORMATION
2:1 Introduction to Health Careers

There are over 200 different health care careers, so it would be impossible to discuss all of them in this unit. A broad overview of a variety of careers is presented however.

1/2 Educational requirements for health careers depend on many factors and can vary from state to state. Basic preparation begins in high school (secondary education) and should include the sciences, social studies, English, and mathematics. General typing and accounting skills are also utilized in many health occupations. Secondary vocational health occupations education (HOE) programs can prepare a student for immediate employment in many health careers or for additional education after graduation. Post-secondary education (after high school) can include training in a vocational-technical school, community college, or university. Some careers require an associate's degree, which is awarded by a vocational-technical school or a community college after completion of a prescribed two-year course of study. Other careers require a bachelor's degree, which is awarded by a college or university after a prescribed course of study that usually lasts for four or more years. In some cases, a master's degree is required. This is awarded by a college or university after completion of one or more years of work beyond a bachelor's degree. Other careers require a doctorate, or doctor's degree, which is awarded by a college or university after completion of two or more years of work beyond a bachelor's or master's degree. Some doctorates can require four to six years of additional study.

Three other terms associated with health careers are *certification, registration,* and *licensure.* These are methods used to ensure the skill and competency of health care personnel and to protect the consumer or patient.

Certification means that a person has fulfilled requirements of education and performance and meets the standards established by the professional organization or government agency that regulates a particular career. A certificate or statement is issued by the organization. Examples of certified positions include certified dental assistant, certified laboratory technician, and certified medical assistant.

Registration is required in some health occupations. This is performed by a regulatory body that administers examinations and maintains a current list ("registry") of qualified personnel in a given health care area. Examples of registered positions include registered dietitian, registered respiratory therapist, and registered animal health technician.

Licensure is a process whereby a government agency authorizes individuals to work in a given occupation. Health occupations requiring licensure can vary from state to state. Obtaining and retaining licensure usually requires that a person complete an approved educational program, pass a state board test, and maintain certain standards. Examples of licensed positions include physician, dentist, physical therapist, registered nurse, and licensed practical/vocational nurse.

Continuing education units (CEUs) are required to renew licenses or maintain certification or registration in many states. An individual must obtain additional hours of education in the specific health career area during a specified period of time. For example, many states require registered nurses to obtain twenty-four to forty-eight CEUs every one to two years in order to renew licenses. Health care workers should be aware of the state requirements regarding CEUs for their given careers.

TRAINING

Generally speaking, training for most health occupations can be categorized into four levels:

1. *Professional*—usually requires four or more years of college and often an advanced degree; an example is a medical doctor; can also apply to a technologist.
2. *Technologist or therapist*—usually requires at least three to four years of college plus work experience; examples include medical technologist and physical therapist.
3. *Technician*—usually requires a two-year associate's degree, special health occupations education, or three to four years of on-the-job training; examples include dental laboratory technician and medical laboratory technician.
4. *Assistant or aide*—usually requires up to one or more years of training combining classoom and/or on-the-job work or experience; examples include dental, medical, and nurse assistants.

A new trend in health occupations is that of the multicompetent or multiskilled worker. Because of high health care costs, smaller facilities and rural areas often cannot afford to hire a specialist for every aspect of care. Therefore, workers are hired who can perform a variety of health care skills. For example, a health care worker may be hired to perform the skills of both an electrocardiograph (ECG or EKG) technician (who records electrical activity of the heart) and an electroencephalographic (EEG) technologist (who records electrical activity of the brain). Another example might involve combining the basic skills of radiology, medical laboratory, and respiratory therapy. At times, workers trained in one field or occupation receive additional education to work in a second and even third occupation. In other cases, educational programs have been established to prepare multicompetent workers.

Another opportunity available in many health occupations is that of entrepreneur. An **entrepreneur** is an individual who organizes, manages, and assumes the risk of a business. Many health occupations allow an individual to become independent; however, even as entrepreneurs, many health professionals must still work under the direction or guidance of doctors. Examples include dental laboratory technician, physical therapist, respiratory therapist, recreational therapist, doctor, dentist, and optometrist. While entrepreneurship involves many risks and requires a certain level of education and ability, it can be an extremely satisfying choice for the individual who is well motivated, self-confident, responsible, creative, and independent.

In the following discussion of health careers, a basic description of the job duties for each career is provided. The various levels in each health occupation are also given. In addition, tables for each career group show educational requirements, job outlook, and average yearly earnings. In order to simplify the information presented in these tables, the highest level of education for each career group is listed. The designations used are as follows: on-the-job training is designated "on-the-job"; a vocational health occupations education program is "HOE program"; a two-year associate's degree is "associate's degree"; a four-year bachelor's degree is "bachelor's degree"; a master's degree with one or more years beyond a bachelor's degree is "master's degree"; and a doctorate with four or more years beyond a bachelor's degree is "doctor's degree." It is important to note that although many health ca-

reers begin with vocational HOE programs, obtaining additional education after graduation from HOE programs allows health care workers to progress in career level to higher-paying positions. The job outlook or expected job growth through the year 2005 is stated in the tables as "below average," "average," or "above average." Average yearly earning is presented as a range of income, because earnings will vary according to geographical location, specialty area, level of education, and work experience.

All career information presented includes a basic introduction. *Because requirements for various health occupations can vary from state to state, it is important for students to obtain information pertinent to their respective states.* More detailed information on any given occupation discussed can be obtained from the sources listed for that occupation's career cluster or from the references listed at the end of this unit.

2:2 INFORMATION Dental Careers

Dental workers focus on the health of the teeth and the soft tissues of the mouth. Care is directed toward preventing dental disease; repairing or replacing diseased or damaged teeth; and treating the gingiva (gums) and other supporting structures of the teeth.

Places of employment include private dental offices, laboratories, and clinics; or dental departments in hospitals, schools, health departments, or government agencies.

Most dental professionals work in general dentistry practices where all types of dental conditions are treated in people of all ages. Some, however, work in specialty areas such as the following:

◆ **Endodontics**—treatment of diseases of the pulp, nerves, blood vessels, and roots of the teeth; often called root canal treatment
◆ **Orthodontics**—alignment or straightening of the teeth
◆ **Oral Surgery**—surgery on the teeth, mouth, and jaw
◆ **Pedodontics**—dental treatment of children and adolescents

◆ Periodontics—treatment and prevention of diseases of the gum

◆ Prosthodontics—replacement of natural teeth with artificial teeth or dentures

Levels of workers in dentistry include dentist, dental hygienist, dental laboratory technician, and dental assistant (see table 2-1).

Dentists are doctors who examine teeth and mouth tissues to diagnose and treat disease and abnormalities; perform surgery on the teeth, gums, and tissues; and work to prevent dental disease. They also supervise the work of other dental workers. Most are entrepreneurs.

Dental hygienists work under the supervision of dentists. They remove stains and deposits from teeth; expose and develop X-rays; and perform other preventative or therapeutic (treatment) services. In some states, dental hygienists can be entrepreneurs.

Dental laboratory technicians make and repair a variety of dental appliances such as dentures, crowns, and orthodontic appliances according to the specifications of dentists. Specialities include dental ceramist and orthodontic technician. Some dental laboratory technicians are entrepreneurs.

Dental assistants, working under the supervision of dentists, prepare patients for examinations; pass instruments; prepare dental materials; take and develop X-rays; teach preventative dental care; sterilize instruments; and/or perform dental receptionist duties such as scheduling appointments and handling accounts. Their duties may be limited by the dental practice laws of the state in which they work.

ADDITIONAL SOURCES OF INFORMATION

◆ American Association of Dental Schools
1625 Massachusetts Avenue, NW
Washington, DC 20036
◆ American Dental Assistants' Association
203 N. Lasalle, Suite 1320
Chicago, IL 60601
◆ American Dental Association
Council on Dental Education
211 E. Chicago Avenue
Chicago, IL 60611

TABLE 2-1 **Dental Careers**

OCCUPATION	EDUCATION REQUIRED	JOB OUTLOOK TO YEAR 2005	AVERAGE YEARLY EARNINGS
Dentist	Doctor of Dental Medicine (DMD) or Doctor of Dental Surgery (DDS); 2 or more years additional education for specialization; licensure in state of practice	Average growth	$65,000–$135,000
Dental Hygienist	Associate's or bachelor's degree; licensure in state of practice	Above average growth	$25,400–$37,500
Dental Laboratory Technician	3–4 years on-the-job or 1–2 years HOE program or associate's degree; certification can be obtained from National Board for Certification in Dental Technology	Average growth	$15,400–$26,600
Dental Assistant and Certified Dental Assistant (CDA)	1–3 years on-the-job or 1–2 years in HOE program or associate's degree; certification can be obtained from Dental Assisting National Board	Above average growth	$12,500–$21,400

◆ American Dental Hygienists' Association
444 N. Michigan Avenue, Suite 3400
Chicago, IL 60611
◆ Dental Assisting National Board, Inc.
216 E. Ontario Street
Chicago, IL 60611
◆ National Association of Dental Laboratories
3801 Mt. Vernon Avenue
Alexandria, VA 22305

2:3 INFORMATION
Diagnostic Services

Health workers in the diagnostic services perform tests or evaluations that aid in the detection, diagnosis, and treatment of disease, injury, or other physical conditions.

Many workers are employed in hospital laboratories, but others work in private laboratories, doctors' offices, clinics, public health agencies, pharmaceutical (drug) firms, and research or government agencies. In some occupations, individuals are entrepreneurs, owning and operating their own businesses.

Many careers fall under the designation of diagnostic services. Some of the more common ones are discussed in this unit. There are various levels of workers in most fields (see table 2-2).

Electrocardiograph (ECG or EKG) technicians operate electrocardiograph machines, which record electrical impulses that originate in the heart. Physicians use the electrocardiogram (EKG/ECG) to help diagnose heart disease and to note changes in the condition of a patient's heart. EKG technicians having more advanced training also perform stress tests (which record the action of the heart during physical activity), Holter monitorings (EKGs lasting 24–48 hours, see figure 2-1), and other specialized cardiac tests that frequently involve the use of computers. An associate's degree leads to a position as a cardiovascular technologist. These individuals assist with cardiac catheterization procedures and angioplasty (a procedure to remove blockages in blood vessels).

An **electroencephalographic (EEG) technologist** operates an instrument called an electroencephalograph, which records the electrical activity of the brain. The record produced, called an electroencephalogram, is used by a variety of physicians, especially neurologists (doctors specializing in nerve and brain diseases), to diagnose and evaluate diseases and disorders of the brain. Electroencephalographic technologists may also operate other monitoring devices involving computers and video equipment. These devices may be used to obtain specific information regarding the function and activities of nerve cells in the brain. Another professional in this field is the EEG technician. These workers perform primarily basic functions and receive on-the-job training or training from HOE programs.

Medical technologists, also called clinical laboratory technologists, work under the supervision of doctors called pathologists. They study tissues, fluids, and cells of the human body to help

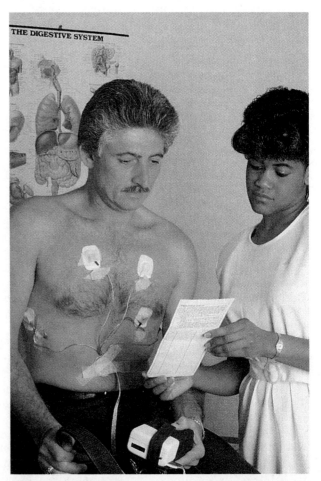

Figure 2-1 Electrocardiograph (ECG or EKG) technicians assist with Holter monitorings of the heart.

TABLE 2-2 **Diagnostic Services**

OCCUPATION	EDUCATION REQUIRED	JOB OUTLOOK TO YEAR 2005	AVERAGE YEARLY EARNINGS
Electrocardiograph (ECG/EKG) Technician	1–12 months on-the-job or 6–12-month HOE program; credentials can be obtained from National Board of Cardiovascular Testing	Below average growth	$14,200–$28,200
Electroencephalographic (EEG) Technologist	Few have 1–2 years on-the-job; 1–2-year HOE program or associate's degree; registration can be obtained from American Board of Registration of EEG Technologists	Above average growth	$17,900–$29,700
Medical Technologist (MT) **Certified Medical Technologist (CMT)**	Bachelor's or master's degree; licensure or registration required in some states; certification can be obtained from National Certification Agency for Medical Laboratory Personnel or American Medical Technologists	Average growth	$24,800–$39,500
Medical Laboratory Technician (MLT) **Certified Laboratory Technician (CLT)**	2-year HOE program or associate's degree; certification can be obtained from National Certification Agency for Medical Laboratory Personnel or American Medical Technologists; licensure or registration required in some states	Average growth	$18,700–$27,300
Medical Laboratory Assistant	1–2-year HOE program; certification can be obtained from the Board of Certified Laboratory Assistants	Average growth	$10,700–$18,100
Phlebotomist	1–2 years on-the-job or HOE program	Average growth	$11,100–$18,600
Radiologic Technologist ARRT (Registered)	Associate's degree or bachelor's degree; licensure required in some states; registration can be obtained from American Registry of Radiologic Technologies	Above average growth	$22,900–$41,700
Biomedical Equipment Technician CBET (certified)	Associate's degree or bachelor's degree; certification can be obtained from Certification Commission for Clinical Engineering and Biomedical Technology	Above average growth	$19,300–$37,400

determine the presence and/or cause of disease. They perform complicated chemical, microscopic, and automated analyzer/computer tests (see figure 2-2). In small laboratories, technologists perform many types of tests. In larger laboratories, they may specialize. Examples of specialization include: biochemistry (chemical analysis of body fluids), blood bank technology (collection and preparation of blood and blood products for transfusions), cytotechnology (study of human body cells and cellular abnormalities), hematology (study of blood cells), histology (study of human body tissue), and microbiology (study of bacteria and other microorganisms).

Medical laboratory technicians, working under the supervision of medical technologists or pathologists, perform many of the routine tests that do not require the advanced knowledge held by a medical technologist. Like the technologist, the technician can specialize in a particular field or perform a variety of tests.

Medical laboratory assistants, working under the supervision of medical technologists, technicians, or pathologists, perform basic laboratory tests; prepare specimens for examination or testing; and perform other laboratory duties such as cleaning and helping to maintain equipment.

Phlebotomists (see figure 2-3), or venipuncture technicians, collect blood and prepare it for testing. In some states, they perform blood tests under the supervision of medical technologists or pathologists.

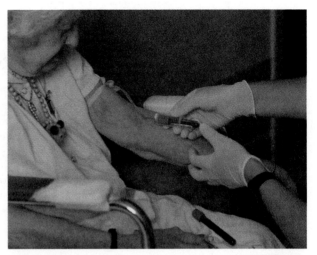

Figure 2-3 Phlebotomists collect blood and prepare it for testing.

Radiologic technologists, working under the supervision of doctors called radiologists, use X-rays, radiation, nuclear medicine, ultrasound, and magnetic resonance to diagnose and treat disease. Most techniques involve examining or treating the internal organs of patients without entering the body. In many cases, recent advances in this field have eliminated the need for surgery and, therefore, offer less risk to patients. Most radiologic technologists operate equipment used to produce images of body parts. This equipment includes X-ray machines, fluoroscopes, ultrasonic scanners, and computerized tomography (CT) scanners (formerly known as computerized axial tomography [CAT] scanners). Many radiologic technologists also provide radiation treatment. Specific job titles exist for technologists who specialize. Radiographers (see figure 2-4) take X-rays of the body for diagnosis purposes. Radiation therapy technologists administer prescribed doses of radiation to treat disease (usually cancer). Nuclear medicine technologists prepare radioactive substances for administration to patients. Once administered, these professionals use films, images on a screen, or body specimens such as blood or urine to determine how the radioactive substances pass through or localize in different parts of the body. This information is used by physicians to detect abnormalities or diagnose disease. Ultrasound technologists, or sonographers, use equipment that sends high frequency sound waves into the body. As the sound waves bounce back from the part being examined, an image of the part is viewed on a screen. This can

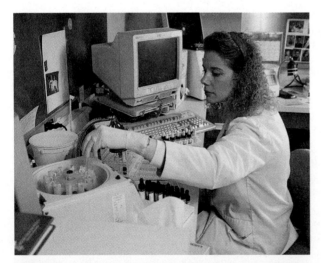

Figure 2-2 Medical technologists perform computerized blood analysis tests. *(Photo by Marcia Butterfield, courtesy of W. A. Foote Memorial Hospital, Jackson, MI)*

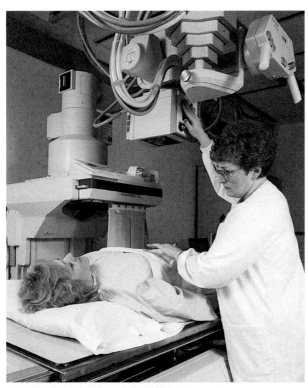

Figure 2-4 Radiologic technologists take X-rays used in the diagnosis of disease. *(Photo by Marcia Butterfield, courtesy of W. A. Foote Memorial Hospital, Jackson, MI)*

be recorded on a printout strip or be photographed. Ultrasound is frequently used to examine the fetus (developing infant) in a pregnant woman and can reveal the sex of the unborn child. Magnetic resonance imaging (MRI) is a new field where superconductive magnets and radio waves are used to produce detailed images of internal anatomy. The information is processed via computer and displayed on a videoscreen. Examples of MRI use include identifying multiple sclerosis and detecting hemorrhaging (bleeding) in the brain. A positron emission scanner (PET), another diagnostic device, uses electrons to scan the body for disease processes.

Biomedical equipment technicians work with the many different machines used to diagnose, treat, and monitor patients. They install, test, service, and repair equipment such as patient monitors, kidney machines, incubators, electrocardiographs, X-ray units, pacemakers, sterilizers, blood-gas analyzers, heart-lung machines, respirators, and other similar devices. Lives depend on the accuracy and proper operation of many of these machines, so constant maintenance and testing for defects is critical. Some biomedical equipment

technicians also teach other staff members how to use biomedical equipment.

ADDITIONAL SOURCES OF INFORMATION

- American College of Cardiology
  9111 Old Georgetown Road
  Bethesda, MD 20814
- American College of Radiology
  1891 Preston White Drive
  Reston, VA 22091
- American Medical Technologists Association
  710 Higgins Road
  Park Ridge, IL 60068
- American Registry of Radiologic Technologists
  1255 Northland Drive
  Mendota Heights, MN 55120
- American Society for Medical Technology
  7910 Woodmont Avenue, Suite 1301
  Bethesda, MD 20814
- American Society of Electroneurodiagnostic Technologists
  204 W. 7th Street
  Carroll, IA 51401
- American Society of Radiologic Technologists
  15000 Central Avenue SE
  Albuquerque, NM 87123
- International Society for Clinical Laboratory Technicians
  818 Olive Street
  St. Louis, MO 63101
- Society of Cardiovascular Technology
  1101 Connecticut Avenue NW, Suite 700
  Washington, DC 20036

INFORMATION
2:4 *Emergency Medical Services*

Emergency medical services personnel (see figure 2-5) provide emergency, prehospital care to victims of accidents, injuries, or sudden illnesses. Although individuals with only basic training in first aid do sometimes work in this field, emergency medical

Figure 2-5 Emergency medical technicians (EMTs) provide emergency, prehospital care to victims of accidents, injuries, or sudden illness.

technician (EMT) training is required for most jobs. Formal EMT training is available in all states and is offered by fire departments, hospitals, vocational schools, and as a nondegree course in technical/community colleges and universities.

Places of employment include fire and police departments; rescue squads; ambulance services; hospital or private emergency rooms; urgent care centers; industry; emergency helicopter services; and the military. Some EMTs are also entrepreneurs. Emergency medical technicians also sometimes serve as volunteers in fire and rescue departments.

Levels of EMT include the EMT ambulance/basic, EMT intermediate, and EMT paramedic (see table 2-3).

Emergency medical technicians ambulance/basic (EMT-A) provide care for a wide range of illnesses and injuries including medical emergencies, bleeding, fractures, airway obstruction, oxygen administration, emergency childbirth, rescue of trapped persons, and transporting of victims.

Emergency medical technician defibrillator (EMT-D) is a new level of EMT-A. It allows EMT-As with additional training and competency in basic life support to administer electrical defibrillation to certain heart attack victims.

Emergency medical technicians intermediate (EMT-I) perform the same tasks as do EMT-As along with assessing patients, managing shock, using intravenous equipment, and inserting esophageal airways.

Emergency medical technicians paramedic (EMT-P) perform all of the basic EMT duties plus in-depth patient assessment, provision of ad-

TABLE 2-3 Emergency Medical Services

OCCUPATION	EDUCATION REQUIRED	JOB OUTLOOK TO YEAR 2005	AVERAGE YEARLY EARNINGS
Emergency Medical Technician Ambulance/Basic (EMT-A)	Usually minimum 100–120-hour approved EMT program plus 10 hours of internship in emergency room; state certification; registration by National Registry of EMTs required in some states	Above average growth	$18,800–$32,300
Emergency Medical Technician Intermediate (EMT-I)	Additional approved training of at least 35–55 hours with clinical experience; state certification; registration required in some states	Above average growth	$20,100–$34,600
Emergency Medical Technician Paramedic (EMT-P)	Additional 3–6 months (700–2,000 hours) approved paramedic training; 6 months experience as paramedic; state certification; registration or licensure required in most states	Above average growth	$23,700–$37,400

vanced life support, EKG interpretation, endotracheal intubation, drug administration, and operation of complex equipment.

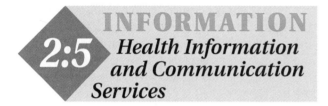

ADDITIONAL SOURCES OF INFORMATION

◆ National Association of Emergency Medical Technicians
9140 Ward Parkway
Kansas City, MO 64114
◆ National Registry of Emergency Medical Technicians
6610 Busch Boulevard
Columbus, OH 43229

INFORMATION
2:5 Health Information and Communication Services

Health information and communication services employ many different types of health workers at all levels. Careers include medical records workers

(who maintain complete accurate patient records), medical illustrators, photographers, writers, and librarians (see table 2-4). Computers are used in almost all of the careers.

Places of employment include hospitals, clinics, research centers, health departments, long-term care facilities, colleges, law firms, and insurance companies.

Medical records administrators plan the systems for storing and obtaining information from records; prepare information for legal actions and insurance claims; compile statistics for organizations and government agencies; manage medical records departments; and supervise and train other personnel. Because computers are used in almost all aspects of the job, it is essential for the medical records administrator to be able to operate and program a computer.

Medical records technicians (see figure 2-6), organize and code patient records; gather statistical or research data; and record information. Computers have simplified many of the duties and are used to organize records; compile and report statistical data; and perform similar tasks. Computer operation is an important part of the education program for medical records technicians. Medical records departments also employ clerks, who organize records. Clerks typically complete a one- or two-year vocational program, or are trained on-the-job.

TABLE 2-4 **Health Information and Communication Services**

OCCUPATION	EDUCATION REQUIRED	JOB OUTLOOK TO YEAR 2005	AVERAGE YEARLY EARNINGS
Medical Records Administrator Registered (RRA)	Bachelor's degree; registration can be obtained from American Medical Record Association	Average growth	$20,300–$47,300
Medical Records Technician Accredited (ART)	2–4 years experience as medical clerk and 30 credit hours in medical records at college level or associate's degree; accreditation (certification) can be obtained from Committee on Allied Health Education and Accreditation of the American Medical Association	Above average growth	$14,200–$25,400
Unit Secretary Ward Clerk Unit Coordinator	1 or more years vocational or technical education program; some have on-the-job training	Below average growth	$10,900–$16,800

Figure 2-6 Medical records technicians organize and code patients' records. *(Courtesy of Hinsdale Hospital, Hinsdale, IL)*

Unit secretaries, ward clerks, or **unit coordinators** are employed in hospitals, extended care facilities, clinics, and other health facilities to record information on records; schedule procedures or tests; answer telephones; order supplies; and work with computers to record or obtain information.

ADDITIONAL SOURCES OF INFORMATION

◆ American Health Information Management Association
919 N. Michigan Avenue, Suite 1400
Chicago, IL 60611
◆ American Medical Association
Division of Allied Health Education and Accreditation
515 N. State Street
Chicago, IL 60610
◆ American Medical Records Association
Suite 1850, 875 N. Michigan Avenue
Chicago, IL 60611

INFORMATION
2:6 Hospital/Health Care Facility Services

Any hospital or large health care facility requires workers to operate the support departments such as administration, the business office, the admis-

sions office, central/sterile supply, and housekeeping. Each department has workers at all levels and with varying levels of education (see table 2-5).

Places of employment include hospitals, clinics, long-term care facilities, health maintenance organizations (HMOs), and public health or governmental agencies.

Health care administrators manage the operation of health care facilities. They are frequently called chief executive officers (CEOs). A health care administrator may be responsible for personnel; supervise department heads; determine budget and finance; establish policies and procedures; perform public relations duties; and coordinate all activities in the facility. Duties depend on the size of the facility.

Admitting officers/clerks work in the admissions department of a health care facility. They are responsible for obtaining all necessary information when a patient is admitted to the facility; assigning rooms; maintaining records; and processing information when the patient is discharged. An admitting department manager is a higher level of worker in this field, usually having an associate's or bachelor's degree.

Central/sterile supply workers (see figure 2-7), are involved in ordering, maintaining, and supplying all of the equipment and supplies used by other departments in a health care facility. They sterilize instruments or supplies, maintain equipment, inventory materials, and fill requisitions from other departments.

Housekeeping workers/sanitary managers help maintain the cleanliness of the health care

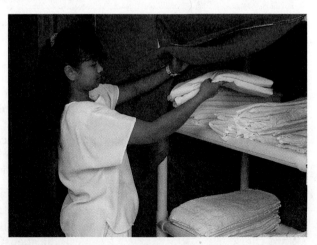

Figure 2-7 Central/sterile supply workers prepare all of the equipment and supplies used by other departments in a health care facility.

TABLE 2-5 **Hospital/Health Care Facility Services**

OCCUPATION	EDUCATION REQUIRED	JOB OUTLOOK TO YEAR 2005	AVERAGE YEARLY EARNINGS
Health Care Administrator	Usually bachelor's or master's, but smaller facilities may accept an associate's degree; licensure required for long-term care facilities; certification can be obtained from American College of Hospital Administrators	Above average growth	$41,200–$196,000
Admitting Officer or Clerk	1–2-year HOE or business/office vocational/technical education; few have on-the-job training	Average growth	$11,300–$21,200
Central/Sterile Supply Technician	On-the-job training or 1–2-year HOE program	Average growth	$10,900–$18,300
Housekeeping Worker Sanitary Manager	On-the-job training or 1-year vocational program	Average growth	$10,900–$18,700

facility in order to provide a pleasant, sanitary environment.

ADDITIONAL SOURCES OF INFORMATION

- American College of Health Care Administrators
  325 S. Patrick Street
  Alexandria, VA 22314
- American Health Care Association
  1201 L Street NW
  Washington, DC 20005
- American Hospital Association
  840 N. Lake Shore Drive
  Chicago, IL 60611

INFORMATION
2:7 *Medical Careers*

Medical careers is a broad category encompassing physicians (doctors) and other individuals who work in any of the varied careers under the supervision of physicians. All such careers focus on di-

agnosing, treating, or preventing diseases and disorders of the human body.

Places of employment include private practices, clinics, hospitals, public health agencies, research facilities (HMOs), government agencies, and colleges or universities.

Levels include physician, physician assistant, and medical assistant (see table 2-6).

Physicians examine patients, order tests, make diagnoses, perform surgery, treat diseases/disorders, and teach preventative health. Several classifications are as follows:

- Doctor of Medicine (M.D.)—Diagnoses, treats, and prevents diseases or disorders; may specialize as noted in table 2-7.
- Doctor of Osteopathy (D.O.)—Treats diseases/disorders, placing special emphasis on the nervous, muscular, and skeletal systems, and the relationship between the body, mind, and emotions; may also specialize.
- Doctor of Podiatric Medicine (D.P.M.)—Examines, diagnoses, and treats diseases/disorders of the feet or of the leg below the knee.
- Doctor of Chiropractic (D.C.)—Focuses on ensuring proper alignment of the spine and optimal operation of the nervous system to maintain health.

Physician assistants, working under the supervision of physicians, take medical histories;

TABLE 2-6 **Medical Careers**

OCCUPATION	EDUCATION REQUIRED	JOB OUTLOOK TO YEAR 2005	AVERAGE YEARLY EARNINGS
Physician	Doctor's degree; 1 or more years postgraduate training, more for specialities; state licensure; certification in specialty area	Above average growth	$95,000–$255,000
Physician Assistant (PA) PAC (certified)	2 or more years of college and often a bachelor's degree; 2 or more years physician assistant program with certificate, associate's, or bachelor's degree; registration, certification, or licensure required in most states; certification from National Commission of Physician's Assistants	Above average growth	$32,400–$65,600
Medical Assistant (MA) CMA (certified) RMA (registered)	1–2-year HOE program or associate's degree; certification can be obtained from American Association of Medical Assistants; registered credentials can be obtained from American Medical Technologists	Above average growth	$10,500–$23,300

TABLE 2-7 **MEDICAL SPECIALITIES**

PHYSICIAN'S TITLE	SPECIALTY
Anesthesiologist	Administration of medications to cause loss of sensation or feeling during surgery
Cardiologist	Diseases of the heart and blood vessels
Dermatologist	Diseases of the skin
Emergency Physician	Acute illness or injury
Endocrinologist	Diseases of the endocrine glands
Family Physician/Practice	Illness or injury in all age groups
Geriatrician	Diseases of elderly individuals
Gynecologist	Diseases of the female reproductive organs
Internist	Diseases of the internal organs (lungs, heart, glands, intestines, kidneys)
Neurologist	Disorders of the brain and nervous system
Obstetrician	Pregnancy and childbirth
Oncologist	Diagnosis and treatment of tumors (cancer)
Ophthalmologist	Diseases and disorders of the eye
Orthopedist	Diseases and disorders of muscles and bones
Otolaryngologist	Disease of the ear, nose, and throat
Pathologist	Diagnose disease by studying changes in organs, tissues, and cells
Pediatrician	Diseases and disorders of children
Plastic Surgeon	Corrective surgery to repair injured or malformed body parts
Proctologist	Diseases of the lower part of the large intestine
Psychiatrist	Diseases and disorders of the mind
Radiologist	Use of X-rays and radiation to diagnose and treat disease
Surgeon	Surgery to correct deformities or treat injuries or disease
Thoracic Surgeon	Surgery of the lungs, heart, or chest cavity
Urologist	Diseases of the kidney, bladder, or urinary system

Figure 2-8 Medical assistants take vital signs and prepare patients for examinations.

perform routine physical examinations and basic diagnostic tests; make preliminary diagnoses; and prescribe and administer appropriate treatments.

Medical assistants, working under the supervision of physicians, prepare patients for examinations; take vital signs and medical histories; assist with procedures and treatments; perform basic laboratory tests; prepare and maintain equipment and supplies; and/or perform secretarial-receptionist duties (see figure 2-8). The type of facility and physician determines the kinds of duties. Assistants working for physicians who specialize are called specialty assistants. For example, an assistant working for a pediatrician is called a pediatric assistant.

ADDITIONAL SOURCES OF INFORMATION

◆ American Academy of Physician Assistants
950 N. Washington Street
Alexandria, VA 22314
◆ American Association of Medical Assistants
20 N. Wacker Drive, Suite 1575
Chicago, IL 60606
◆ American Chiropractic Association
1701 Clarendon Boulevard
Arlington, VA 22209
◆ American Medical Association
515 North State Street
Chicago, IL 60610

◆ American Osteopathic Association
142 East Ontario Street
Chicago, IL 60611
◆ American Podiatric Medical Association
9312 Old Georgetown Road
Bethesda, MD 20814
◆ American Society of Podiatric Assistants
2124 S. Austin Boulevard
Cicero, IL 60650
◆ Registered Medical Assistants of American Medical Technologists
710 Higgins Road
Park Ridge, IL 60068

INFORMATION

2:8 Mental and Social Services

Mental services professionals focus on helping people with mental or emotional disorders or those who are mentally retarded. Social workers help people deal with illnesses, employment, or community problems. Workers in both fields try to help individuals function to their maximum capacities.

Places of employment include hospitals; psychiatric hospitals or clinics; home health care agencies; public health departments; government agencies; and long-term care facilities.

Levels of employment range from psychiatrist (a physician) who diagnoses and treats mental illness, to psychologist and psychiatric technician. There are also various levels (including assistant) employed in the field of social work (see table 2-8).

Psychiatrists are physicians who specialize in diagnosing and treating mental illness. Specialties include child or adolescent psychiatry, geriatric psychiatry, and drug/chemical abuse.

Psychologists study human behavior and use this knowledge to help individuals deal with problems of everyday living. Many specialize in specific aspects of psychology, which include child psychology, adolescent psychology, geriatric psychology, behavior modification, drug/chemical abuse, and physical/sexual abuse.

Psychiatric/mental health technicians, working under the supervision of psychiatrists or psychologists, help patients and their families follow treatment and rehabilitation plans. They provide understanding and encouragement; assist with

TABLE 2-8 **Mental and Social Services**

OCCUPATION	EDUCATION REQUIRED	JOB OUTLOOK TO YEAR 2005	AVERAGE YEARLY EARNINGS
Psychiatrist	Doctor's degree; 2–7 years postgraduate specialty training; state licensure; certification in psychiatry	Average growth	$95,500–$205,000
Psychologist PsyD (Doctor of Psychology)	Bachelor's or master's degree; doctor of psychology required for some positions; licensure or certification required in all states	Above average growth	$22,700–$76,200 or more with doctorate
Psychiatric/Mental Health Technicians	Associate's degree; licensure required in some states; certification available from National Commission for Human Service Workers	Average growth	$11,200–$34,300
Social Workers/ Sociologists	Bachelor's or master's degree or Doctor of Philosophy or Social Work (DSW); licensure or registration required in all states	Above average growth	$19,200–$53,800

physical care; observe and report behavior; and help teach patients constructive social behavior. Assistants or aides who have completed one or more years in an HOE program are also employed in this field.

Social workers, also called sociologists, case managers, or counselors (see figure 2-9), aid people who have difficulty coping with various problems by helping such people make adjustments in their lives and/or by referring them to community resources for assistance. Specialties include child welfare, geriatrics, family, correctional (jail), and occupational social work. Many areas employ assistants or technicians who have one or more years of an HOE program.

Figure 2-9 Social workers help people make life adjustments and refer patients to community resources for assistance.

ADDITIONAL SOURCES OF INFORMATION

◆ American Psychiatric Association
1400 K Street NW
Washington, DC 20005
◆ American Psychology Association
750 1st Street NE
Washington, DC 20036
◆ American Sociological Association
1722 N Street NW
Washington, DC 20036

INFORMATION
2:9 Nursing Careers

Those in the nursing careers provide care for patients as directed by physicians. Care focuses on the mental, emotional, and physical needs of the patient.

Hospitals are the major places of employment, but nursing workers are also employed in long-term care facilities, rehabilitation centers, physicians' offices, clinics, public health agencies, home health care agencies, health maintenance organizations (HMOs), schools, and industry.

Levels include registered nurse, licensed practical/vocational nurse, and nurse assistant/technician (see table 2-9).

Registered nurses (RNs) (see figure 2-10), work under the direction of physicians and provide total care to patients. The RN observes patients; assesses patients' needs; reports to other health care personnel; administers prescribed medications and treatments; teaches health care; and supervises other nursing personnel. The type of facility determines specific job duties. Registered nurses with an advanced education can specialize. Examples include nurse practitioner (CRNP), nurse midwifes (CNM), nurse educator, and nurse anesthetist. Nurse practitioners take health histories; perform basic physical examinations; order laboratory tests and other procedures; refer patients to physicians; help establish treatment plans; treat common

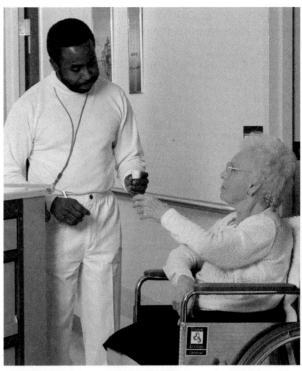

Figure 2-10 Registered nurses (RNs) administer prescribed medications to patients.

TABLE 2-9 **Nursing Careers**

OCCUPATION	EDUCATION REQUIRED	JOB OUTLOOK TO YEAR 2005	AVERAGE YEARLY EARNINGS
Registered Nurse (RN)	2–3-year diploma program in hospital school of nursing, or associate's degree or bachelor's degree; master's or doctor's for some administrative/educational positions; licensure in state of practice	Above average growth	$24,500–$62,700
Licensed Practical/ Vocational Nurse (LPN/LVN)	1–2-year state-approved HOE practical/vocational nurse program; licensure in state of practice	Above average growth	$16,400–$31,700
Nurse Assistant Geriatric Aide Home Health Care Assistant Certified Nurse Technician	6–18 months HOE program; certification or registration required in all states for long-term care facilities—obtained by completing state-approved program	Average growth; above average in geriatric or home care	$10,500–$22,300
Surgical Technician/ Technologist CST (certified)	1–2-year HOE program; associate's degree; certification can be obtained from Association of Surgical Technologists	Above average growth	$18,100–$27,300

illnesses such as colds or sore throats; and teach and promote optimal health. Nurse midwives provide total care for normal pregnancies. The nurse midwife examines the pregnant woman at regular intervals; performs routine tests; teaches childbirth and childcare classes; monitors the infant and mother during childbirth; delivers the infant; and refers any problems to a physician. Nurse educators teach in HOE programs; schools of nursing; colleges and universities; wellness centers; and health care facilities. Nurse anesthetists administer anesthesia, monitor patients during surgery, and assist anesthesiologists (who are physicians).

Licensed practical/vocational nurses (LPNs/LVNs), working under the supervision of physicians or RNs, provide patient care requiring technical knowledge but not the level of education required of RNs. The type of care is determined by the work environment, which can include the home, hospital, long-term care facility, adult day-care center, physician's office, clinic, wellness center, and health maintenance organization. Care provided by LPN/LVNs is also determined by state laws regulating the extent of duties.

Nurse assistants (also called nurse aides, nurse technicians, or orderlies) work under the supervision of RNs or LPNs/LVNs. They provide patient care such as baths, bedmaking, and feeding; assist in transfer and ambulation; and administer basic treatments. **Geriatric aides/assistants** acquire additional education to provide care for the elderly in work environments such as extended care facilities, nursing homes, retirement centers, adult day care agencies, and other similar agencies. **Home health care assistants** are trained to work in the patient's home and may perform additional duties such as meal preparation or cleaning.

OBRA Each nursing assistant working in a long-term care facility is now required under federal law to complete a mandatory, state-approved training program and pass a written and/or competency exam to obtain certification or registration. Health workers in these environments should check the requirements of their respective states.

Surgical technicians/technologists, also called operating room technicians (see figure 2-11), working under the supervision of RNs or physicians, prepare patients for surgery; set up instruments, equipment, and sterile supplies in the operating room; and assist during surgery by passing instruments and supplies to the surgeon. Although most surgical technicians/technologists work in hospital

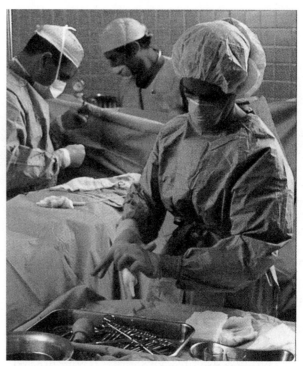

Figure 2-11 Surgical technicians assist by passing instruments and supplies to the surgeon. *(Photo courtesy of the U.S. Army)*

operating rooms, some are employed in outpatient surgical centers, emergency rooms, urgent care centers, physicians' offices, and other facilities.

ADDITIONAL SOURCES OF INFORMATION

◆ American Health Care Association
1201 L Street NW
Washington, DC 20005
◆ American Nurses' Association
600 Maryland Avenue SW
Washington, DC 20024
◆ Association of Surgical Technologists
7108-C S. Alton Way
Englewood, CO 80112
◆ Foundation for Hospice and Homecare
519 C Street NE
Washington, DC 20002
◆ National Association for Practical Nurse Education
1400 Spring Street, Suite 310
Silver Springs, MD 20910

◆ National League for Nursing
350 Hudson Street
New York, NY 10014

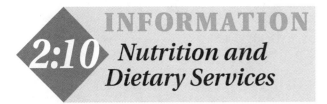

2:10 INFORMATION *Nutrition and Dietary Services*

Workers employed in the nutrition and dietary services recognize the importance of proper nutrition to good health. Using knowledge of nutrition, they promote wellness and optimum health by providing dietary guidelines used to treat various diseases, teaching proper nutrition, and preparing foods for health care facilities.

Places of employment include hospitals; long-term care facilities; child and adult day care facilities; wellness centers; schools; home health care agencies; public health agencies; clinics; and offices.

Levels include dietitian, dietetic technician, and dietetic assistant (see table 2-10).

Dietitians (see figure 2-12) manage food service systems; assess patients'/residents' nutritional needs; plan menus; teach others proper nutrition and special diets; purchase food and equipment; enforce sanitary and safety rules; and supervise and/or train other personnel.

Dietetic technicians, working under the supervision of dietitians, plan menus; order foods; stan-

Figure 2-12 Dietitians manage food service systems, assess nutritional needs, and plan menus according to prescribed diets.

dardize and test recipes; assist with food preparation; and provide basic dietary instruction.

Dietetic assistants, also called **food service workers,** work under the supervision of dietitians and assist with food preparation and service; help patients select menus; clean work areas; and assist other dietary workers.

TABLE 2-10 **Nutrition and Dietary Services**

OCCUPATION	EDUCATION REQUIRED	JOB OUTLOOK TO YEAR 2005	AVERAGE YEARLY EARNINGS
Dietitian, RD (registered)	Bachelor's degree; registration can be obtained from American Dietetic Association; licensure, certification, or registration required in many states	Average growth	$25,300–$43,400
Dietetic Technician	Associate's degree	Average growth	$15,400–$23,600
Dietetic Assistant	6–12 months on-the-job; 1 or more years HOE or food service vocational program	Average growth	$9,500–$16,400

ADDITIONAL SOURCES OF INFORMATION

◆ American Dietetic Association
216 W. Jackson Boulevard, Suite 800
Chicago, IL 60606

INFORMATION
2:11 *Therapeutic Services*

Workers in the therapeutic services use a variety of treatments to help patients who are injured; physically or mentally disabled; or emotionally disturbed. All treatment is directed toward allowing patients to function at maximum capacity.

Places of employment include rehabilitation facilities, hospitals, clinics, mental health facilities, long-term care facilities, home health care agencies, schools, and government agencies.

Most therapeutic occupations include levels of therapist, technician, and assistant/aide (see table 2-11).

Occupational therapists (OTs) (see figure 2-13) help people with physical or emotional disabilities to overcome, correct, or adjust to their particular

Figure 2-13 Occupational therapists (OTs) help patients with disabilities to overcome, correct, or adjust to the disabilities. *(Courtesy March of Dimes-Birth Defects Foundation)*

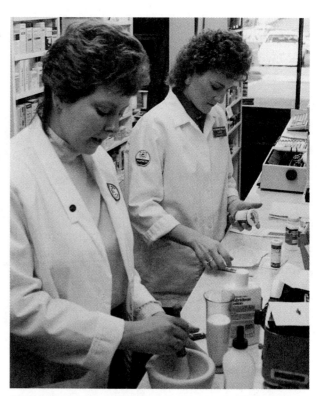

Figure 2-14 Pharmacists dispense medications and provide information on drugs. *(Courtesy of the Michigan Pharmacists Association and the Michigan Society of Pharmacy Technicians)*

problems. The occupational therapist uses various activities to assist the patient in learning skills or activities of daily living (ADL), adapting job skills, or preparing for return to work. Treatment is directed toward helping patients acquire independence, regain lost functions, adapt to disabilities, and lead useful and constructive lives.

Occupational therapy assistants, working under the guidance of occupational therapists, help patients carry out programs of prescribed treatment. They direct patients in arts and crafts projects, recreation, or social events; teach and help patients carry out projects; use games to develop balance and coordination; assist patients trying to master the activities of daily living; and inform therapists of patients' responses and progress.

Pharmacists (see figure 2-14) dispense medications per written orders from physicians, dentists, and others authorized to prescribe medications. They also provide information on drugs and correct ways to use them; order and dispense other health care items such as surgical and sickroom supplies; recommend nonprescription items to customers/

TABLE 2-11 **Therapeutic Services**

OCCUPATION	EDUCATION REQUIRED	JOB OUTLOOK TO YEAR 2005	AVERAGE YEARLY EARNINGS
Occupational Therapist (OT) OTR (Registered)	Bachelor's degree; licensure required in most states; certification (registration) can be obtained from American Occupational Therapy Association	Above average growth	$25,500–$49,600
Occupational Therapy Assistant COTA (certified)	1–2-year HOE program or associate's degree; licensure or certification required by some states; certification can be obtained from American Occupational Therapy Association	Above average growth	$11,200–$24,700
Pharmacist (Pharm D)	5–6-year college program with Bachelor or Doctor of Pharmacy degree; licensure by state required	Above average growth	$31,600–$62,400
Pharmacy Technician	1 or more years on-the-job or 1–2-year HOE program or associate's degree	Above average growth	$11,200–$29,300
Physical Therapist (PT)	Bachelor's or master's degree; licensure by state	Above average growth	$25,000–$53,500
Physical Therapy Assistant	1–2-year HOE program or associate's degree; licensure required in most states	Above average growth	$12,500–$26,800
Recreational Therapist	Associate's or bachelor's degree; licensure or certification required in a few states; certification can be obtained from National Council for Therapeutic Recreation Certification	Above average growth	$18,000–$34,600
Recreational Therapist Assistant	1–2-year HOE program or certificate or associate's degree; certification can be obtained from National Council for Therapeutic Recreation Certification	Above average growth	$10,500–$24,600
Respiratory Therapist, RT RRT (registered)	Associate's or bachelor's degree; licensure or certification required in most states; registration can be obtained from National Board for Respiratory Care	Above average growth	$21,500–$48,200

TABLE 2-11 **Therapeutic Services** *(continued)*

OCCUPATION	EDUCATION REQUIRED	JOB OUTLOOK TO YEAR 2005	AVERAGE YEARLY EARNINGS
Respiratory Therapy Technician RTT CRTT (certified)	1–2-year HOE program; licensure or certification required in many states; certification can be obtained from National Board for Respiratory Care	Above average growth	$12,500–$26,800
Speech-Language Therapist and/or Audiologist	Master's degree; licensure in many states; certification from American Speech-Language-Hearing Association	Above average growth	$26,500–$46,800
Art, Music, Dance Therapist	Bachelor's or master's degree	Average growth	$18,800–$32,500
Athletic Trainer ATC (certified)	Bachelor's or master's degree; licensure required in some states; certification can be obtained from National Athletic Trainers Association	Above average growth	$15,600–$31,200
Dialysis Technician	1–2-year HOE program or associate's degree	Average growth	$10,500–$24,300
Perfusionist	1–2-year HOE program and/or 1–4 years college; licensure required in some states	Above average growth	$18,500–$44,400

patients; ensure drug compatibility; maintain records on medications dispensed; and perform other similar duties. Pharmacists can also either be entrepreneurs or work for one of the many drug manufacturers involved in researching, manufacturing, and selling drugs.

Pharmacy technicians, working under the supervision of pharmacists, help prepare medications for dispensing to patients; label medications; perform inventories and order supplies; prepare intravenous solutions; help maintain records; and perform other duties as directed by pharmacists.

Physical therapists (PTs), see figure 2-15, provide treatment to improve mobility and prevent or limit permanent disability of patients with disabling injuries or diseases. Treatment may include exercise, massage, and/or applications of heat, cold, water, light, electricity, or ultrasound. Therapists assess the functional abilities of patients and use this information to plan treatment programs. They also promote health and prevent injuries by developing proper exercise programs and teaching patients correct use of muscles. Some physical therapists are entrepreneurs.

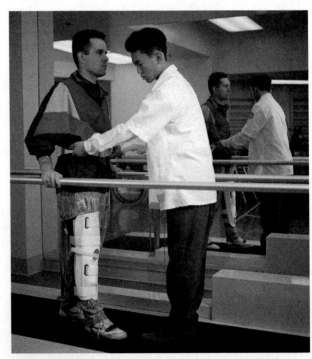

Figure 2-15 Physical therapists (PTs) provide treatment to improve mobility of patients with disabling injuries or diseases.

Physical therapy assistants, working under the supervision of physical therapists, help carry out prescribed plans of treatment. They perform exercises; administer applications of heat, cold, and/or water; assist patients to ambulate with canes, crutches, or braces; inform therapists of patients' responses and progress; and perform other duties, as directed by therapists.

Recreational therapists use recreational and leisure activities as forms of treatment to minimize patients' symptoms and improve physical, emotional, and mental well-being. Activities might include organized athletic events; dances; arts and crafts; musical activities; field trips to shopping centers or other places of interest; movies; or poetry or book readings. All activities are directed toward allowing the patient to gain independence, build self-confidence, and relieve anxiety. Some recreational therapists are entrepreneurs.

Recreational therapy assistants work under the supervision of recreational therapists. They assist in carrying out the activities planned by therapists, and, at times, arrange activities or events. They note and inform therapists of patients' responses and progress.

Respiratory therapists (RTs), under physicians' orders, treat patients with heart and lung diseases by administering oxygen, gases, or medications; using exercise to improve breathing; and performing diagnostic respiratory function tests (see figure 2-16). Some respiratory therapists are entrepreneurs.

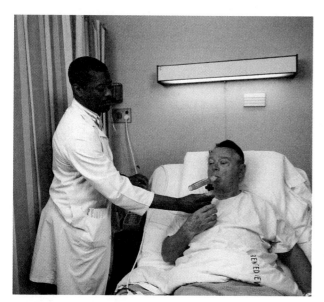

Figure 2-16 Respiratory therapists (RTs) provide treatments to patients with heart and lung diseases.

Respiratory therapy technicians work under the supervision of respiratory therapists, and administer respiratory treatments; perform basic diagnostic tests; clean and maintain equipment; and note and inform therapists of patients' responses and progress.

Speech-language therapists identify, evaluate, and treat patients with speech and language disorders. They help patients communicate as effectively as possible, and also teach patients to cope with the problems created by speech impairments.

Audiologists provide care to individuals who have hearing problems. They test hearing, diagnose problems, and prescribe treatment, which may include hearing aids, auditory training, or instruction in speech or lip reading. They also test noise levels in workplaces and develop hearing protection programs.

Art, music, and **dance therapists** use the arts to help patients deal with social, physical, or emotional problems. Therapists usually work with individuals who are emotionally disturbed, mentally retarded, or physically disabled, but they may also work with adults and children who have no disabilities in an effort to promote physical and mental wellness.

Athletic trainers prevent and treat athletic injuries and provide rehabilitative services to athletes. The athletic trainer frequently works with a physician who specializes in sports medicine. Athletic trainers teach proper nutrition; assess the physical condition of athletes; give advice regarding exercises to increase strength and flexibility or correct weaknesses; put tape or padding on players to protect body parts; treat minor injuries; administer first aid for serious injuries; and help carry out any rehabilitation treatment prescribed by sports medicine physicians or other therapists.

Dialysis technicians operate the kidney dialysis machines used to treat patients with limited or no kidney function. Careful patient monitoring is critical during the dialysis process. The dialysis technician must also provide emotional support for the patient and teach proper nutrition (because many patients must follow restricted diets).

Perfusionists operate the heart-lung machines used in coronary bypass surgery (surgery on the coronary arteries in the heart). This field is expanding to include new advances such as artificial hearts. Monitoring and operating these machines correctly is critical because the patient's life depends on the machines.

ADDITIONAL SOURCES OF INFORMATION

◆ American Association for Respiratory Care
11030 Ables Lane
Dallas, TX 75229
◆ American Association of Colleges of Pharmacy
1426 Prince Street
Alexandria, VA 22314
◆ American Athletic Trainers Association
2952 Stemmons, Suite 200
Dallas, TX 75247
◆ American Physical Therapy Association
1111 N. Fairfax Street
Alexandria, VA 22314
◆ American Occupational Therapy Association
1383 Piccard Drive, P.O. Box 1725
Rockville, MD 20849
◆ American Society of Hospital Pharmacists
4630 Montgomery Avenue
Bethesda, MD 20814
◆ American Speech-Language-Hearing Association
10801 Rockville Pike
Rockville, MD 20852
◆ National Athletic Trainers Association
1001 East 4th Street
Greenville, NC 27858
◆ National Therapeutic Recreation Society
2775 S. Quincy Street, Suite 300
Arlington, VA 22206

INFORMATION
2:12 Veterinary Careers

Veterinary careers focus on providing care to all types of animals—from house pets to livestock to wildlife.

Places of employment include animal hospitals; veterinarian offices; laboratories; zoos; farms; drug or animal food companies; and fish and wildlife services.

Levels of employment include veterinarian, animal health technician, and assistant (see table 2-12).

Veterinarians (DVMs or VMDs) work to prevent, diagnose, and treat diseases and injuries in animals. Specialties include surgery, small animal care; livestock; fish and wildlife; and research.

Animal health technicians, working under the supervision of veterinarians, assist with the handling and care of animals; collect specimens; assist with surgery; perform laboratory tests; and maintain records.

Veterinary assistants are hired in some places of employment to feed and bathe animals; prepare animals for treatment; assist with examinations; clean cages; and maintain records.

ADDITIONAL SOURCES OF INFORMATION

◆ American Association for Laboratory Animal Science
70 Timber Creek Drive, Suite 5
Cordova, TN 93018
◆ American Veterinary Medical Association
1931 N. Meacham Road, Suite 100
Schaumburg, IL 60173
◆ Animal Caretakers Information
The Humane Society of the U.S.
5430 Grosvenor Lane
Bethesda, MD 20814

INFORMATION
2:13 Vision Services

Workers in the vision services provide care to prevent and treat vision disorders. Places of employment include offices, optical shops, department stores, hospitals, schools, health maintenance organizations (HMOs), government agencies, and clinics.

Levels include ophthalmologist (a medical doctor specializing in diseases and disorders of the eye), optometrist; optometric technician and assistant; optician; and optical laboratory technician (see table 2-13). Many individuals in this field are entrepreneurs.

Ophthalmologists are medical doctors specializing in diseases and disorders of the eyes. They diagnose and treat disease; perform surgery; and correct vision problems or defects.

Optometrists (OD), doctors of optometry, examine eyes for vision problems and defects; pre-

TABLE 2-12 **Veterinary Careers**

OCCUPATION	EDUCATION REQUIRED	JOB OUTLOOK TO YEAR 2005	AVERAGE YEARLY EARNINGS
Veterinarian DVM or VMD	4 years preveterinary college; 4 years veterinary college and Doctor of Veterinary Medicine degree; state licensure	Above average growth	$28,300–$72,400 or more
Animal Health Technician ATR (registered)	Certificate or associate's degree; registration, certification, or licensure required in many states	Above average growth	$13,200–$23,500
Veterinary Assistant	1–2 years on-the-job or 1–2-year HOE program	Average growth	$9,500–$15,200

TABLE 2-13 **Vision Services**

OCCUPATION	EDUCATION REQUIRED	JOB OUTLOOK TO YEAR 2005	AVERAGE YEARLY EARNINGS
Ophthalmologist (MD)	Doctor's degree; 2–7 years postgraduate specialty training; state licensure; certification in ophthalmology	Average growth	$85,000–$190,000
Optometrist OD	2–4 years preoptometric college; 4 years at college of optometry; state licensure	Average growth	$42,500–$78,600
Optometric Technician OptTR (registered)	Associate's degree; registration can be obtained from National Paraoptometric Registry; certification can be obtained from Joint Commission on Allied Health Personnel in Ophthalmology	Average growth	$12,300–$24,600
Optometric Assistant	Some on-the-job training; 1-year HOE program	Average growth	$9,800–$16,400
Optician	2–4 years on-the-job or 1–2-year HOE program or associate's degree; licensure or certification required in some states; certification can be obtained from American Board of Opticianry	Above average growth	$15,200–$34,000
Ophthalmic Laboratory Technician	2–3 years on-the-job or 1-year HOE certificate program	Average growth	$11,600–$24,200

scribe corrective lenses or eye exercises; and, in some states, use drugs for diagnosis and/or treatment. If eye disease is present or if eye surgery is needed, the optometrist refers the patient to an ophthalmologist.

Optometric technicians and assistants (see figure 2-17) work under the supervision of ophthalmologists or optometrists. Assistants prepare patients for exams, perform receptionist duties, help patients with frame selection, order lenses, and teach proper care and use of contact lenses. Technicians can perform the same duties, but also may administer basic vision tests or teach eye exercises.

Opticians make and fit the eye glasses or lenses prescribed by ophthalmologists and optometrists. Some specialize in contact lenses.

Ophthalmic laboratory technicians grind, finish, polish, and mount the lenses used in eye glasses and contact lenses.

ADDITIONAL SOURCES OF INFORMATION

◆ American Optometric Association
243 N. Lindbergh Boulevard
St. Louis, MO 63141
◆ Commission on Opticianry Accreditation
10111 Martin Luther King Jr. Highway, Suite 100
Bowie, MD 20720
◆ Joint Commission on Allied Health Personnel in Ophthalmology
2025 Woodlane Drive
St. Paul, MN 55125
◆ Opticians Association of America
10341 Democracy Lane
Fairfax, VA 22030

STUDENT *Go to the workbook and complete the assignment sheet for Unit 2, Careers in Health Care.*

Figure 2-17 Optometric technicians perform basic vision tests and teach eye exercises. *(Courtesy of the American Optometric Association, St. Louis, MO)*

UNIT *2* SUMMARY

Over 200 different careers in health care provide individuals with opportunities to find occupations they enjoy. Each health care career differs somewhat in the type of duties performed; the education required; the standards that must be met and maintained; and the salary earned.

This unit has described some of the major health care careers. For each career group, levels of workers, basic job duties, educational requirements, anticipated need for workers through the year 2005, and average yearly salaries were provided. Use this unit to evaluate the different health careers, and request additional information on specific careers from sources listed at the end of the respective career sections. In this way, you can research various occupational opportunities and determine which health care career is most appropriate for your interests and abilities.

UNIT 2 SUGGESTED REFERENCES

American Medical Association. *Allied Health Education Directory.* Chicago, IL: American Medical Association, 1995–96.

Career Information Center. *Volume 7: Health.* 3rd ed. Peoria, IL: Glencoe Publishers, 1987.

Center for Nursing and Health Careers. *Health Careers.* Toledo, OH: Center for Nursing and Health Careers, 1994.

McCutcheon, Maureen. *Exploring Health Careers.* Albany, NY: Delmar Publishers, 1993.

National Health Council. *200 Ways to Put Your Talent to Work in the Health Field.* New York, NY: National Health Council, Nd.

U. S. Department of Labor. *Occupational Outlook Handbook.* Washington, D.C.: U. S. Government Printing Office, updated annually.

Williams, Catherine, and Jim Zukowski. *Basic Allied Health Education Core.* Austin, TX: EIMC, University of Texas at Austin, 1992.

UNIT 3

Personal Qualities of a Health Care Worker

UNIT OBJECTIVES

After completing this unit of study, you should be able to:

◆ Create a characteristic profile of a health care worker that includes at least eight personal/professional traits or attitudes

◆ Explain how diet, rest, exercise, good posture, and avoiding tobacco, alcohol, and drugs contribute to good health

◆ Demonstrate the standards of a professional appearance as they apply to uniforms, clothing, shoes, nails, hair, jewelry, and makeup

◆ Define, pronounce, and spell all of the key terms

KEY TERMS

acceptance of criticism
competence
   (kom´-peh-tense)
dependability
discretion

empathy
   (em´-path-ee″)
enthusiasm
honesty
patience

personal hygiene
responsibility
self-motivation
tact
willingness to learn

INTRODUCTION

Although health care workers are employed in many different career areas and in a variety of facilities, certain personal/professional characteristics, attitudes, and rules of appearance apply to all health care professionals. This unit discusses these basic requirements.

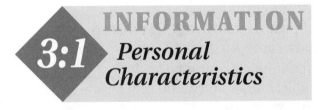

INFORMATION
3:1 *Personal Characteristics*

Many personal/professional characteristics and attitudes are required in the health occupations. As a health care worker, you should make every effort to develop the following characteristics and attitudes and to incorporate them into your personality.

Empathy: Empathy means being able to identify with and understand another person's feelings, situation, and motives. As a health care worker, you may care for persons of all ages—from the newborn infant to the elderly individual. In order to be successful in this, you must be sincerely interested in working with people. You must care about others and be able to communicate and work with them. Understanding the needs of people and learning effective communication is one way to develop empathy. This topic is covered in greater detail in Unit 7 of this text.

Honesty: Truthfulness and integrity are important in any career field. Others must be able to trust you at all times. You must be willing to admit mistakes so they can be corrected.

Dependability: Employers and patients rely on you, so you must accept the responsibility required in your position. You must be prompt in reporting to work, and maintain a good attendance record

(figure 3-1). You must perform assigned tasks on time and accurately.

Willingness to learn: You must be willing to learn and to adapt to changes. The field of health care changes because of research, new inventions, and many other factors. Change often requires learning new techniques or procedures. At times, additional education may be required to remain competent in a particular field.

Patience: You must be tolerant and understanding. You must learn to control your temper and "count to ten" in difficult situations. Learning to deal with frustration and overcome obstacles is important.

Acceptance of criticism: Patients, employers, coworkers, and others may criticize you. Some criticism will be constructive and allow you to improve your work. Instead of becoming resentful, you must be willing to accept criticism and learn from it.

Enthusiasm: You must enjoy your work and display a positive attitude. Enthusiasm is contagious; it helps you do your best and encourages others to do the same. If you do not like some as-

Figure 3-1 A health care worker must report to work on time and maintain a good attendance record.

pects of your job, concentrating on the positive points can help diminish the importance of the negative points.

Self-motivation: Self-motivation is the ability to begin or to follow through with a task. You should be able to determine things that need to be done and do them without constant direction.

Tact: Being tactful means having the ability to say or do the kindest or most fitting thing in a difficult situation. It requires constant practice. Tactfulness implies a consideration for the feelings of others. It is important to remember that all individuals have a right to their respective feelings, and that these feelings should not be judged as right or wrong.

Competence: Being competent means that you are qualified and capable of performing a task. You follow instructions, use approved procedures, and strive for accuracy in all you do. You know your limits and ask for help or guidance if you do not know how to perform a procedure.

Responsibility: Responsibility implies being willing to be held accountable for your actions. Others can rely on you and know that you will meet your obligations.

Discretion: You must always use good judgment in what you say and do. In any health care career, you will have access to confidential information. This information should not be told to anyone without proper authorization. A patient is entitled to confidential care; you must be discrete and ensure that the patient's rights are not violated.

Each of the preceding characteristics and attitudes must be practiced and learned. Some take more time to develop than do others. By being aware of these characteristics and striving constantly to improve, however, you will provide good patient/resident care and be a valuable asset to your employer and other members of the health care team.

3:2 INFORMATION
Personal Appearance

As a worker in any health career, it is important to present an appearance that inspires confidence and a positive self-image. Although the rules of suitable appearance may vary, certain professional standards apply to most health careers and should be observed.

GOOD HEALTH

Health care involves promoting health and preventing disease. The worker should present a healthy appearance. Five main factors contribute to good health:

◆ *Diet*—Eating well-balanced meals and nutritious foods provides the body with the materials needed for optimum health. Foods from each of the five major food groups (milk; meat; vegetables; fruits; and bread, cereals, rice, and pasta) should be eaten daily.

◆ *Rest*—Adequate rest and sleep help provide energy and the ability to deal with stress. The amount of sleep required varies from individual to individual.

◆ *Exercise*—Exercise maintains circulation and improves muscle tone. It also helps mental attitude and contributes to more restful sleep. Individuals should choose the form of exercise best suited to their own needs, but should exercise daily.

◆ *Good Posture*—Good posture helps prevent fatigue and puts less stress on muscles. Basic principles include standing straight with stomach muscles pulled in, shoulders relaxed, and weight balanced equally on each foot.

◆ *Avoid Use of Tobacco, Alcohol, and Drugs*—The use of tobacco, alcohol, and drugs can seriously affect good health. Tobacco affects the function of the heart, circulatory system, lungs, and digestive system. In addition, the odor of smoke is offensive to many individuals. For these reasons, many health care facilities are "smoke-free" environments. The use of alcohol and drugs impairs mental function, decreases ability to make decisions, and adversely affects many body systems. The use of alcohol or drugs can also result in job loss. Avoiding tobacco, alcohol, and drugs helps prevent damage to the body systems and contributes to good health.

PROFESSIONAL APPEARANCE

When you obtain a position in a health career, it is important to learn the rules or standards that have been established by your place of employment.

Abide by the rules, and make every effort to maintain a neat, clean, and professional appearance.

Uniform

Many health occupations require uniforms. A uniform should always be neat, well fitting, clean, and free from wrinkles (figure 3-2). Some agencies require a white uniform, but others allow pastel colors. In some facilities, the colors identify groups of workers. If white uniforms are required, white or neutral undergarments should be worn. A large variety of uniform styles is available. Extreme styles in any type of uniform should be avoided. It is important that the health care worker learn what type and color uniform is required or permitted and follow the standards established by the place of employment.

Clothing

If regular clothing is worn in place of a uniform, the clothing must be clean, neat, and in good repair (figure 3-3). The style should allow for freedom of body movement and should be appropriate for the job. For example, while clean, neat jeans might be appropriate at times for a recreational therapist, they are not proper attire for most other health professionals. Washable fabrics are usually best because frequent laundering is necessary.

Name Badge

Most health care facilities require personnel to wear name badges or photo identification tags at all times. The badge usually states the name, title, and department of the health care worker. In some health care settings, such as long-term care facilities, workers are required by law to wear identification badges.

Shoes

Although white shoes are frequently required, many occupations allow other types of shoes. Any shoes should fit well and provide good support to prevent fatigue. Low heels are usually best because they help prevent fatigue and accidents. Avoid wearing tennis shoes or sandals, unless they are standard dress for a particular occupation. Shoes should be cleaned daily. If shoelaces are part of the shoes, these must also be cleaned or replaced frequently. Women should wear white or beige pantyhose with uniforms; colored or patterned pantyhose should be avoided. Men should wear white socks under white uniforms.

Figure 3-2 Uniform styles may vary, but a uniform should always be neat, well fitting, clean, and free from wrinkles.

Figure 3-3 If regular clothing is worn in place of a uniform, the clothing should reflect a professional appearance.

Personal Hygiene

Good **personal hygiene** is essential. Because health care workers typically work in close contact with others, body odor must be controlled. A daily bath or shower; use of deodorant or antiperspirant; good oral hygiene; and clean undergarments all help prevent body odor. Strong odors caused by tobacco, perfumes, scented hairsprays, and aftershave lotions can be offensive. The use of these products should be avoided when working with patients and coworkers.

Nails

Nails should be kept short and clean. If fingernails are long and/or pointed, they can injure patients. They can also transmit germs, because dirt can collect under long nails. In addition, health care workers are now required to wear gloves for many procedures. Long nails can tear or puncture gloves. The use of colored nail polish is discouraged because the color can conceal any dirt that may collect under the nails. Further, because frequent handwashing causes polish to chip, germs can collect on the surfaces of nails. Finally, the flash of bright colors may bother a person who does not feel well. If nail polish is worn, it should be clear or colorless, and the nails must be kept scrupulously clean. Hand cream or lotion should be used to keep the hands from becoming chapped and dry from frequent handwashing.

Hair

Hair should be kept clean and neat. It should be styled attractively and be easy to care for. Fancy or extreme hairstyles and hair ornaments should be avoided. If the job requires close contact with patients, long hair must be pinned back and kept off the collar. This prevents the hair from touching the patient/resident; falling on a tray or on equipment; or blocking necessary vision during procedures.

Jewelry

Jewelry is usually not permitted with a uniform because it can cause injury to the patient and transmit germs or pathogens. Exceptions sometimes include a watch, wedding ring, and small, pierced earrings. When a uniform is not required, jewelry should still be limited. Excessive jewelry can interfere with patient care and detracts from the professional appearance of the health care worker.

Makeup

Excessive makeup should be avoided. The purpose of makeup is to create a natural appearance and add to the attractiveness of a person.

STUDENT *Go to the workbook and complete the assignment sheet for Unit 3, Personal Qualities of a Health Care Worker.*

UNIT 3 SUMMARY

Certain personal characteristics, attitudes, and rules of appearance apply to health care workers in all health careers. Every health care worker must constantly strive to develop the necessary characteristics and to present a professional appearance.

Personal characteristics such as honesty, dependability, patience, enthusiasm, responsibility, discretion, and competence are essential. In addition, health care workers must be willing to learn and to accept criticism. These characteristics must be practiced and learned.

A professional appearance helps inspire confidence and a positive self-image. Good health is an important part of appearance. By eating correctly, obtaining adequate rest, exercising daily, observing the rules of good posture, and avoiding the use of tobacco, alcohol, and drugs, a health care worker can strive to maintain good health. Wearing the appropriate uniform or appropriate clothing and shoes is essential to projecting the proper image. Proper hair and nail care; good personal hygiene; and limited makeup also help create a professional appearance.

Health care workers must learn and follow the standards and requirements established by the health care facility in which they are employed.

UNIT 3 SUGGESTED REFERENCES

Milliken, Mary Elizabeth. Understanding Human Behavior: *A Guide for Health Care Providers.* 5th ed. Albany, NY: Delmar Publishers, 1993.

Townsend, Carolynn E. *Nutrition and Diet Therapy.* 6th ed. Albany, N Y: Delmar Publishers, 1994.

UNIT 4

Legal Responsibilities

UNIT OBJECTIVES

After completing this unit of study, you should be able to:

◆ Provide one example of a situation that might result in legal action for each of the following: malpractice; negligence; assault and battery; invasion of privacy; false imprisonment; abuse; and defamation

◆ Describe how contract laws affect health care

◆ Define *privileged communications* and explain how they apply to health care

◆ State the legal regulations that apply to health care records

◆ List at least six basic rules of ethics for health care personnel

◆ List at least six rights of the patient who is receiving health care

◆ Justify at least eight professional standards by explaining how they help meet legal/ethical requirements

◆ Define, pronounce, and spell all of the key terms

KEY TERMS

abuse
agent
assault and battery
civil law
confidentiality
   (con"-fih-den-chee"-ahl´-ih-tee)
contract
criminal law
defamation
   (deff"-ah-may´-shun)

Durable Power of Attorney (POA)
ethics
   (eth-iks)
false imprisonment
health care records
informed consent
invasion of privacy
legal
legal directives
legal disability
libel   *(ly´-bull)*

living wills
malpractice
negligence
   (neg´-lih-gents)
Patient Self-Determination Act
   (PSDA)
patients' rights
privileged communications
slander
torts

INTRODUCTION

In every aspect of life, there are certain laws and legal responsibilities formulated to protect you and society. An excellent example is the need to obey traffic laws when driving a motor vehicle. A worker in any health career also has certain responsibilities. Being aware of and following legal regulations is important for your own protection, the protection of your employer, and the safety and well-being of the patient.

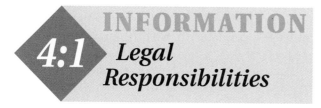

INFORMATION
4:1 *Legal Responsibilities*

Legal responsibilities are those that are authorized or based on law. This can include **civil law,** which focuses on legal relationships between people and the protection of a person's rights, and **criminal law,** which focuses on wrongs against a person, property, or society. Although health care is mainly affected by civil law, especially those aspects involving contracts and **torts** (wrongful acts that do not involve contracts), criminal laws can also apply. Examples of such criminal laws include practicing in a health profession without having the required license, misuse of narcotics, theft, and murder. In addition, *health care professionals/workers are also required to know and follow the state laws that regulate their respective licenses or registrations or set standards for their respective professions.*

TORTS

Failure to meet your legal responsibilities can result in legal action against you and your employer. Many different types of torts, or civil wrongs (as opposed to crimes), can lead to legal action. These offenses may be quite complex and may be open to different legal interpretations. Some of the more common torts include the following:

Malpractice: Malpractice can be interpreted as "bad practice" and is commonly called "professional negligence." It can be defined as the failure of a professional to use the degree of skill and learning commonly expected in that individual's profession, resulting in injury, loss, or damage to the person receiving care. Examples might include a physician not administering a tetanus injection when a patient has a puncture wound, or a nurse performing minor surgery without having any training.

Negligence: Negligence can be described as failure to give care that is normally expected of a person in a particular position, resulting in injury to another person. Examples include falls and injuries that occur when siderails are left down; using or not reporting defective equipment; infections caused by the use of nonsterile instruments and/or supplies; and burns caused by improper heat or radiation treatments.

Assault and battery: Assault includes a threat or attempt to injure, and battery includes the unlawful touching of another person without consent. They are closely related and often used together. It is important to remember that patients must give consent for any care and that they have the right to refuse care. Some procedures or practices require written consent from the patient. Examples can include surgery, certain diagnostic tests, experimental procedures, treatment of minors (individuals below legal age, which varies from state to state), and even simple things such as siderail releases for a patient who wants siderails left down when other factors indicate siderails should be up to protect the patient. Verbal consent is permitted in other cases, but the law states that this must be "informed consent." **Informed consent** is permission granted voluntarily by a person who is of sound mind after the procedure and all risks involved have been explained in terms the person can understand. It is important to remember that a person has the right to withdraw consent at any time. Therefore, all procedures must be explained to the patient, and no procedure should be performed if the patient does not give consent. Examples of assault and battery include performing a procedure after a patient has refused to give permission and improper handling or rough treatment of a patient while providing care.

Invasion of privacy: Invasion of privacy includes unnecessarily exposing an individual or revealing personal information about an individual without that person's consent. Examples include improperly draping or covering a patient during a procedure so that other patients or personnel can see the patient exposed; sending information regarding a patient to an insurance company without the patient's written permission; or informing the news media of a patient's condition without the patient's permission.

False imprisonment: False imprisonment refers to restraining an individual or restricting an individual's freedom. Examples include keeping patients hospitalized against their will, or applying physical restraints without proper authorization or with no justification.

Abuse: Abuse includes any care that results in physical harm, pain, or mental anguish. Examples include denial of rights, mistreatment, deprivation of services, mental intimidation, and unnecessary restraint. Many of the other torts can lead to charges of abuse, or a charge of abuse can occur alone. Abuse is sometimes classified as physical; verbal or mental; or sexual. Physical abuse includes hitting; forcing people against their will; restraining movement; depriving people of food or water; and not providing physical care. Verbal abuse includes talking harshly; swearing or shouting; teasing or ridiculing; and intimidating. Sexual abuse includes any unwanted sexual touching or act. Laws in all states require that any form of abuse be reported to the proper authorities.

Defamation: Defamation occurs when false statements either cause a person to be ridiculed or damage the person's reputation. Incorrect information given out in error can result in defamation. If the information is spoken, it is **slander;** if it is written, it is **libel.** Examples include reporting that a patient has an infectious disease to a government agency when lab results are inaccurate, or telling others that a person has a drug problem when another medical condition actually exists.

CONTRACTS

In addition to tort laws, contract laws also affect health care. A **contract** is an agreement between two or more parties. Most contracts have three parts: an offer, an acceptance, and a consideration. The offer occurs when a competent individual enters into a relationship with a health care provider and offers to be a patient. The acceptance occurs when the health care provider gives an appointment or examines or treats the patient. The consideration is the payment made by the patient for the services provided.

Contracts in health care are implied or expressed. Implied contracts are those obligations that are understood without verbally expressed terms. For example, when a qualified health worker prepares a medication and a patient takes the medication, it is implied that the patient accepts this treatment. Expressed contracts are stated in distinct and clear language, either orally or in writing. An example is a surgery permit. Promises of care must be kept. Therefore, all risks associated with treatment must be explained completely to the patient (figure 4-1).

All parties entering into a contract must be free of **legal disability.** A person who has a legal disability does not have the legal capacity to form a contract. Examples of legal disabilities include minors (individuals under legal age), mentally incompetent persons, individuals under the influence of drugs that alter the mental state, and semiconscious or unconscious people. In such cases, parents, guardians, or others permitted by law must form the contract for the individual.

A contract requires that certain qualities of care be provided by competent, qualified individuals. If

Figure 4-1 All risks of treatment must be explained to a patient before asking the patient for permission to administer treatment.

the contract is not performed according to agreement, the contract is breached. Failure to provide care and/or giving improper care on the part of the health provider, or failure on the part of the patient to pay according to the consideration can be considered breach of contract and cause for legal action.

A final important consideration in contract law is the role of the agent. When a person works under the direction or control of another person, the employer is called the principal, and the person working under the employer is called the agent. The principal is responsible for the actions of the agent and can be required to pay or otherwise compensate people who have been injured by the agent. For example, if a dental assistant tells a patient "your dentures will look better than your real teeth," the dentist may have to compensate the patient financially should this statement prove false. Health care workers should therefore be aware of their role as agents to their employers and work to protect the interests of their employers.

PRIVILEGED COMMUNICATIONS

Privileged communications are another important aspect of legal responsibility. Privileged communications comprise all information given to health care personnel by a patient; by law, this information must be kept confidential. It cannot be told to anyone else without the written consent of the patient. The consent should state what information is to be released, to whom the information should be given, and any applicable time limits. Certain information is exempt by law and must be reported. Examples of exempt information are births and deaths; injuries caused by violence (such as assault and battery, abuse, stabbings) that may require police involvement; drug abuse; communicable diseases; and sexually transmitted diseases.

Health care records are also considered privileged communications. Such records contain information on the care provided to the patient. While such records belong to the health care provider (for example, the physician, dentist, hospital, long-term care facility), the patient has a right to obtain a copy of any information in the record. Health care records can be used as legal records in a court of law. Erasures are therefore not allowed on such records. Errors should be crossed out with a single line so material is still readable. Correct information should then be inserted, initialed, and dated. If necessary, an explanation for the correction should also be provided. Health care records must be properly maintained, kept confidential, and retained for the amount of time required by state law (figure 4-2). When records are destroyed after the legal time for retention, they should be burned or shredded to maintain confi-

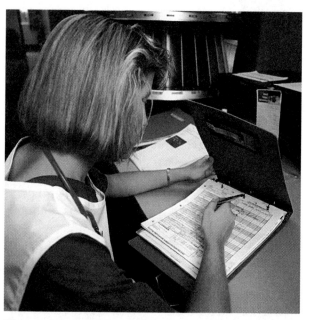

Figure 4-2 Confidentiality must be maintained with regard to health care records.

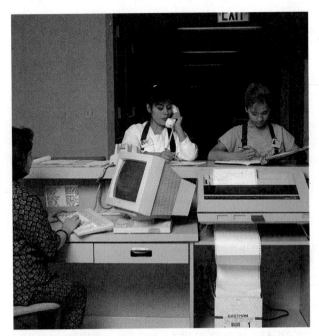

Figure 4-3 The growing use of computerized records has created the need for limiting access to computers in order to maintain confidentiality.

dentiality. The growing use of computerized records has amounted to somewhat of a dilemma in maintaining confidentiality (figure 4-3). In a large health care facility such as a hospital, many different individuals may have access to a patient's records. For this reason, many health care providers are creating safeguards to maintain computer confidentiality. Some examples include limiting personnel who have access to such records; using codes to prevent access to certain information; requiring passwords in order to access specific information on records; and constantly monitoring and evaluating computer use.

Legal responsibilities are important aspects of health care. All states have rules and regulations governing health care. In addition, most health care agencies have specific rules, regulations, and standards that determine activities performed by individuals holding different positions of employment. Standards can vary from state to state, and even from agency to agency. It is important to remember that you are liable, or legally responsible, for your own actions regardless of what anyone tells you or what position you hold. Therefore, when you undertake a particular position of employment in a health agency, *it is your responsibility to learn exactly what you are legally permitted to do, and to familiarize yourself with your exact responsibilities.*

INFORMATION
4:2 *Ethics*

Legal responsibilities are determined by law. **Ethics** are a set of principles relating to what is morally right or wrong. Ethics provide a standard of conduct or code of behavior. This allows a health care provider to analyze information and make decisions based on what people believe is right and good conduct. Modern health care advances, however, have created many ethical dilemmas for health care providers. Some of these dilemmas include:

Is euthanasia (assisted death) justified in certain patients?

Should a patient be told that a health care provider has AIDS?

Should aborted fetuses be used for research?

When should life support be discontinued?

Do parents have a religious right to refuse a life-saving blood transfusion for their child?

Can a health care facility refuse to provide expensive treatment such as a bone marrow transplant if a patient cannot pay for the treatment?

Who decides whether a 75-year-old patient or a 56-year-old patient gets a single kidney available for transplant?

Should people be allowed to sell organs for use in transplants?

If a person can benefit from marijuana, should a physician be allowed to prescribe it as a treatment?

Although there are no easy answers to any of these questions, some guidelines are provided by an ethical code. Most of the national organizations affiliated with the different health care occupations have established ethical codes for personnel in their respective occupations. Although such codes differ slightly, most contain the same basic principles.

A basic rule of ethics for health care personnel is to put the saving of life and the promotion of health above all else. This can be very difficult when caring for either the dying patient or the patient having little chance for a long and productive life. The health care worker must, however, make every effort to keep the patient as comfortable as possible and to preserve life whenever possible unless prohibited by a living will.

Another rule is to treat all patients equally, regardless of race; religion; social or economic status; sex; or nationality. Bias, prejudice, and discrimination have no place in health care. You must provide care for *all* individuals to the best of your ability.

Health care workers must maintain a competent level of skill consistent with their particular occupations. They should stay informed and up to date and pursue continuing education as necessary.

C **Confidentiality** and respect for the privacy of others must always be maintained. Information obtained from patients should not be repeated or used for personal gain. If patients reveal information that has a bearing on their well-being or care, this information should be reported to the immediate supervisor. Gossiping about patients is ethically wrong.

Refraining from immoral, unethical, and illegal practices is another basic ethical rule. If health care workers observe others taking part in illegal actions, they should report such actions to the proper authorities.

Health care workers must show loyalty to patients, coworkers, and employers. This requires avoiding negative or derogatory statements and always expressing a positive attitude.

Finally, it is important to be sincere, honest, and caring. Treat others as you want to be treated. Show respect and concern for the feelings, dignity, and rights of others.

When you enter a health occupation, learn the code of ethics for that occupation. Make every effort to abide by the code so as to become a competent and ethical health care worker. In doing so, you will earn the respect and confidence of patients, coworkers, and employers.

INFORMATION
4:3 *Patients' Rights*

OBRA Many health care agencies have written policies concerning **patients' rights,** or the factors of care that patients can expect to receive. Agencies expect all personnel to respect and honor these rights.

The American Hospital Association has affirmed a "Patient's Bill of Rights" that is recognized and honored by many health care facilities. This bill of rights states, in part, that a patient has the right to:

1. considerate and respectful care;
2. obtain complete, current information concerning diagnosis, treatment, and prognosis (expected outcome);
3. receive information necessary to give informed consent prior to the start of any procedure or treatment;
4. refuse treatment to the extent permitted under law (figure 4-4);
5. privacy concerning a medical-care program;
6. confidential treatment of all communications and records;
7. reasonable response to a request for services;
8. obtain information regarding any relationship of the hospital to other health care and educational institutions;
9. be advised of and have the right to refuse to participate in any research project;
10. expect reasonable continuity of care;
11. examine bills and receive an explanation of all charges;
12. be informed of any hospital rules or regulations.

OBRA Residents in long-term care facilities are guaranteed certain rights under the Omnibus Budget Reconciliation Act (OBRA) of

Figure 4-4 Patients have the right to refuse treatment.

1987. Every long-term care facility must inform residents or their guardians of these rights and a copy must be posted in each facility. This is often called a "Resident's Bill of Rights" and states, in part, that a resident has a right to:

1. free choice regarding physician, treatment, care, and participation in research;
2. freedom from abuse and chemical or physical restraints;
3. privacy and confidentiality of personal and clinical records;
4. accommodation of needs and choice regarding activities, schedules, and health care;
5. voice grievances without fear of retaliation or discrimination;
6. organize and participate in family/resident groups and in social, religious, and community activities;
7. information on medical benefits, medical records, survey results, deficiencies of the facility, and advocacy groups including the ombudsman program (state representative who checks on resident care and violation of rights);
8. manage personal funds and use personal possessions;
9. unlimited access to immediate family or relatives and to share a room with his or her spouse, if both are residents (figure 4-5);

Figure 4-5 A married couple in a long-term care facility has the legal right to share a room if both members of the couple are residents in the facility.

10. remain in the facility and not be transferred or discharged except for medical reasons; the welfare of the resident or others; failure to pay; or if the facility either cannot meet the resident's needs or ceases to operate.

All states have adopted these rights, and some have added additional rights. It is important to check state law and obtain a list of rights established in your state. Health care workers can face job loss, fines, and even imprisonment if they do not follow and grant established patients' or residents' rights. By observing these rights, the health care worker helps ensure the patient's safety, privacy, and well-being, and provides quality care at all times.

INFORMATION
4:4 Legal Directives for Health Care

Legal directives for health care, also known as advance directives, are legal documents that allow individuals to state what medical treatment they want or do not want in the event that they become incapacitated and are unable to express their wishes regarding medical care. Two main directives are a living will and a Durable Power of Attorney (POA) for Health Care.

Living wills (figure 4-6) are documents that allow individuals to state what measures should or should not be taken to prolong life when their conditions are terminal (death is expected). Most states now have laws that allow the withholding of life-sustaining procedures and that honor living wills. A living will frequently results in a do not resuscitate (DNR) order for a terminally ill individual.

A **Durable Power of Attorney (POA)** for Health Care is a document that permits an individual (known as a principal) to appoint another person (known as an agent) to make any decisions regarding health care if the principal should become unable to make decisions. This includes providing or withholding specific medical or surgical procedures; hiring or dismissing health care providers; spending or withholding funds for health care; and having access to medical records. Although they are most frequently given to spouses or adult children, POAs can be given to any qualified adult.

Society for the Right to Die

250 West 57th Street/New York, NY 10107

Living Will Declaration

T₀ My Family, Doctors, and All Those Concerned with My Care

INSTRUCTIONS
Consult this column for help and guidance.

This declaration sets forth your directions regarding medical treatment.

I, _____, being of sound mind, make this statement as a directive to be followed if I become unable to participate in decisions regarding my medical care.

If I should be in an incurable or irreversible mental or physical condition with no reasonable expectation of recovery, I direct my attending physician to withhold or withdraw treatment that merely prolongs my dying. I further direct that treatment be limited to measures to keep me comfortable and to relieve pain.

You have the right to refuse treatment you do not want, and you may request the care you do want.

These directions express my legal right to refuse treatment. Therefore I expect my family, doctors, and everyone concerned with my care to regard themselves as legally and morally bound to act in accord with my wishes, and in so doing to be free of any legal liability for having followed my directions.

You may list specific treatment you do not want. For example:

Cardiac resuscitation
Mechanical respiration
Artificial feeding/fluids by tube

Otherwise, your general statement, top right, will stand for your wishes.

I especially do not want: _____

_____

_____

_____

_____

_____

_____

You may want to add instructions for care you do want—for example, pain medication; or that you prefer to die at home if possible.

Other instructions/comments: _____

_____

_____

_____

If you want, you can name someone to see that your wishes are carried out, but you do not have to do this.

Proxy Designation Clause: Should I become unable to communicate my instructions as stated above, I designate the following person to act in my behalf:

Name_____

Address_____

If the person I have named above is unable to act in my behalf, I authorize the following person to do so:

Name_____

Address_____

Sign and date here in the presence of two adult witnesses, who should also sign.

Signed: _____ Date:_____

Witness: _____ Witness: _____

Keep the signed original with your personal papers at home. Give signed copies to doctors, family, and proxy. Review your Declaration from time to time; initial and date it to show it still expresses your intent.

Figure 4-6 A living will is a legal document that allows an individual to state what measures should or should not be taken to prolong life. *(Reprinted by permission of Choice in Dying, 200 Varick Street, New York, New York 10014)*

A federal law called the Patient Self-Determination Act (PSDA), which went into effect in 1991, requires that all health care facilities receiving any type of federal aid provide patients with information regarding and assistance in preparing advance directives. Under this law, patients must be told about their right-to-die options according to state laws. The facilities must note any legal directives on medical records and must have procedures in place to comply with the directives. In this way, patients are informed of their rights and have the opportunity to determine the care they will receive.

All health care workers must be aware of and honor legal or advance directives. In addition, health care workers should give serious consideration to preparing their own legal directives.

INFORMATION 4:5 Professional Standards

Legal responsibilities, ethics, patients' rights, and legal directives all help determine the type of care provided by health care workers. By following certain standards at all times, you can protect yourself, your employer, and the patient. Some of the basic standards are as follows:

1. **Perform only those procedures for which you have been trained and are legally permitted to do.** Never perform any procedure unless you are qualified. The necessary training may be obtained from an educational facility, from your employer, or in special classes provided by an agency. If you are asked to perform any procedure for which you are not qualified, it is your responsibility to state that you have not been trained and to refuse to do it until you receive the required instruction. If you are not legally permitted to either perform a procedure or to sign documents, it is your responsibility to refuse to do so because of legal limitations.

2. **Use approved, correct methods while performing any procedure.** Follow specific methods taught by qualified instructors in educational facilities or observe and learn procedures from your employer or authorized personnel. Most health care agencies have an approved procedure manual that explains the step-by-step methods for performing tasks. Use this manual or read the manufacturer's instructions on specific equipment or supplies.

3. **Obtain proper authorization before performing any procedure.** In some health careers, you will obtain authorization directly from the doctor, therapist, or individual in charge of a patient's care. In other careers, you will obtain authorization by checking written orders (figure 4-7). In careers where you have neither access to patients' records nor direct contact with the individuals in charge of care, an immediate supervisor will interpret orders and then direct you to perform procedures.

4. **Identify the patient and obtain the patient's consent before performing any procedure.** In some health care agencies, patients wear identification bands. If this is the case, check this name band (figure 4-8). In addition, state the patient's name clearly, repeating it if necessary. For example, say "Miss Jones?" followed by "Miss Sandra Jones?" to be sure you have the correct patient. Always explain a procedure briefly or state what you are going to do, and obtain the patient's consent. It is best to avoid statements such as "Can I take your blood

Figure 4-7 Obtain proper authorization before performing any procedure on a patient.

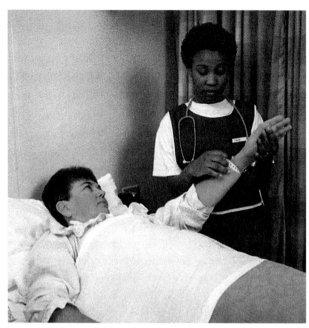

Figure 4-8 If a name band is present, use it to identify the patient.

pressure?" because the patient can say "No." By stating, "The doctor would like me to check your blood pressure," you are identifying the procedure and obtaining consent by the patient's acceptance and/or lack of objection. If a patient refuses to allow you to perform a procedure, check with your immediate supervisor. Some procedures require written consent from the patient. Follow the agency policy with regard to such procedures. Never sign your name as a witness to any written consent or document unless you are authorized to do so.

5. **Observe all safety precautions.** Handle equipment carefully. Be alert to all aspects of safety to protect the patient. Know and follow safety rules and regulations. Be alert to safety hazards in any area and make every effort to correct or eliminate such hazards as quickly as possible.

6. **Keep all information confidential.** This includes oral and written information. Ensure that you do not place patient records in any area where they can be seen by unauthorized individuals. Do not reveal any information contained in the records without proper authorization and patient consent. If you are reporting specific information about a patient to your immediate supervisor, ensure that your conversation cannot be heard by others. Avoid discussing patients with others at home, in social situations, in public places, or anywhere outside the agency.

7. **Think before you speak and carefully consider everything you say.** Do not reveal information, such as a blood pressure reading, to the patient unless you are specifically instructed to do so.

8. **Treat all patients equally regardless of race; religion; social or economic status; sex; or nationality.** Provide care for *all* individuals to the best of your ability.

9. **Accept no tips or bribes for the care you provide.** You receive a salary for your services, and the care you provide should not be influenced by the amount of money a patient can afford to pay. A polite refusal such as "I'm sorry, I am not allowed to accept tips," is usually the best way to handle this situation.

10. **If any error occurs or you make a mistake, report it immediately to your supervisor.** Never try to hide or ignore an error. Make every effort to correct the situation as soon as possible, and take responsibility for your actions.

11. **Behave professionally in dress, language, manners, and actions.** Take pride in your occupation and in the work you do. Promote a positive attitude at all times.

Even when standards are followed, errors leading to legal action sometimes still occur. Liability insurance constitutes an additional form of protection in such cases. Many insurance companies offer policies at reasonable cost for health care workers and students. Some companies will even issue liability protection under a homeowner's policy or through a liability policy that protects the person against all liabilities, not just those related to occupation.

Again, remember that it is your responsibility to understand the legal and ethical implications of your particular health career. Never hesitate to ask specific questions or to request written policies from your employer. Contact your state board of health or state board of education to obtain information regarding regulations and guidelines for your occupation. By obtaining this information and by following the basic standards listed, you will protect yourself, your employer, and the patient to whom you provide health care.

STUDENT *Go to the workbook and complete the assignment sheet for Unit 4, Legal Responsibilities.*

UNIT 4 SUMMARY

All health care workers have legal and ethical responsibilities that exist to protect the health care worker and employer, and to provide for the safety and well-being of the patient.

Legal responsibilities in health care usually involve torts and contracts. Torts are wrongful acts that do not involve contracts. Examples of torts that can lead to legal action include malpractice; negligence; assault and battery; invasion of privacy; false imprisonment; and defamation. A contract is an agreement between two or more parties. Contracts create obligations that must be met by all involved individuals. If a contract is not performed according to agreement, the contract is breached, and legal action can occur.

Understanding privileged communications is another important aspect of legal responsibilities. A health care worker must be aware that all information given by a patient is confidential and should not be told to anyone else without the written consent of the patient. Health care records are also privileged communications and can be used as legal records in a court of law.

Ethical responsibilities are based not on law but, rather, on what is morally right or wrong. Most health care occupations each have an established code of ethics that provides a standard of conduct or code of behavior. Health care workers should make every effort to abide by the codes of ethics established for their given professions.

Health care workers must respect patients' rights. Health care agencies have written policies concerning the factors of care that patients can expect to receive. All personnel must respect and honor these rights.

Legal directives for health care are legal documents that allow individuals to state what medical treatment they want or do not want in the event that they become incapacitated. Two main examples are a living will and a Durable Power of Attorney for Health Care. As a result of a federal law called the Patient Self-Determination Act, any health care facility receiving federal funds must provide patients with information regarding and assistance in preparing legal directives.

Professional standards of care help provide guidelines for meeting legal responsibilities, ethics, and patients' rights. Every health care worker should follow these standards at all times. In addition, all health care workers should know and follow the state laws that regulate their respective occupations.

UNIT 4 SUGGESTED REFERENCES

Cooper, Marian G., and David E. Cooper. *The Medical Assistant.* 6th ed. New York, NY: McGraw-Hill, 1993.

Edge, Raymond. *The Ethics of Health Care: A Guide for Clinical Practice.* Albany, NY: Delmar Publishers, 1994.

Flight, Myrtle R. *Law, Liability and Ethics for Medical Office Personnel.* 2nd ed. Albany, NY: Delmar Publishers, 1993.

Hegner, Barbara, and Esther Caldwell. *Nursing Assistant: A Nursing Process Approach.* 7th ed. Albany, NY: Delmar Publishers, 1995.

Keir, Lucille, Connie Krebs, and Barbara A. Wise, *Medical Assisting: Administrative and Clinical Competencies.* 3rd ed. Albany, NY: Delmar Publishers, 1993.

Quill, Timothy. *Death and Dignity.* New York, NY: W.W. Norton and Co., 1993.

Williams, Catherine, and Jim Zukowski. *Basic Allied Health Education Core.* Austin, TX: EIMC, University of Texas at Austin, 1992.

UNIT 5

Medical Terminology

C

UNIT OBJECTIVES

After completing this unit of study, you should be able to:

◆ Identify basic medical abbreviations selected from a standard list
◆ Define prefixes, suffixes, and word roots selected from a list of words
◆ Spell and pronounce medical terms correctly
◆ Define, pronounce, and spell all of the key terms

KEY TERMS

abbreviations
prefix

suffix

word roots

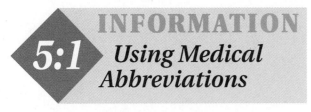

INFORMATION
5:1 Using Medical Abbreviations

As a health care worker, you will see many abbreviations. You will be expected to recognize the most common abbreviations. This section provides a basic list of these abbreviations.

Abbreviations are shortened forms of words, usually just letters. Common examples are A.M., which means morning, and P.M., which means afternoon or evening.

Abbreviations are used in many health fields. Sometimes they are used by themselves; other times, several abbreviations are combined to give orders or directions. Consider the following examples:

> BR c̄ BRP, FFl qh, VS qid
> NPO 8 PM, To Lab for CBC, BUN,
> and FBS.

These examples are short forms for giving directions. The first example is interpreted as follows: bedrest with bathroom privileges, force fluids every hour, vital signs four times a day. The second example is interpreted as follows: nothing by mouth after eight o'clock in the evening, to the laboratory for a complete blood count, blood urea nitrogen, and fasting blood sugar. As these examples illustrate, it is much easier to write using abbreviations than it is to write the corresponding detailed messages.

A sample list of abbreviations and symbols follows. This list contains some of the most commonly used abbreviations. Different abbreviations may be used in different facilities and in different parts of the country, however. It is the responsibility of health care workers to learn the meanings of the abbreviations used in the agencies where they are employed.

NOTE: There is a growing trend toward eliminating periods from most abbreviations. Although the following list does not show periods, you may work in an agency that chooses to use them. When in doubt, follow the policy of your agency.

NOTE: Learn the abbreviations in the following way:

1. Use a set of index cards to make a set of flashcards of the abbreviations found on the abbreviation list. Print one abbreviation in big letters on each card. Put the abbreviation on the front of the card and the meaning on the back of the card.

2. Use the flashcards to study the abbreviations. A realistic goal is to learn all abbreviations for one letter per week. For example, learn all of the *A*s the first week, all of the *B*s the second week, all of the *C*s the third week, and so on until all are learned.

3. Prepare for weekly tests on the abbreviations. The tests will be cumulative. They will cover the letter of the week plus any letters learned in previous weeks.

A

@—at
A&D—admission and discharge
A&P—anterior and posterior or anatomy and physiology
a̅a̅—of each
abd—abdomen or abdominal
ABG—arterial blood gas
ac—before meals
AD—right ear
ad lib—as desired
ADL—activities of daily living
adm—admission
AHA—American Hospital Association
AIDS—acquired immune deficiency syndrome
am or AM—morning, before noon
AMA—American Medical Association or against medical advice
amal—amalgam
amb—ambulate, walk
amt—amount
ANA—American Nurses' Association
ant—anterior
AP—apical pulse
approx—approximately
aq or aqua—aqueous (water base)

ARC—AIDS-related complex
ART—accredited records technician
AS—left ear
as tol—as tolerated
ASA—aspirin
ASAP—as soon as possible
ASCVD—arteriosclerotic cardiovascular disease
ASHD—arteriosclerotic heart disease
AU—both ears
av—average
AV—arteriovenus, atrioventricular
Ax—axilla, axillary, or armpit

B

Ba—barium
bacti—bacteriology
B&B—bowel and bladder training
BBB—bundle branch block
B&C—biopsy and conization
BE—barium enema
bid—twice a day
bil—bilateral
Bl—blood
Bl Wk—blood work
BM—bowel movement
BMR—basal metabolic rate
BP—blood pressure
BR—bed rest
BRP—bathroom privileges
BS—blood sugar
BSC or bsc—bedside commode
BUN—blood urea nitrogen
Bx or bx—biopsy

C

°C—degrees Celsius (Centigrade)
c̄ or w/—with
Ca—calcium
CA—cancer
cal—calorie
Cap—capsule
CAT—computerized axial tomography
Cath—catheter
CBC—complete blood count
CBET—certified biomedical equipment technician

CBR—complete bedrest
cc—cubic centimeter
CC—chief complaint
CCU—coronary care unit or critical care unit
CDA—certified dental assistant
CDC—Centers for Disease Control
CEO—chief executive officer
CHD—coronary heart disease
CHF—congestive heart failure
CHO—carbohydrate
chol—cholesterol
CICU—cardiac intensive care unit
ck—check
Cl—chloride or chlorine
cl liq—clear liquids
cm—centimeter
CMA—certified medical assistant
CNP—certified nurse practitioner
CNS—central nervous system
co or c/o—complains of
CO—carbon monoxide or coronary occlusion
CO_2—carbon dioxide
Comp—complete or compound
cont—continued
COPD—chronic obstructive pulmonary disease
COTA—certified occupational therapy assistant
CP—cerebral palsy
CPK—creatine phosphokinase (cardiac enzyme)
CPR—cardiopulmonary resuscitation
CPT—current procedure terminology
CRTT—certified respiratory therapy technician
CS—central supply or service
C&S—culture and sensitivity
CSF—cerebral spinal fluid
CSR—central supply room
CST—certified surgical technologist
CT—computerized tomography
Cu—copper
CVA—cerebral vascular accident (stroke)
Cx—cervix, complications, or complaints

D

d—day
D&C—dilatation and curettage
DA—dental assistant
DAT—diet as tolerated
DC—doctor of chiropractic

D/C, disc, or dc—discontinued or discharge
DDS—doctor of dental surgery
DEA—Drug Enforcement Agency
del—delivery
Dept—department
DH—dental hygienist
DHHS—Department of Health and Human Services
Diff—differential white blood cell count
dil—dilute or dissolve
DMD—doctor of dental medicine
DMS—diagnostic medical sonography
DNR—do not resuscitate
DO—doctor of osteopathy
DOA—dead on arrival
DOB—date of birth
DON—director of nursing
DPM—doctor of podiatric medicine
DPT—diptheria, pertussis, tetanus
Dr—doctor
dr—dram or drainage
DRG—diagnostic related group
drg or drsg—dressing
D/S—dextrose in saline
DSD—dry sterile dressing
DT—delirium tremors
DVM—doctor of veterinary medicine
DW—distilled water
D/W—dextrose in water
Dx or dx—diagnosis

E

ea—each
EEG—electroencephalogram
EENT—ear, eye, nose, and throat
EKG or ECG—electrocardiogram
elix—elixir
EMG—electromyogram
EMS—emergency medical services
EMT—emergency medical technician
ENT—ear, nose, throat
EPA—Environmental Protection Agency
ER—emergency room
ESR—erythrocyte sedimentation rate
etiol or et—etiology (cause of disease)
Ex or exam—examination
Exc—excision
Exp—exploratory
ext—extract, extraction, or external

F

°F—degrees Fahrenheit
FBS—fasting blood sugar
FBW—fasting blood work
FC—Foley catheter
FDA—Food and Drug Administration
Fe—iron
FF or FFl—force fluids
FH or FHB—fetal heart beat
Fl or fl—fluid
Fr or Fx—fracture
ft—foot
FUO—fever of unknown origin

G

GA—gastric analysis
gal—gallon
GB—gallbladder
Gc—gonococcus, gonorrhea
GI—gastrointestinal
Gm or g—gram
gr—grain
gt, gtt, or gtts—drop, drops
GTT—glucose tolerance test
GU—genitourinary
Gyn—gynecology

H

H—hydrogen
H_2O—water
H_2O_2—hydrogen peroxide
H, (h), or hypo—hypodermic injection
HA—hearing aid or headache
HBV—hepatitis B virus
HCl—hydrochloric acid
hct—hematocrit
HDL—high density lipoproteins (healthy type of cholesterol)
Hg—mercury
Hgb or Hb—hemoglobin
HHA—home health assistant/aide
HIV—human immunodeficiency virus (AIDS virus)
HMO—health maintenance organization

HOB—head of bed
HOH—hard of hearing
HOSA—Health Occupations Students of
  America
Hr, hr, H, or h—hour, hours
HS—hour of sleep (bedtime)
Ht—height
Hx or hx—history
hypo—hypodermic injection or under
Hyst—hysterectomy

I

I&D—incision and drainage
I&O—intake and output
ICD—international classification of diseases
ICU—intensive care unit
IH—infectious hepatitis
IM—intramuscular
in—inch
inf—infusion, inferior, or infection
ing—inguinal
inj—injection
int—internal, interior
IPPB—intermittent positive pressure breathing
irr or irrig—irrigation
Isol or isol—isolation
IUD—intrauterine device
IV—intravenous
IVP—intravenous pyelogram

J

jt—joint

K

K—potassium
KCl—potassium chloride
Kg or kg—kilogram
KUB—kidney, ureter, bladder X-ray

L

L—lumbar
L&D—labor and delivery

L&W—living and well
(L), lt, or lft—left
L or l—liter (1,000 cc)
Lab—laboratory
Lap—laparotomy
lat—lateral
lb—pound
LDH—lactose dehydrogenase (cardiac enzyme)
LDL—low density lipoprotein (unhealthy type
  of cholesterol)
lg—large
liq—liquid
LLQ—left lower quadrant
LMP—last menstrual period
LOC—laxative of choice or level of
  consciousness
LP—lumbar puncture
LPN—licensed practical nurse
LS—lumbar sacral
LUQ—left upper quadrant
LVN—licensed vocational nurse

M

m—minim
MA—medical assistant
Mat—maternity
mcg—microgram
MD—medical doctor, muscular dystrophy, or
  myocardial disease
Med—medical, medicine
mEq—milliequivalent
mg—milligram
Mg—magnesium
MI—myocardial infarction (heart attack)
min—minute
mL or ml—milliliter
MLT—medical laboratory technician
mm—millimeter
MN—midnight
mod—moderate
MOM—milk of magnesia
MRI—magnetic resonance imaging
MS—multiple sclerosis or mitral stenosis
MT—medical technologist

N

N—nitrogen
Na—sodium

NA—nurse aide or assistant
NaCl—sodium chloride (salt)
NB—newborn
neg—negative, none
Neur—neurology
NG or ng—nasogastric tube
NIH—National Institute of Health
nil—none
no—number
NO—nursing office
noc, noct—at night, night
NP—nurse practitioner
NPN—nonprotein nitrogen
NPO—nothing by mouth
N/S—normal saline
Nsy—nursery
N/V or N&V—nausea and vomiting
NVS—neurological vital signs

O

O_2—oxygen
O&P—ova and parasites
Ob or Obs—obstetrics
od—overdose
OD—right eye, occular dextro
oint—ointment
OJ—orange juice
OOB—out of bed
OPD or OPC—outpatient department or clinic
opp—opposite
OR—operating room
Ord—orderly
Orth—orthopedics
os—mouth
OS—left eye, occular sinistra
OT—occupational therapy, occupational therapist
OU—each eye
OV—office visit
oz—ounce

P

p̄—after
P—pulse or phosphorus
PA—physician's assistant
PAC—premature atrial contraction
PAP—Papanicolaou test (smear)
Path—pathology

Pb—lead
PBI—protein bound iodine
pc—after meals
PCA—patient controlled analgesia
PCP—patient care plan
PDR—Physicians' Desk Reference
PE—physical exam or pulmonary edema
Peds—pediatrics
per—by or through
PET—positron emission tomography
pH—measure of acidity/alkalinity
Pharm—pharmacy
PID—pelvic inflammatory disease
PKU—phenylketonuria
PM or pm—after noon
PMC—postmortem (after death) care
PMS—premenstrual syndrome
PNS—peripheral nervous system
po—by mouth
PO—phone order
post—posterior or after
post-op—after an operation
PP—postpartum (after delivery)
PPO—preferred provider organization
pre—before
pre-op—before an operation
prep—prepare
prn—whenever necessary, as needed
Psy—psychology or psychiatry
pt—patient or pint (500 mL or cc)
Pt—prothrombin time
PT—physical therapy, physical therapist
PTT—partial thromboplastin time
PVC—premature ventricular contraction
PVD—peripheral vascular disease
Px—prognosis (expected outcome) or physical exam

Q

q—every
qd—every day
qh—every hour
q2h—every 2 hours
q3h—every 3 hours
q4h—every 4 hours
qhs—every night at bedtime
qid—four times a day
qns—quantity not sufficient
qod—every other day
qs—quantity sufficient
qt—quart

R

R—respiration or rectal
(R) or Rt—right
Ra—radium
RBC—red blood cell or count
RDA—recommended daily allowance
REM—rapid eye movement
RHD—rheumatic heart disease
RLQ—right lower quadrant
RN—registered nurse
R/O—rule out
ROM—range of motion
RR—recovery room
RRT—registered respiratory therapist or
   registered radiologic technologist
RT—respiratory therapist
RUQ—right upper quadrant
Rx—prescription, take, treatment

S

S—sacral
S&A—sugar and acetone
s̄ or w/o—without
SA—sino atrial
sc or SC—subcutaneous
SGOT or SGPT—transaminase test
SICU—surgical intensive care unit
SIDS—sudden infant death syndrome
Sig—give the following directions
sm—small
SOB—short of breath
Sod (Na)—sodium
sol—solution
sos—if necessary
spec—specimen
SpGr or sp gr—specific gravity
SPN—student practical nurse
spt—spirits, liquor
s̄s̄—one half
SSE or SS enema—soap solution enema
staph—staphylococcus infection
stat—immediately (at once)
STD—sexually transmitted disease
strep—streptococcus infection
sup—superior
supp—suppository

Surg—surgery, surgical
susp—suspension
Sx—symptom, sign
syp—syrup

T

T&A—tonsillectomy and adenoidectomy
T or Temp—temperature
tab—tablet
TB—tuberculosis
tbsp—tablespoon
TCDB—turn, cough, and deep breathe
TIA—transient ischemic attack
tid—three times a day
TLC—tender loving care
TO—telephone order
tol—tolerated
TPN—total parental nutrition
TPR—temperature, pulse, and respiration
tr or tinct—tincture
tsp—teaspoon
TUR—transurethral resection
TWE—tap water enema
tx—traction, treatment, or transplant

U

UA or U/A—urinalysis
ung—ointment
Ur or ur—urine
URI—upper respiratory infection
UTI—urinary tract infection
UV—ultraviolet

V

Vag—vaginal
VD—venereal disease
VDRL—serology for syphillis
VICA—Vocational Industrial Clubs of America
VO—verbal order
Vol—volume
VS—vital signs (TPR and BP)

W

WBC—white blood cell or count
WC—ward clerk or secretary
w/c—wheelchair
WHO—World Health Organization
W/P—whirlpool
wt—weight

X

x—times (example: 2x means do two times)
x-match—cross match
XR—X-ray

Z

Zn—zinc

MISCELLANEOUS SYMBOLS

>—greater than
<—less than
↑—higher, elevate, or up
↓—lower or down
#—pound or number
ʒ—dram
℥—ounce
'—foot or minute
"—inch or second
°—degree
♀ or F—female
♂ or M—male
I or *i* or Ī—one
II or *ii* or ĪĪ—two
V—five
X—ten
L—fifty
C—one hundred
D—five hundred
M—one thousand

STUDENT *Go to the workbook and complete the assignment and evaluation sheets for 5:1, Using Medical Abbreviations.*

INFORMATION
5:2 *Interpreting Word Parts*

Medical dictionaries have been written to include the many words used in health occupations. It would be impossible to memorize all such words. By breaking the words into parts, however, it is sometimes possible to figure out their meanings. This section provides basic information on doing just that.

A word is often a combination of different parts. The parts include prefixes and suffixes (see figure 5-1).

A **prefix** can be defined as a syllable or word placed at the beginning of a word. A **suffix** can be defined as a syllable or word placed at the end of the word.

The meanings of prefixes and suffixes are set. For example, the suffix *itis* means "inflammation of." *Tonsillitis* means "an inflammation of the tonsils," and *appendicitis* means "an inflammation of the appendix." Note that the meaning of the suffix is usually placed first when the word is defined.

Word roots can be defined as main words or parts to which prefixes and suffixes can be added. In the example *appendicitis*, the word root is *appendix*. By adding the prefix *pseudo*, which means "false," and the suffix *itis*, which means "inflammation of," the word becomes *pseudoappendicitis*. This is interpreted as a "false inflammation of the appendix."

The prefix usually serves to further define the word root. The suffix usually describes what is happening to the word root.

By learning basic prefixes, suffixes, and word roots, you will frequently be able to interpret the meaning of a word even when you have never before encountered the word. A list of common prefixes, suffixes, and word roots follows.

NOTE: Learn the prefixes, suffixes, and words root in the following way:

1. Use a set of index cards to make flashcards of the word parts found on the prefix, suffix, and

Figure 5-1 Prefixes, suffixes, and word roots can be used to interpret the meaning of a word.

word root list. Place one prefix, suffix, or word root on each card. Put the word part on the front of the card and the meaning of the word part on the back of the card. Ensure that each is spelled correctly.

2. Use the flashcards to learn the meanings of the word parts. A realistic goal is to learn one letter per week. For example, learn all word parts starting with the letter *A* the first week, all of those starting with *B* the second week, all of those starting with *C* the third week, and so on until all are learned. Practice correct spelling of all of the word parts.

3. Prepare for weekly tests on the word parts. The tests will be cumulative. They will cover the letter of the week plus any letters learned in previous weeks. Words will be presented that use the various word parts. In order to be considered correct, you must spell the words correctly.

A

a-, an-: without, not
ab-: from, away
-able: capable of
-ac, -ic: pertaining to
acr-, acro-: extremities (arms and legs)
ad-: to, toward
aden-, adeno-: gland, glandular
adren-, adreno-: adrenal gland
aer-, aero-: air
-al: like, similar, pertaining to
alges-, algesi-: oversensitivity to pain
-algia: pain
ambi-: both, both sides
an-, ano-: anus (opening to rectum)
angi-, angio-: vessel

ankyl-: crooked, looped; immovable, fixed
ante-: before
antero-: in front of, ahead of
anti-: against
append-, appendo-: appendix
arter-, arterio-: artery
arthr-, arthro-: joint
-ase: enzyme
-asis: condition of
-asthenia: weakness, lack of strength
ather-, athero-: fatty, lipid
audi-, audio-: sound, hearing, dealing with the ear
aur-: ear
auto-: self

B

bi, bis-: twice, double, both
bio-: life
-blast: germ cell, embryonic cell
blephar-, blepharo-: eyelid
brachi-: arm
brachy-: short
brady-: slow
bronch-, bronchi-: air tubes in the lungs (bronchi)
bucc-, bucca-: cheek

C

calc-, calculus-: stone
carcin-, carcino-: cancer, malignancy
cardi-, cardia-, cardio-: pertaining to the heart
carp-, carpo-: wrist
-cele: swelling, tumor, cavity, or hernia

cent-, centi-: one hundred
-centesis: surgical puncture to remove fluid
cephal-, cephalo-: head, pertaining to the head
cerebro-: brain
cerv-, cervic-: neck, neck of uterus
cheil-, cheilo-: lip
chem-, chemo-: drug, chemical
chir-, chiro-: hand
chlor-, chloro-: green
chol-, chole-, cholo-: bile or gall; gallbladder
chondi-, chondr-, chondri-: cartilage
chrom-, chromo-: color
-cide: causing death
circum-: around, about
-cise: cut
-clysis: washing or irrigation
-coccus: round
coele-: chamber, enlarged space
col-, colo-: colon, bowel, large intestine
colp-, colpo-: vagina
con-, co-: with, together
contra-: against, counter
costa-, costo-: rib
crani-, cranio-: pertaining to the skull
-crine: secrete
cryo-: cold
crypt-: hidden
cut-: skin
cyan-, cyano-: blue
cyst-, cysto-, cysti-: bladder, bag, sac
-cyte, cyt-, cyto-: cell

D

dacry-: tear duct, tear
dactyl-, dactylo-: finger, toe
dec-, deca-, deci-: ten
demi-: half
dent-, dento-: tooth
derm-, derma-, dermo-, dermat-: pertaining to skin
-desis: surgical union or fixation
dextro-: to the right
di-, diplo-: double, twice
dia-: through, between, or part
dis-, disto-: separation, away from
dorsi-, dorso-: to the back, back
duoden-, duodeno-: duodenum (first part of small intestine)
-dynia, -dynic: pain
dys-: difficult, painful, bad

E

e-, ec-: without
-eal: pertaining to
ec-, ecto-: outside, external
-ectasis: expansion, dilation, stretching
-ectomy: surgical removal of
electr-, electro-: electrical
-emesis: vomit
-emia: blood
encephal-, encephalo-: brain, pertaining to the brain
endo-: within, innermost
enter-, entero-: intestine, pertaining to the intestine
epi-: upon, over, or upper
erythro-: red
-esis: condition of
-esthesia, aesthesio-: sensation, perception, feel
eu-: well, easy
ex-, exo-: outside of, beyond

F

-fascia: fibrous band
-ferous: producing
fibr-, fibro-: fiber, fibrous, connective tissue
fore-: in front of
-form: having the form of, shape
-fuge: driving away or expelling

G

galacto-: milk, galactose (milk sugar)
gasti-, gastro-: stomach
-genesis: development, production, creation
-genetic, -genic: origin, producing, causing
genito-: organs of reproduction
-genous: kind or type
geront-, geronto-: old age, elderly
gingiv-: gums, gingiva
gloss-, glosso-: tongue
gluc-, gluco-: sweetness, sugar, glucose
gly-, glyco-: sugar
-gram: tracing, picture, record
-graph: diagram or instrument for recording
gyn-, gynec-, gyno-: women, female

H

hem-, hema-, hemo-, hemato-: blood
hemi-: half
hepato-: liver
herni-: rupture
hetero-: other, unlike, different
hist-, histo-: tissue
homo-, homeo-: same, like
hydro-: water
hyper-: excessive, high, over, increased, or more than normal
hypno-: sleep
hypo-: decreased, deficient, less than normal, low, or under
hyster-, hystero-: uterus

I

-ia, -iasis: condition of, abnormal or pathological state
-ic, -ac: pertaining to
idio-: peculiar to an individual, self-originating
ile-, ileo-: ileum (last part of small intestine)
infra-: beneath, below
inter-: between or among
intra-: within, into, inside
-ism: condition, theory, state of being
iso-: equal, alike, same
-itis: inflammation, inflammation of

K

kerat-, kerato-: cornea of the eye
-kinesis, kinetic-: motion

L

labi-, labia-, labio-: lip
lacrima-: tears
lact-, lacto-: milk
lapar-, laparo-: abdomen, abdominal wall
laryng-, laryngo-: larynx (voicebox)
latero-: side
-lepsy: seizure, convulsion

leuco-, leuko-: white
lingua-, linguo-: tongue
lip-, lipo-: fat, lipids
lith-, litho-: stone, calculus
-logy, -ology: study of, science of
lymph-, lympho-: lymph tissue
-lys, -lysis, -lyso: destruction, dissolving of

M

macro-: large
mal-: bad, abnormal, disordered, poor
malac-, -malacia: softening of a tissue
mamm-, mammo-: breast, mammary glands
-mania: insanity, mental disorder
mast-, masto-: breast
med-, medi-: middle, midline
-megaly, mega-, megalo-: large, enlarged
melan-, melano-: black
mening-, meningo-: membranes covering the brain and spinal cord
meno-: monthly, menstruation
mes-, meso-: middle, midline
-meter: measuring instrument, measure
-metry: measurement
micro-: small
mono-: one, single
-mortem: death
muc-, muco-: mucus, secretion of mucous membrane
multi-: many, much, a large amount
my-, myo-: muscle
myc-, myco-: fungus
myel-, myelo-: bone marrow, spinal cord
myring-, myringo-: eardrum, tympanic membrane

N

narc-, narco-: sleep, numb, stupor
nas-, naso-: nose
-natal: birth
necr-, necro-: death
neo-: new
neph-, nephro-: kidney
neur-, neuro-: nerve or nervous system
noct-, nocti-: night, at night
non-: no, none

O

ocul-, oculo-: eye
-ode, -oid: form, shape; like or resembling
odont-, odonto-: tooth
olig-, oligo-: few, less than normal, or small
-ologist: person who does, person who studies
-ology: study of, science of
-oma: tumor, a swelling
onco-: mass, bulk, tumor
oophor-, oophoro-: ovary, female egg cell
ophthalm-, ophthalmo-: eye
-opia: vision
-opsy: to view
opt-, optic-: vision, eye
or-, oro-: mouth
orch-, orchido-: testicle, testes
-orrhea, -rrhea: flow, discharge
orth-, ortho-: normal, straight
os-, oste-, osteo-: bone
-oscopy: diagnostic examination
-osis: condition, state, process
-ostomy: creation of an opening by surgery
ot-, oto-: ear
-otic: pertaining to a condition
-otomy: cutting into
-ous: full of, pertaining to, condition,
    or material
ovi-, ovario-: egg, female sex gland, ovary

phag-, phago-: eat, ingest
-phage, -phagia: to eat, consuming, swallow
pharyng-, pharyngo-: pharynx, throat
-phas, -phasia, -phaso: speech
-phil, -philia, -philic: affinity for, attracted to,
    "loves"
phleb-, phlebo-: vein
-phobia: fear
phon-, phono-: sound, voice
-phylaxis: protection, preventative
-plasty: surgical correction or repair
-plegia: paralysis
pleuro-: side or rib
-pnea: breathing
pneum-, pneumo-: lung, pertaining to the
    lungs; air
pod-, podo-: foot
poly-: many, much
post-: after, behind
pre-: before, in front of
pro-: in front of, forward
proct-, procto-: rectum, rectal, anus
psora-: itch
psuedo-: false
psych-, psycho-: pertaining to the mind
-ptosis: drooping down, sagging, downward
    displacement
pulmon-, pulmono-: lung
py-, pyo-: pus
pyel-, pyelo-: renal pelvis (of kidney)
pyr-, pyro-: heat, fever

P

pan-: all, complete, entire
pancreat-, pancreato-: pancreas
para-: near, beside, beyond, abnormal, or lower
    half of the body
-paresis: paralysis
-partum: birth, labor
path-, patho-, pathy, -pathia: disease, abnormal
    condition
ped-, pedia-: child
-penia: lack of, abnormal reduction in number,
    deficiency
pent-, penta-: five
-pepsia, -pepsis: digestion
per-: through, by, or excessive
peri-: around
-pexy: fixation

Q

quad-, quadri-: consisting of four

R

radi-, radio-: X-rays, radiation
re-: back, again
rect-, recto-: rectum
ren-, reno-: kidney
retro-: backward, in back, behind
rhin-, rhino-: nose, pertaining to the nose
-rraphy: suture of, sewing up of a gap or defect
-rrhagia: sudden or excessive flow
-rrhea: flow, discharge
-rrhexis: rupture of

S

salpingo-: tube, fallopian tube
sanguin-, sanguino-: blood
sarc-, sarco-: malignant (cancer) connective
   tissue
-sarcoma: tumor, cancer
scler-, sclero-: hardening
-sclerosis: dryness or hardness
-scope, -scopy: examining instrument;
   observation
-sect: cut
semi-: half, part
sep-, septi-: poison, rot, infection
sinistr-, sinistro-: left
soma-, somat-: body
somni-, somno-: sleep
son-, sono-: sound
-spasm: involuntary contraction
sperm-, spermato-: spermatoza, male
   germ (sex) cell
splen-, spleno-: spleen
-stasis: stoppage; maintaining a
   constant level
steno-: contracted, narrow
stern-, sterno-: sternum, breast bone
stoma-, stomat-: mouth
stomy: artificial opening
sub-: less, under, below
super-, supra-: above, upon, over, or
   higher in position
sym-, syn-: joined or fused, together

T

tacho-, tachy-: rapid, fast
tendo-, teno-: tendon
tetra-: four
-therapy: treatment
therm-, thermo-, -thermy: heat
thorac-, thoraco-: thorax, chest
thromb-, thrombo-: clot, thrombus
thym-, thymo-: thymus gland
thyr-, thyro-: thyroid gland
-tome: instrument that cuts
-tox, -toxic: poison
trache-, trachi-, tracho-: trachea, windpipe
trans-: across, over, or beyond
tri-: three

trich-, tricho-: hair
-trips, -tripsy: crushing by rubbing or
   grinding
-trophy: nutrition, growth or development
tympan-, tympano-: eardrum, tympanic
   membrane

U

ultra-: beyond, excess
uni-: one
ur-, uro-: urine, urinary tract
ureter-, uretero-: ureter (tube from kidney
   to bladder)
urethr-, urethro-: urethra (tube from bladder
   to urinary meatus [outside])
-uria: urine
uter-, utero-: uterus, womb

V

vas-, vaso-: vessel, duct
ven-, vena-: vein
ventro-: to the front; abdomen
vertebr-, vertebro-: spine, vertebrae
vesic-, vesico-: urinary bladder
viscer-, viscero-: internal organs
vit-, vita-: necessary for life

X

xanth-, xantho-: yellow

Z

zoo-: animal

STUDENT *Go to the workbook and complete the assignment and evaluation sheets for 5:2, Interpreting Word Parts.*

UNIT 5 SUMMARY

Medical abbreviations and terminology are used in all health care occupations and facilities. In order to communicate effectively, health care workers must be familiar with common abbreviations and terminology.

Medical abbreviations are shortened forms of words, usually just letters. Sometimes, they are used by themselves; other times, several abbreviations are combined to give orders or directions.

Medical terminology consists of the use of prefixes, suffixes, and word roots to create words. Entire dictionaries have been written to include the terminology used in health care. It would be impossible to memorize the meaning of every word. By learning common prefixes, suffixes, and word roots, however, health care worker can break a word into parts and thereby figure out the meaning of the word.

UNIT 5
SUGGESTED REFERENCES

Applegate, April, and Valerie Overton. *The Elements of Medical Terminology*. Albany, NY: Delmar Publishers, 1995.

Dennerll, Jean Tannis. *Medical Terminology Made Easy*. Albany, NY: Delmar Publishers, 1993.

DeSousa, Luis. *Common Medical Abbreviations*. Albany, NY: Delmar Publishers, 1995.

Ehrlich, Ann. *Introduction to Dental Terminology, Charting, and Procedures*. 2nd ed. Champaign, IL: Colwell Co., 1995.

Ehrlich, Ann. *Medical Terminology for Health Professions*. 2nd ed. Albany, NY: Delmar Publishers, 1994.

Kinn, Mary E. *Medical Terminology: Building Blocks for Health Careers*. Albany, NY: Delmar Publishers, 1990.

Kinn, Mary E. *Medical Terminology Review Challenge*. Albany, NY: Delmar Publishers, 1987.

Layman, Dale. *The Medical Language: A Programmed, Body-Systems Approach*. Albany, NY: Delmar Publishers, 1995.

Rice, Jane. *Medical Terminology with Human Anatomy*. 3rd ed. Norwalk, CT: Appleton-Lang, 1994.

Rice, Jane. *Spellright: A Medical Word Book*. Norwalk, CT: Appleton-Lang, 1991.

Sanders, W. B. *Dorland's Pocket Medical Dictionary*. 28th ed. Philadelphia, PA: W. B. Sanders, 1991.

Smith, Genevieve L., Phyllis E. Davis, and Jean Tannis Dennerll. *Medical Terminology: A Programmed Text*. 7th ed. Albany, NY: Delmar Publishers, 1996.

Sormunen, Carolee, and Marie Moisio. *Terminology for Allied Health Professionals*. 3rd ed. Albany, NY: Delmar Publishers, 1995.

Thomas, Clayton L., ed. *Taber's Cyclopedic Medical Dictionary*. 17th ed. Philadelphia, PA: F. A. Davis, 1993.

UNIT 6

Anatomy and Physiology

UNIT OBJECTIVES

After completing this unit of study, you should be able to:

◆ Apply the appropriate terminology to major organs and systems of the human body
◆ Identify the major functions of the body systems
◆ Compare the interrelationship of the body systems
◆ Describe the basic diseases affecting each of the body systems
◆ Define, pronounce, and spell all of the key terms

KEY TERMS

abdominal

anatomy

cell

circulatory

digestive

endocrine
 (en´-doe-krin)

excretory
 (ex´-kreh-tor″-ee)

integumentary
 (in-teg-u-men´-tah-ree)

lymphatic
 (lim-fat´-ik)

muscular

nervous

organ

physiology
 (fizz-ee-ahl″-oh-gee)

reproductive

respiratory
 (res´-peh-reh-tor″-ee)

skeletal

system

thoracic
 (tha-rass´-ik)

tissue

urinary

Note: *This unit is meant to serve as a brief introduction to anatomy and physiology. For more detailed information, refer to the references listed at the end of the unit.*

6:1 Basic Structure of the Human Body

Objectives

After completing this section, you should be able to:

◆ Label a diagram of the main parts of a cell
◆ Describe the basic function of each part of a cell
◆ Compare the four main types of tissue by describing the basic function of each type
◆ Explain the relationship between cells, tissues, organs, and systems
◆ Define, pronounce, and spell all of the key terms

KEY TERMS

anatomy

cell

cell membrane

centrosome
 (sen´-troh-sohm)

chromatin
 (crow´-ma-tin)

connective tissue

cytoplasm
 (sy´-toe-pla-z-em)

dehydration

edema
 (eh-dee´-mah)

endoplasmic reticulum
 (en´-doe-plaz-mik
 re-tik´-you-lum)

epithelial tissue
 (ep´-eh-thiel″-e-al
 tish´-u)

Golgi apparatus
 (gawl´-jee ap-a-rat´-
 us)

lysosomes
 (ly´-sah-soms)

meiosis

mitochondria
 (my-toe-con´-dree-
 ah)

mitosis
 (my-toe´-sis)

muscle tissue

nerve tissue

nucleolus
 (new″-klee-oh´-lus)

nucleus

organ

organelles

pathophysiology

physiology
 (fizz-ee-all´-oh-gee)

pinocytic vesicles

protoplasm
 (pro´-toe-plaz-um)

system

tissue

6:1 INFORMATION

The human body is often described as an efficient, organized machine. When this machine does not function correctly, disease occurs. Before understanding the disease processes, however, the health worker must first understand the normal functioning of the body. A basic understanding of anatomy and physiology is therefore necessary. Anatomy is the study of the form and structure of an organism. Physiology is the study of the processes of living organisms, or why and how they work. Pathophysiology is the study of how disease occurs and the responses of living organisms to disease processes.

The basic substance of all life is protoplasm. This material makes up all living things. Although protoplasm is composed of ordinary elements such as carbon, oxygen, hydrogen, sulfur, nitrogen, and phosphorus, scientists are unable to combine such elements to create that characteristic called *life*.

CELLS

Protoplasm forms the basic unit of structure and function in all living things: the cell. Cells are microscopic structures that carry on all the functions of life. They take in food and oxygen; produce heat and energy; move and adapt to their environment; eliminate wastes; perform special functions; and reproduce to create new, identical cells. The human body contains trillions of cells. These cells vary in shape and size and perform many different functions.

Most cells have the following basic parts (see figure 6-1):

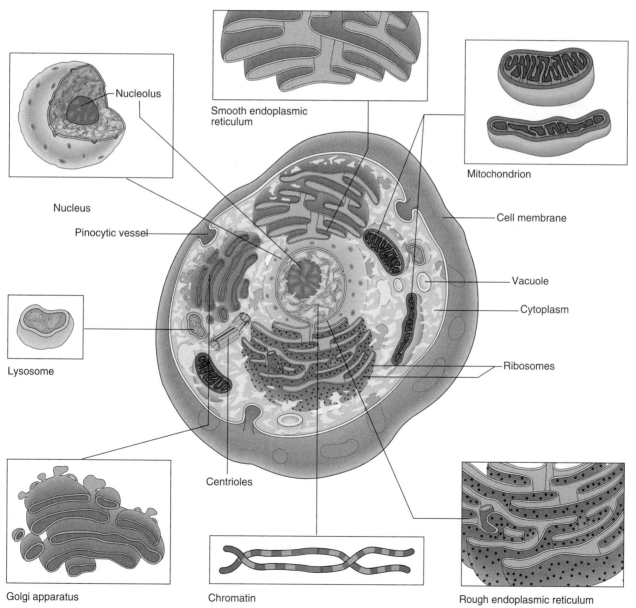

Nucleolus

Smooth endoplasmic reticulum

Mitochondrion

Nucleus

Cell membrane

Pinocytic vessel

Vacuole

Cytoplasm

Lysosome

Ribosomes

Centrioles

Golgi apparatus

Chromatin

Rough endoplasmic reticulum

Figure 6-1 Basic parts of a cell.

◆ **Cell membrane**—the outer protective covering of the cell. It is semipermeable, which means that it allows certain substances to enter and leave the cell while preventing the passage of other substances.

◆ **Cytoplasm**—a semi fluid inside the cell. It contains water, proteins, lipids (fats), carbohydrates, minerals, and salts. It is the site for all chemical reactions that take place in the cell. **Organelles,** or cell structures that help a cell to function, are located in the cytoplasm. The main organelles are the nucleus, mitochondria, ribosomes, lysosomes, centrioles, Golgi apparatus, and endoplasmic reticulum.

◆ **Nucleus**—a mass in the cytoplasm. It is often called the "brain" of the cell because it controls many cell activities and is important in cell division.

◆ **Nucleolus**—located inside the nucleus, and important in cell reproduction. Ribosomes, made of ribonucleic acid (RNA) and protein, are manufactured in the nucleolus. The ribosomes move from the nucleus to the cytoplasm, where they aid in the synthesis (production) of protein. They can exist freely in the cytoplasm or be attached to the endoplasmic reticulum.

◆ **Chromatin**— located in the nucleus and made of deoxyribonucleic acid (DNA) and protein. During cell reproduction, the chromatin condenses to form chromosomes. A human cell has forty-six chromosomes or twenty-three pairs. The chromosomes contain the genes, which carry inherited characteristics. Each gene has a specific and unique sequence of approximately 1,000 base pairs of DNA; the DNA sequence carries the genetic coding that allows for exact duplication of the cell. Since the DNA sequence on genes is unique for each individual, it is sometimes used as an identification tool similar to fingerprints, but much more exact.

◆ **Centrosome**—located in the cytoplasm and near the nucleus. It contains two centrioles, which are important during cell reproduction.

◆ **Mitochondria**—rod-shaped organelles located throughout the cytoplasm. These are often called the "furnaces" or "powerhouses" of the cell because they produce adenosine triphosphate (ATP), the major energy source of the cell.

◆ **Golgi apparatus**—a stack of membrane layers located in the cytoplasm. This structure produces, stores, and packages secretions for discharge from the cell.

◆ **Endoplasmic reticulum**—a fine network of tubular structures located in the cytoplasm. This network allows for the transport of materials in and out of the nucleus, and also aids in the synthesis and storage of proteins. Rough endoplasmic reticulum contains ribosomes while smooth endoplasmic reticulum does not.

◆ **Lysosomes**—found throughout the cytoplasm. These structures contain digestive enzymes that digest and destroy old cells, bacteria, and foreign materials.

◆ **Pinocytic vesicles**—pocketlike folds in the cell membrane. These folds allow large molecules such as proteins and fats to enter the cell. When such molecules are inside the cell, the folds close to form vacuoles or bubbles in the cytoplasm.

Cell Reproduction

Most cells reproduce by dividing into two identical cells. This process is called **mitosis,** a form of asexual reproduction (see figure 6-2). Some specialized cells, such as nerve cells in the brain and spinal cord and muscle cells, do not reproduce after birth. When such cells are damaged or destroyed, others are not formed to replace them.

Prior to mitosis, the chromatin material in the nucleus condenses to form chromosomes, and an exact duplicate of each chromosome is made. Each chromosome then consists of two identical strands, called *chromatids,* joined together by a structure called a *centromere.* When mitosis begins, the two centrioles in the centrosome move to opposite ends of the cell. A spindle of threadlike fibers trails from the centrioles. The nuclear membrane disappears, and the pairs of duplicated chromosomes attach to the spindles at the center of the cell. The chromatids then split from their duplicated halves and move to opposite ends of the cell. Each end now has forty-six chromosomes or twenty-three pairs. The cytoplasm divides, and a new cell membrane forms to create two new identical cells.

Sex cells (gametes) divide by a process known as **meiosis.** This form of cell division produces ovum and sperm that each contain only twenty-three chromosomes. When an ovum and sperm join to create a new life, the zygote, or new cell, has forty-six chromosomes: twenty-three from the ovum and twenty-three from the sperm. Thus, the zygote has twenty-three pairs of chromosomes, the normal number for all body cells except the sex cells.

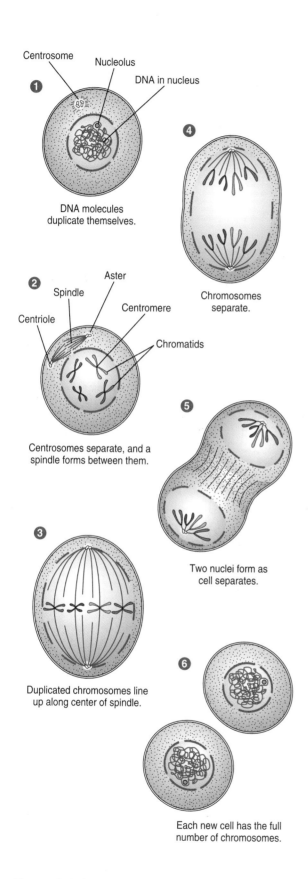

Figure 6-2 Mitosis is a form of asexual reproduction where a cell divides into two identical cells.

TISSUE

Although most cells contain the same basic parts, cells vary greatly in shape, size, and special function. When cells of the same type join together for a common purpose, they form a tissue. Tissues are 60 percent to 99 percent water with various dissolved substances. This water is slightly salty in nature and is called *tissue fluid*. If there is an insufficient amount (not enough) tissue fluid, a condition called dehydration occurs. When there is an excess amount (too much) tissue fluid, a condition called edema, or swelling of the tissues, occurs.

There are four main groups of tissues: epithelial, connective, nerve, and muscle (see figure 6-3).

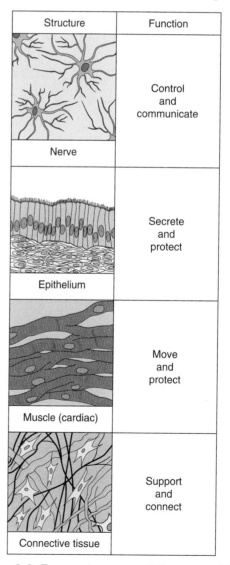

Figure 6-3 Four main groups of tissues and their functions.

Epithelial tissue covers the surface of the body and is the main tissue in the skin. It forms the lining of the intestinal, respiratory, and urinary tracts, as well as that of other body cavities. It also forms the body glands.

Connective tissue is the supporting fabric of organs and other body parts. There are two main classes of connective tissue: soft and hard. Soft con-

nective tissue includes adipose, or fatty, tissue (which stores fat as a food reserve [or source of energy], insulates the body, and acts as padding) and fibrous connective tissue, such as ligaments and tendons (which help hold body structures together). Hard connective tissue includes cartilage and bone. Cartilage is a tough, elastic material that is found between the bones of the spine and at the end of

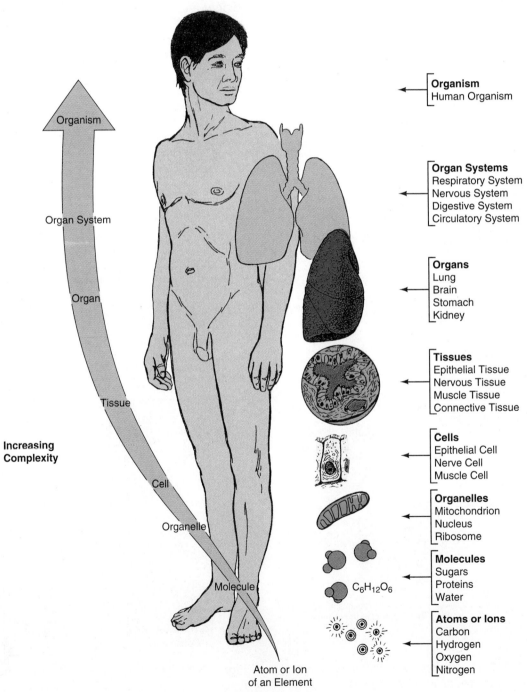

Figure 6-4 The levels of complexity in the human organism.

long bones and that acts as a shock absorber. It is also found in the nose, ears, and larynx, or "voice box." Bone is similar to cartilage but has calcium salts, nerves, and blood vessels; it is frequently called *osseous tissue.* Bone helps form the rigid structure of the human body. Blood and lymph are classified as liquid connective tissue. Blood carries nutrients and oxygen to the body cells and carries metabolic waste away from cells. Lymph transports tissue fluid, proteins, fats, and other materials from the tissues to the circulatory system.

Nerve tissue is made up of special cells called *neurons.* It transmits messages throughout the body and composes the nerves, brain, and spinal cord.

Muscle tissue produces power and movement by contraction of muscle fibers. There are three main types of muscle tissue: skeletal, cardiac, and visceral (smooth). Skeletal muscle attaches to the bones and provides for movement of the body. Cardiac muscle causes the heart to beat. Visceral muscle is present in the walls of many organs such as the stomach, intestine, and blood vessels.

ORGANS AND SYSTEMS

Two or more tissues joined together to perform a specific function are called an **organ.** Examples of organs include the heart, stomach, and lungs.

Organs and other body parts joined together to perform a particular function are called a **system.** The basic systems (discussed in more detail in succeeding sections) are the integumentary, skeletal, muscular, circulatory, lymphatic, nervous, respiratory, digestive, urinary (or excretory), endocrine, and reproductive.

In summary, cells combine to form tissues, tissues combine to form organs, and organs and other body parts combine to form systems. These systems working together help create the miracle called the human body (see figure 6-4.)

STUDENT *Go to the workbook and complete the assignment sheet for 6:1, Basic Structure of the Human Body.*

6:2 Body Planes, Directions, and Cavities

Objectives

After completing this section, you should be able to:

◆ Label the names of the planes and the directional terms related to these planes on a diagram of the three planes of the body
◆ Label a diagram of the main body cavities
◆ Identify the main organs located in each body cavity
◆ Locate the nine abdominal regions
◆ Define, pronounce, and spell all of the key terms

KEY TERMS

abdominal cavity
abdominal regions
anterior

body cavities
body planes

caudal
  (kaw´-doll)
cranial
  (kray´-nee-al)
cranial cavity
distal
dorsal
dorsal cavity
frontal (coronal) plane
inferior
lateral
  (lat´-eh-ral)
medial
  (me´-dee-al)
midsagittal (median)
  plane
  (mid-saj´-ih-tahl)

pelvic cavity
posterior
proximal
  (prox´-ih-mahl)
spinal cavity
superior
thoracic cavity
  (tho-rass´-ik)
transverse plane
ventral
ventral cavity

6:2 ## INFORMATION

Because terms such as *south* and *east* would be difficult to apply to the human body, other directional terms have been developed. These terms are used to describe the relationship of one part of the body to another part.

BODY PLANES

Body planes are imaginary lines drawn through the body at various parts to separate the body into sections. Directional terms are created by these planes. The three main body planes are the transverse, midsagittal, and frontal (see figure 6-5).

The **transverse plane** is a horizontal plane that divides the body into a top half and a bottom half. Body parts above other parts are termed **superior,** and body parts below other parts are termed **inferior.** For instance, the shin is superior to the ankle- but inferior to the knee. Two other directional terms related to this plane include **cranial,** which means body parts located near the head, and **caudal,** which means body parts located near the sacral region of the spinal column (also known as the "tail").

The **midsagittal,** or **median, plane** divides the body into right and left sides. Body parts close to the midline, or plane, are called **medial,** and body parts away from the midline are called **lateral.**

The **frontal,** or **coronal, plane** divides the body into a front section and a back section. Body parts in front of the plane, or on the front of the body, are called **ventral,** or **anterior.** Body parts on the back of the body are called **dorsal,** or **posterior.**

Two other directional terms are **proximal** and **distal.** These are used to describe the location of the extremities (arms and legs) in relation to the main trunk of the body, generally called the *point of reference*. Body parts close to the point of reference are called proximal, and body parts distant from the point of reference are called distal. For example, in describing the relationship of the wrist and elbow to the shoulder (or point of reference), the wrist is distal and the elbow is proximal to the shoulder.

BODY CAVITIES

Body cavities are spaces within the body that contain vital organs. There are two main body cavities; the dorsal, or posterior, cavity and the ventral, or anterior, cavity (see figure 6-6).

The **dorsal cavity** is one long, continuous cavity located on the back of the body. It is divided into two sections: the **cranial cavity,** which contains the brain, and the **spinal cavity,** which contains the spinal cord.

The **ventral cavities** are larger than the dorsal cavities. The ventral cavity is separated into two distinct cavities by the dome-shaped muscle called the *diaphragm*, which is important for respiration (breathing). The **thoracic cavity** is located in the chest and contains the heart, lungs, and large blood vessels. The **abdominal cavity** is divided into an upper part and a lower part. The upper abdominal cavity contains the stomach, small intes-

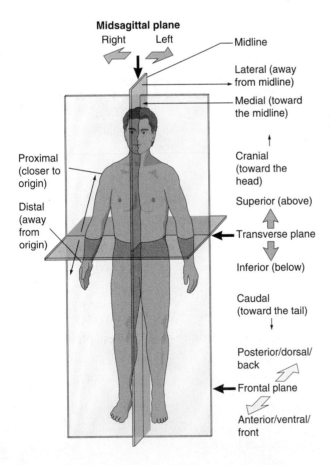

Figure 6-5 Body planes and directional terms.

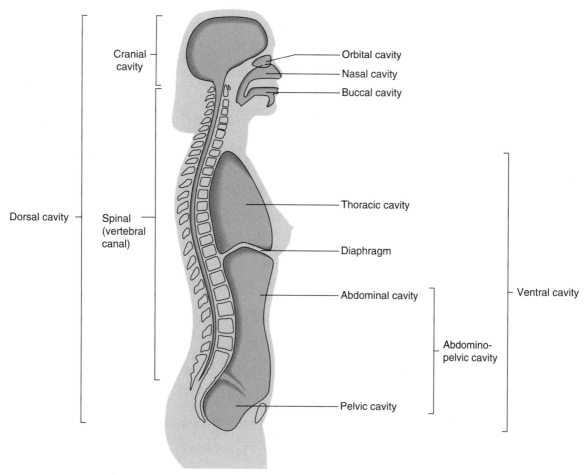

Figure 6-6 Body cavities.

tine, most of the large intestine, liver, gallbladder, pancreas, and spleen. The lower abdominal cavity, or **pelvic cavity,** contains the urinary bladder, the reproductive organs, and the last part of the large intestine.

Three small cavities are the orbital cavity (for the eyes), the nasal cavity (for the nose structures), and the buccal, or mouth, cavity.

ABDOMINAL REGIONS

The abdominal cavity is so large that it is divided into regions or sections. One method of division is into quadrants, or four sections. As shown in figure 6-7, this results in a right upper quadrant (RUQ),

left upper quadrant (LUQ), right lower quadrant (RLQ), and left lower quadrant (LLQ). Another method of division is into nine **abdominal regions** (see figure 6-8). The center regions are the epigastric (above the stomach), umbilical (near the umbilicus, or belly button), and hypogastric, or pelvic (below the stomach). On either side of the center the regions are the hypochondriac (below the ribs), lumbar (near the large bones of the spinal cord), and iliac, or inguinal (near the groin).

The terms relating to body planes, directions, and cavities are used frequently in the study of human anatomy.

STUDENT   *Go to the workbook and complete the assignment sheet for 6:2, Body Planes, Directions, and Cavities.*

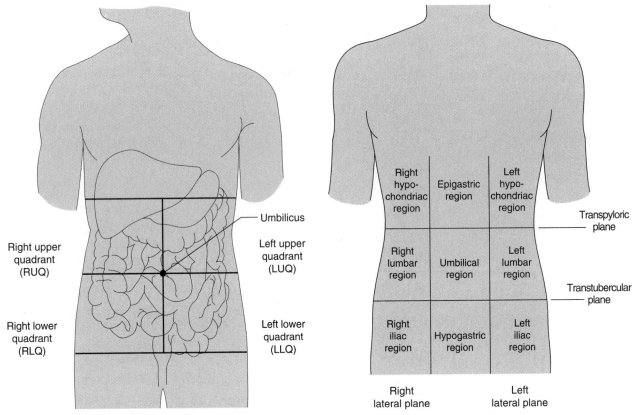

Figure 6-7 Abdominal quadrants.

Figure 6-8 Nine abdominal regions.

6:3 Integumentary System

Objectives

After completing this section, you should be able to:

◆ Label a diagram of a cross section of the skin
◆ Differentiate between the two types of skin glands
◆ List six functions of the skin
◆ Provide the correct names for three abnormal colors of the skin and identify the cause of each abnormal color
◆ Describe at least four skin eruptions
◆ Describe at least four diseases of the integumentary system
◆ Define, pronounce, and spell all of the key terms

KEY TERMS

constrict
  (kun-strict´)
crusts
cyanosis
  (sy˝-eh-noh´-sis)
dermis
dilate
  (die´-late)
epidermis
  (eh-pih-der´-mis)
erythema
  (err-ih-thee´-ma)

integumentary
jaundice
  (jawn´-diss)
macules
  (mack´-youlz)
papules
  (pap´-youlz)
pustules
  (pus´-tyoulz)
sebaceous glands
  (seh-bay´-shus)

subcutaneous fascia
  (hypodermis)
  *(sub-q-tay´-nee-us
  fash´-ee-ah)*
sudoriferous glands
  (sue-de-rif´-eh-rus)

vesicles
  (ves´-i-kulz)
wheals

6:3 INFORMATION

The integumentary system, or skin, has been called both a membrane, because it covers the body, and an organ, because it contains several kinds of tissues. Most anatomy courses, however, refer to it as a system because it has organs and other parts that work together to perform a particular function.

Three main layers of tissue make up the skin (see figure 6-9):

◆ Epidermis—the outermost layer of skin. This layer is actually made of five to six smaller layers but no blood vessels. Two main layers are the *stratum corneum* and the *stratum germinativum*. The cells of the stratum corneum are constantly shed and replaced by new cells from the stratum germinativum.

◆ Dermis—also called *corium,* or "true skin." This layer has a framework of elastic connective tissue and contains blood vessels; nerves; involuntary muscle; sweat and oil glands; and hair follicles. The top of the dermis is covered with papillae, which fit into ridges on the stratum germinativum of the epidermis. These ridges form lines, or striations, on the skin. Because the pattern of ridges is unique to each individual, fingerprints and footprints are often used as methods of identification.

◆ Subcutaneous fascia or hypodermis—the innermost layer. It is made of elastic and fibrous connective tissue and adipose (fatty) tissue, and connects the skin to underlying muscles.

The integumentary system has two main types of glands: sudoriferous and sebaceous. The sudoriferous glands (sweat glands) are coiled tubes that extend through the dermis and open on the surface of the skin at pores. The sweat, or perspiration, eliminated by these glands contains water, salts, and some body wastes. The sebaceous glands are oil glands that usually open onto hair follicles. They produce sebum, an oil that keeps the skin and

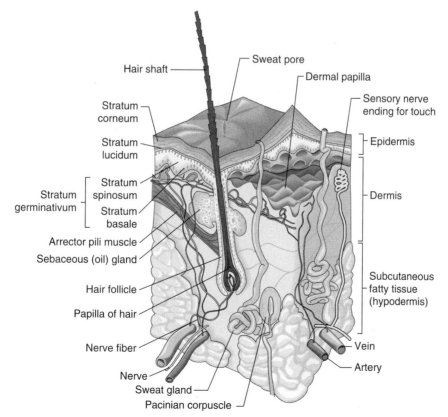

Figure 6-9 Cross section of skin.

hair from becoming dry and brittle. When an oil gland becomes plugged, the accumulation of dirt and oil results in a blackhead or pimple.

Two other parts of the integumentary system are the hair and nails. Each hair consists of a root (which grows in a hollow tube, called a *follicle*) and a hair shaft. Hair helps protect the body. Nails are made of dead epithelial cells packed closely together to form a thick, dense surface. They are formed in the nailbed. If lost, nails can be replaced, if the nailbed is not damaged.

FUNCTIONS

The integumentary system performs the following important functions:

◆ *Protection*—It serves as a barrier to the sun's ultraviolet rays and the invasion of pathogens, or germs. It also holds moisture in and prevents deeper tissues from drying out.
◆ *Sensory perception*—The nerves in the skin help the body respond to pain, pressure, temperature (heat and cold), and touch sensations.
◆ *Body temperature regulation*—The blood vessels in the skin help the body retain or lose heat. When the blood vessels **dilate** (get larger), excess heat from the blood can escape through the skin. When the blood vessels **constrict** (get smaller), the heat is retained in the body. The sudoriferous glands also help cool the body.
◆ *Storage*—The skin has tissues for temporary storage of fat, glucose (sugar), water, vitamins, and salts. Adipose (fatty) tissue in the subcutaneous fascia is a source of energy.
◆ *Absorption*—Certain substances can be absorbed through the skin, but this is limited. Examples include motion sickness or heart disease medications that are placed on transdermal patches and applied to the skin.
◆ *Excretion*—The skin helps the body eliminate salt, a minute amount of waste, and excess water through perspiration.
◆ *Production*—The skin produces vitamin D by combining ultraviolet rays from the sun with skin compounds.

PIGMENTATION

Skin color is determined by pigments in the epidermis of the skin. Melanin, a brownish-black pigment, absorbs ultraviolet light to tan the skin. Small areas of melanin pigment form freckles. Carotene, a yellowish-red pigment, also helps determine skin color. Abnormal colors of the skin can indicate disease. **Erythema** is a reddish color of the skin that can be caused by either burns or a congestion of blood in the vessels. **Jaundice,** a yellow discoloration of the skin, can indicate bile in the blood as a result of liver or gallbladder disease. Jaundice also occurs in conjunction with certain diseases that involve the destruction of red blood cells. **Cyanosis** is a bluish discoloration of the skin caused by insufficient oxygen. It can be associated with heart, lung, and circulatory diseases or disorders. Chronic poisoning may cause a gray or brown skin discoloration.

SKIN ERUPTIONS

Skin eruptions can also indicate disease. **Macules** (macular rash) are flat spots on the skin, such as freckles. **Papules** (papular rash) are firm, raised areas such as pimples and the eruptions seen in some stages of chickenpox and syphilis. **Vesicles** are blisters, or fluid-filled sacs, such as those seen in chickenpox. **Pustules** are pus-filled sacs such as those seen in acne, or pimples. **Crusts,** areas of dried pus and blood, are commonly called "scabs." **Wheals** are itchy, elevated areas with an irregular shape; hives and insect bites are examples.

DISEASES

Acne vulgaris is an inflammation of the sebaceous glands. Although the cause is unknown, acne usually occurs at adolescence. Hormonal changes and increased secretion of sebum are probably underlying causes. Symptoms include papules, pustules, and blackheads. These occur when the hair follicles become blocked with dirt, cosmetics, excess oil, and/or bacteria. Treatment methods include frequent, thorough skin washing; avoiding creams and heavy makeup; antibiotic or vitamin A ointments; oral antibiotics; and/or ultraviolet light treatments.

Athlete's foot is a contagious fungus infection that usually affects the feet. The skin itches, blisters, and cracks into open sores. Treatment involves applying an antifungal medication and keeping the area clean and dry.

Cancer of the skin takes in different forms such as basal cell carcinoma, squamous cell carcinoma, and malignant melanoma. Frequently, skin cancer develops from a mole or nevus that changes in color, shape, size, or texture. Bleeding or itching of a mole can also indicate cancer. Exposure to the sun, irritating chemicals, or radiation are the usual causes of skin cancer. Treatment involves surgical removal of the cancer.

Dermatitis, an inflammation of the skin, can be caused by many factors and is frequently an allergic reaction to detergents, cosmetics, pollen, or certain foods. Contact dermatitis is caused by contact with poison ivy, poison sumac, or poison oak (see figure 6-10). Symptoms include dry skin, erythema, itching, edema, macular-papular rashes, and scaling. Treatment is directed at eliminating the cause, especially in the case of allergens. Anti-inflammatory ointments, antihistamines, and/or steroids are also used in treatment.

Eczema is a noncontagious, inflammatory skin disorder caused by an allergen or irritant. Diet, cosmetics, soaps, medications, and emotional stress can all cause eczema. Symptoms include erythema, edema, itching, vesicles, crusts, and scaling. Treatment involves removing the irritant and applying corticosteroids to reduce the inflammatory response.

Impetigo is a highly contagious skin infection usually caused by streptococci or staphylococci organisms. Symptoms include erythema, oozing vesicles, pustules, and the formation of a yellow crust. Lesions should be washed with soap and water and kept dry. Antibiotics, both topical and oral, are also used in treatment.

Figure 6-10 A contact dermatitis caused by contact with poison oak. *(Courtesy of Timothy Berger, MD, Associate Clinical Professor, University of California, San Francisco).*

Psoriasis is a chronic, noncontagious, inherited skin disease. Symptoms include thick, red areas covered with white or silver scales. Although there is no cure, treatment methods include coal/tar or cortisone ointments; ultraviolet light; and/or scale removal.

Verrucae, or warts, are caused by a viral infection of the skin. A rough, hard, elevated, rounded surface forms on the skin. Some warts disappear spontaneously, but others must be removed with electricity, liquid nitrogen, acid, or chemicals.

STUDENT *Go to the workbook and complete the assignment sheet for 6:3, Integumentary System.*

6:4 Skeletal System

Objectives

After completing this section, you should be able to:

◆ List five functions of bones
◆ Label the main parts of a bone on a diagram of a long bone
◆ Name the two divisions of the skeletal system

and the main groups of bones in each division
◆ Identify the main bones of the skeleton
◆ Compare the three classifications of joints by describing the type of motion allowed by each
◆ Give one example of each joint classification
◆ Describe at least four diseases of the skeletal system
◆ Define, pronounce, and spell all of the key terms

appendicular skeleton
  (ap-pen-dick´-u-lar)
axial skeleton
carpals
clavicles
  (klav´-ih-kulz)
cranium
diaphysis
  (dy-af´-eh-sis)
endosteum
  (en-dos´-tee-um)
epiphysis
  (ih-pif´-eh-sis)
femur
  (fee´-mur)
fibula
  (fib´-you-la)
fontanels
foramina
  (for-ahm´-e-nah)
humerus
  (hue´-mer-us)
joints
ligaments
medullary canal
  (med´-hue-lair-ee)

metacarpals
  (met-ah-car´-pulz)
metatarsals
  (met-ah-tar´-sulz)
os coxae
  (ahs cock´-see)
patella
  (pa-tell´-ah)
periosteum
  (per-ee-os´-tee-um)
phalanges
  (fa-lan´-jeez)
radius
red marrow
ribs
scapula
sinuses
  (sigh´-nuss-ez)
sternum
sutures
tarsals
tibia
ulna
vertebrae
  (vur´-teh-bray)
yellow marrow

INFORMATION

6:4

The skeletal system is made of organs called *bones.* An adult human has 206 bones. These bones work as a system to perform the following functions:

◆ *Framework*—The bones form a framework to support the body's muscles, fat, and skin.
◆ *Protection*—Bones surround vital organs to protect them. Examples include the skull, which surrounds the brain, and the ribs, which protect the heart and lungs.
◆ *Levers*—Muscles attach to bones to help provide movement.
◆ *Production of blood cells*—Bones help produce both red and white blood cells.

◆ *Storage*—Bones store most of the calcium supply of the body.

Bones vary in shape and size depending on their locations within the body. Bones of the extremities (arms and legs) are called *long bones.* The basic parts of these bones are shown in figure 6-11. The long shaft is called the diaphysis, and the two extremities, or ends, are each called an epiphysis. The medullary canal is a cavity in the diaphysis. It is filled with yellow marrow, which is mainly fat cells. The endosteum is a membrane that lines the medullary canal and keeps the yellow marrow intact. It also produces some bone growth. Red marrow is found in certain bones such as the vertebrae, ribs, sternum, and cranium, and in the proximal ends of the humerus and femur. It produces red blood cells (erythrocytes), platelets, and some white blood cells. Because bone marrow is important in the manufacture of blood cells and is involved with

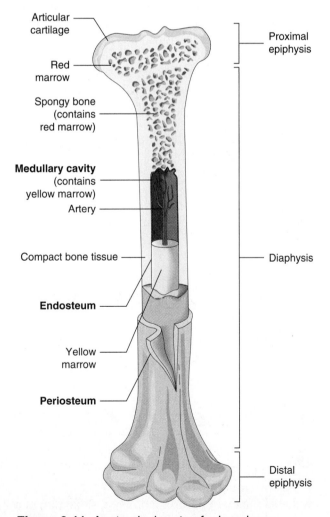

Figure 6-11 Anatomical parts of a long bone.

the body's immune response, the red marrow is used to diagnose blood diseases and is sometimes transplanted in people with defective immune systems. The outside of bone is covered with a tough membrane, called the periosteum, which is necessary for bone growth, repair, and nutrition. A thin layer of articular cartilage covers the epiphysis and acts as a shock absorber when two bones meet to form a joint.

The skeletal system is divided into two sections: the axial skeleton and the appendicular skeleton. The axial skeleton forms the main trunk of the body and is composed of the skull, spinal column, ribs, and breastbone. The appendicular skeleton forms the extremities and is composed of the shoulder girdle, arm bones, pelvic girdle, and leg bones.

The skull is composed of the cranium and facial bones (see figure 6-12). The cranium is the spherical structure that surrounds and protects the brain. It is made of eight bones: one frontal, two parietal, two temporal, one occipital, one ethmoid, and one sphenoid. At birth, the cranium is not solid bone. Spaces called fontanels, or "soft spots," allow for the enlargement of the skull as brain growth occurs. The fontanels are made of membrane and cartilage and turn into solid bone by approximately eighteen months of age. There are fourteen facial bones: one mandible (lower jaw), two maxilla (upper jaw), two zygomatic (cheek), two lacrimal (inner aspect of eyes), five nasal, and two palatine. Sutures are areas where the cranial bones have joined together. Sinuses are air spaces in the bones of the skull that act as resonating chambers for the voice. They are lined with mucous membranes. Foramina are openings in bones that allow nerves and blood vessels to enter or leave the bone.

The spinal column is made of twenty-six bones called vertebrae (see figure 6-13). These bones protect the spinal cord and provide support for the head and trunk. They include seven cervical (neck), twelve thoracic (chest), five lumbar (waist), one sacrum (back of pelvic girdle), and one coccyx (tailbone). Pads of cartilage tissue, called *intervertebral disks,* separate the vertebrae. The disks act as shock absorbers and permit bending and twisting movements of the vertebral column.

There are twelve pairs of ribs, or costae. They attach to the thoracic vertebrae on the dorsal surface of the body. The first seven pairs are called *true ribs* because they attach directly to the sternum, or breastbone, on the front of the body. The next five pairs are called *false ribs.* The first three pairs of false ribs attach to the cartilage of the rib above. The last two pairs of false ribs are called *floating ribs* because they have no attachment on the front of the body.

The sternum or breastbone is the last bone of the axial skeleton. It consists of three parts: the

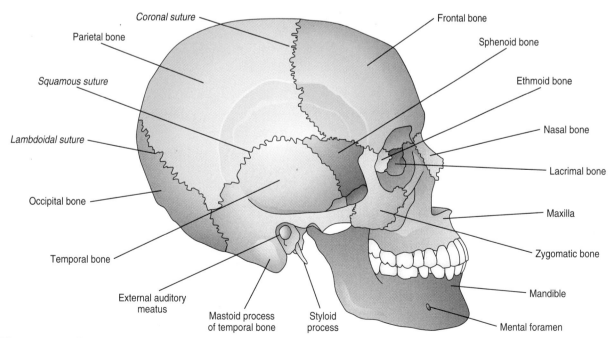

Figure 6-12 Bones of the skull.

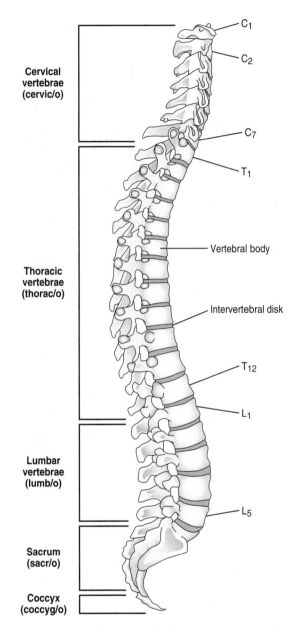

Figure 6-13 Lateral view of the vertebral, or spinal, column.

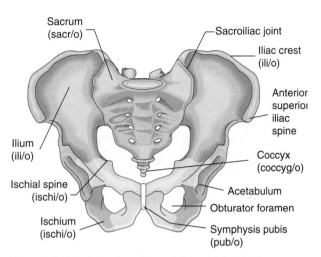

Figure 6-14 Anterior view of the pelvic girdle.

manubrium (upper region), the body, and the xiphoid process (a small piece of cartilage at the bottom). The two collarbones, or clavicles, are attached to the manubrium by ligaments. The ribs are attached to the sternum with costal cartilages to form a "cage" that protects the heart and lungs.

The shoulder, or pectoral, girdle is made of two clavicles (collarbones) and two scapulas (shoulder bones). The scapulas provide for attachment of the upper arm bones.

Bones of each arm include one humerus (upper arm), one radius (lower arm on thumb side), one ulna (larger bone of lower arm with a projection called the *olecranon process* at its upper end, forming the elbow), eight carpals (wrist), five metacarpals (palm of the hand), and fourteen phalanges (fingers).

The pelvic girdle is made of two os coxae (coxal, or hip, bones), which join with the sacrum on the dorsal part of the body (see figure 6-14). Each os coxae is made of three regions: the ilium, the ischium, and the pubis. The pelvic girdle contains two recessed areas, or sockets. These sockets, called *acetabulums,* provide for the attachment of the leg bones.

Each leg consists of one femur (thigh); one patella (kneecap); one tibia and one fibula (lower leg); seven tarsals (ankle); five metatarsals (instep of foot); and fourteen phalanges (toes). The heel is formed by the large tarsal bone called the *calcaneous.* The bones of the skeleton are shown in figure 6-15.

Joints are areas where two or more bones join together. Connective tissue bands, called ligaments, help hold long bones together at joints. Joints are classified as either freely movable (ball-and-socket joints of the shoulder and hip, and hinge joints of the elbow and knee), slightly movable (vertebrae), or immovable (the cranium).

DISEASES

Arthritis is actually a group of diseases involving inflammation of the joints. Two main types are osteoarthritis and rheumatoid arthritis. Osteoarthritis, the most common form, is a chronic dis-

SKULL Cranium
Zygomatic bone
Maxilla
Mandible
SHOULDER GIRDLE

Parietal
Occipital

Clavicle
Scapula

Acromion process
Scapula

Xiphoid process
THORAX
Sternum
Ribs

Costal cartilage
VERTEBRAL COLUMN

UPPER EXTREMITY
Humerus

VERTEBRAL COLUMN
Olecranon process

Ilium
Ulna
Radius
Carpals

PELVIC GIRDLE

Sacrum
Pubis
Ischium

Coccyx

Symphysis pubis

Metacarpals Phalanges

Femur
LOWER EXTREMITY

Femur

Femur
Patella
Tibia
Fibula

Lateral condyle
Medial condyle

Tarsals
Metatarsals
Phalanges

Lateral maleolus
Medial maleolus

Calcaneus

Figure 6-15 Bones of the skeleton.

ease that usually occurs as a result of aging. It frequently affects the hips and knees. Symptoms include joint pain, stiffness, aching, and limited range of motion. Although there is no cure, rest; applications of heat and cold; aspirin; injection of steroids into the joints; and special exercises are used to relieve the symptoms. Rheumatoid arthritis is a chronic, inflammatory disease affecting the connective tissues and joints. It is three times more common in women than in men and onset often occurs between the ages of thirty-five and forty-five. Progressive attacks can cause scar tissue formation and atrophy of bone and muscle tissue, which result in permanent deformity and immobil-

ity. Early treatment is important to reduce pain and limit damage to joints. Rest, prescribed exercise, anti-inflammatory medications such as aspirin, and careful use of steroids are the main forms of treatment. Surgery to replace damaged joints, such as those in the hips and knees, is sometimes performed when severe joint damage has occurred.

Bursitis is an inflammation of the bursae, small, fluid-filled sacs surrounding the joints. It frequently affects the shoulders, elbows, hips, or knees. Symptoms include severe pain, limited movement, and fluid accumulation in the joint. Treatment consists of administering pain medications; injecting steroids and anesthetics into the affected joint; rest; and aspirating (withdrawing fluid with a needle) the joint.

A *fracture* is a crack or break in a bone. A crack in a bone is called a *greenstick fracture*. A complete break with no damage to the skin is called a *simple fracture*. A bone break that pierces or ruptures through the skin is called a *compound fracture*. When the bone is splintered or crushed and bone fragments are present, the fracture is termed *comminuted*. If a severe head injury causes a piece of the skull bone to move inward, a *depressed fracture* results. A severe twisting of a bone resulting in one or more breaks (common in skiing and skating accidents) is called a *spiral fracture*. Before a fracture can heal, the bone must be put back into its proper alignment. This process is called *reduction*. *Closed reduction* involves positioning the bone in correct alignment, usually with traction, and applying a cast or splint to maintain the position until the fracture heals. *Open reduction* involves surgical repair of the bone. In some cases, special pins, plates, or other devices are surgically implanted to maintain correct position of the bone.

A *dislocation* is when a bone is forcibly displaced from a joint. It frequently occurs in shoulders, fingers, knees, and hips. After the dislocation is reduced (the bone is replaced in the joint), the dislocation is immobilized with a splint, a cast, or traction.

A *sprain* is when a twisting action tears the ligaments at a joint. The wrists and ankles are common sites for sprains. Symptoms include pain, swelling, discoloration, and limited movement. Treatment methods include rest; elevation; immobilization with an elastic bandage or splint; and/or cold applications.

Osteomyelitis is a bone inflammation usually caused by a pathogenic organism. The infectious organisms cause the formation of an abscess within the bone and an accumulation of pus in the medullary canal. Symptoms include pain at the site, swelling, chills, and fever. Antibiotics are used to treat the infection.

Osteoporosis, or increased porosity or softening of the bones, is a metabolic disorder caused by a hormone deficiency (especially estrogen in females), prolonged lack of calcium in the diet, and a sedentary lifestyle. The loss of calcium and phosphate from the bones causes the bones to become porous, brittle, and prone to fracture. Treatment methods include increased intake of calcium and vitamin D; exercise; and/or estrogen replacement.

Abnormal curvatures of the spinal column include *kyphosis, scoliosis,* and *lordosis* (see figure 6-16). Kyphosis, or "hunchback," is a rounded bowing of the back at the thoracic area. Scoliosis is a side-to-side, or lateral, curvature of the spine. Lordosis, or "swayback," is an abnormal inward curvature of the lumbar region. Poor posture, structural defects of the vertebrae, malnutrition, and degeneration of the vertebrae can all be causes of these defects. Therapeutic exercises, firm mattresses, and/or braces are the main forms of treatment. Severe deformities may require surgical repair.

STUDENT   *Go to the workbook and complete the assignment sheet for 6:4, Skeletal System.*

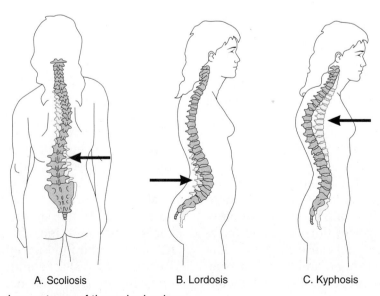

A. Scoliosis   B. Lordosis   C. Kyphosis

Figure 6-16 Abnormal curvatures of the spinal column.

6:5 Muscular System

Objectives

After completing this section, you should be able to:

◆ Compare the three main kinds of muscle by describing the action of each

◆ Differentiate between voluntary muscle and involuntary muscle

◆ List at least three functions of muscles

◆ Describe the two main ways muscles attach to bones

◆ Demonstrate the five major movements performed by muscles

◆ Describe at least three diseases of the muscular system

◆ Define, pronounce, and spell all of the key terms

KEY TERMS

abduction
  (ab-duck´-shun)
adduction
  (ah-duck´-shun)
cardiac muscle
contract
  (con-trackt´)
contractibility
contracture
  (con-track´-shur)
elasticity
excitability
extensibility
extension

fascia
  (fash´-ee"-ah)
flexion
  (flek´-shun)
insertion
involuntary
muscle tone
origin
rotation
skeletal muscle
tendons
visceral(smooth)
  muscle
voluntary

6:5 INFORMATION

Over 600 muscles make up the system known as the muscular system. Muscles are bundles of muscle fibers held together by connective tissue. All muscles have certain properties or characteristics. Excitability, or irritability, is the ability to respond to a stimulus such as a nerve impulse. A second property is contractibility. When muscle fibers are stimulated by nerves, they contract, or become short and thick. This contraction causes movement. Another property is extensibility, or the ability to be stretched. A final property is elasticity. This allows the muscle to return to its original shape after it has contracted or stretched.

There are three main kinds of muscle: cardiac, visceral, and skeletal (see figure 6-17). Cardiac muscle forms the walls of the heart and contracts to circulate blood. Visceral, or smooth, muscle is found in the internal organs of the body such as those of the digestive and respiratory systems, and the blood vessels and eyes. Visceral muscle contracts to cause movement in these organs. Cardiac muscle and visceral muscle are involuntary, meaning they function without conscious thought or control. Skeletal muscle is attached to bones and causes body movement. Skeletal muscle is voluntary because a person has control over its action. Because cardiac muscle and visceral muscle are discussed in sections on other systems, the following concentrates on skeletal muscle.

Skeletal muscles perform important functions: they attach to bones to provide voluntary movement; during contraction, they produce heat and energy for the body; they help maintain posture; and some protect internal organs.

Skeletal muscles attach to bones in different ways. Some attach by tendons, strong, tough connective-tissue cords. An example is the gastrocnemius muscle on the calf of the leg, which attaches to the heelbone by the achilles tendon. Other muscles attach by fascia, a tough, sheetlike membrane that covers and protects the tissue. Examples include the deep muscles of the trunk and back, which are surrounded by the lumbodorsal fascia. When a muscle attaches to a bone, the end that does not move is called the origin. The end that moves when the muscle contracts is called the insertion.

A variety of different actions or movements performed by muscles are shown in figure 6-18 and are described as follows:

Figure 6-17 Three main kinds of muscles.

Figure 6-18 Types of muscle movements.

◆ **Adduction**—moving a body part toward the midline

◆ **Abduction**—moving a body part away from the midline

◆ **Flexion**—decreasing the angle between two bones, or bending a body part

◆ **Extension**—increasing the angle between two bones, or straightening a body part

◆ **Rotation**—turning a body part on its axis by a circular motion

The major muscles of the body are shown in figure 6-19; the locations and actions of the major muscles are noted in table 6-1.

Muscles are partially contracted at all times, even when not in use. This state of partial contraction is called **muscle tone** and is sometimes de-

scribed as a state of readiness to act. Loss of muscle tone can occur in severe illness such as paralysis. When muscles are not used for a long period of time, they can atrophy (shrink in size and lose strength). Lack of use can also result in a **contracture,** a severe tightening of a flexor muscle resulting in bending of a joint. Foot drop is a common contracture, but the fingers, wrists, knees, and other joints can also be affected.

DISEASES

Muscular dystrophy is actually a group of inherited diseases that lead to chronic, progressive muscle atrophy. Muscular dystrophy usually appears in

Anterior Surface Muscles

Posterior Surface Muscles

Figure 6-19 Major muscles of the body.

TABLE 6-1 **Locations and Functions of Major Muscles of the Body**

MUSCLE	LOCATION	FUNCTION
Sternocleidomastoid	Side of neck	Turns and flexes head
Trapezius	Upper back and neck	Turns head, moves shoulder
Deltoid	Shoulder	Abducts arm, injection site
Biceps brachii	Upper arm	Flexes lower arm
Triceps brachii	Upper arm	Extends lower arm
Pectoralis major	Upper chest	Adducts upper arm
Intercostals	Between ribs	Moves ribs for breathing
Rectus abdominus	Ribs to pubis (pelvis)	Compresses abdomen
Latissimus dorsi	Spine around to chest	Extends and adducts upper arm
Gluteus maximus	Buttocks	Extends thigh, injection site
Sartorius	Front of thigh	Abducts thigh, flexes leg
Quadriceps femoris	Front of thigh	Extends leg
Tibialis anterior	Front of lower leg	Flexes and inverts foot
Gastrocnemius	Back of lower leg	Flexes sole of the foot

early childhood; most types result in total disability and early death. Although there is no cure, physical therapy is used to slow the progress of the disease.

Myasthenia gravis is a chronic condition where nerve impulses are not properly transmitted to the muscles. This leads to progressive muscular weakness and paralysis. If the condition affects the respiratory muscles, it can be fatal. While the cause is unknown, myasthenia gravis is thought to be an autoimmune disease, with antibodies attacking the body's own tissues. There is no cure, and treatment is supportive.

Muscle spasms, or cramps, are sudden, painful, involuntary muscle contractions. They usually occur in the legs or feet and may result from overexer-tion, low electrolyte levels, or poor circulation. Gentle pressure and stretching of the muscle is used to relieve the spasm.

A *strain* is an overstretching of or injury to a muscle and/or tendon. Frequent sites include the back, arms, and legs. Prolonged or sudden muscle exertion is usually the cause. Symptoms include myalgia (muscle pain), swelling, and limited movement. Treatment methods include rest; muscle relaxants or pain medications; elevating the extremity; and alternating hot and cold applications.

STUDENT *Go to the workbook and complete the assignment sheet for 6:5, Muscular System.*

Circulatory System

Objectives

After completing this section, you should be able to:

◆ Label the layers, chambers, valves, and major blood vessels on a diagram of the heart

◆ Differentiate between systole and diastole by explaining what happens in the heart during each phase

◆ List the three major types of blood vessels and the action of each type

◆ Compare the three main types of blood cells by describing the function of each

◆ Describe at least five diseases of the circulatory system

◆ Define, pronounce, and spell all of the key terms

KEY TERMS

aortic valve
(ay-or´-tick)
arteries
blood
capillaries
(cap´-ih-lair-eez)
diastole
(dy-az´-tah-lee")
endocardium
(en-doe-car´-dee-um)
erythrocytes
(eh-rith´-row-sitez)
hemoglobin
(hee´-mow-glow"-bin)
left atrium
(ay´-tree-um)
left ventricle
(ven´tri"-kul)
leukocytes
(lew´-coh-sitez")

mitral valve
(my´-tral)
myocardium
pericardium
plasma
(plaz´-ma)
pulmonary valve
right atrium
right ventricle
septum
systole
(sis´-tah-lee")
thrombocytes
(throm´-bow-sitez)
tricuspid valve
veins

INFORMATION

6:6

The **circulatory** system, also known as the cardiovascular system, is often referred to as the "transportation" system of the body. It consists of the heart, blood vessels, and blood. It transports oxygen and nutrients to the body cells, and carbon dioxide and metabolic materials away from the body cells.

The heart is a muscular, hollow organ often called the "pump" of the body (see figure 6-20). It is approximately the size of a closed fist and is located in the mediastinal cavity, between the lungs, behind the sternum, and above the diaphragm. Three layers of tissue form the heart. The **endocardium** is a smooth layer of cells that lines the inside of the heart and is continuous with the inside of blood vessels. It allows for the smooth flow of blood. The thickest layer is the **myocardium,** the muscular middle layer. The **pericardium** is a double-layered membrane, or sac, that covers the outside of the heart.

The **septum** is a muscular wall that separates the heart into a right side and a left side. It prevents blood from moving between the right and left sides of the heart. The upper part of the septum is called the *interatrial septum,* and the lower part is called the *interventricular septum.*

HEART CHAMBERS

The heart is divided into four parts or chambers. The two upper chambers are called *atria,* and the two lower chambers are called *ventricles.* The **right atrium** receives blood as it returns from the body cells. The **right ventricle** receives blood from the right atrium and pumps the blood into the pulmonary artery, which carries the blood to the lungs for oxygen. The **left atrium** receives oxygenated blood from the lungs. The **left ventricle** receives blood from the left atrium and pumps the blood into the aorta for transport to the body cells.

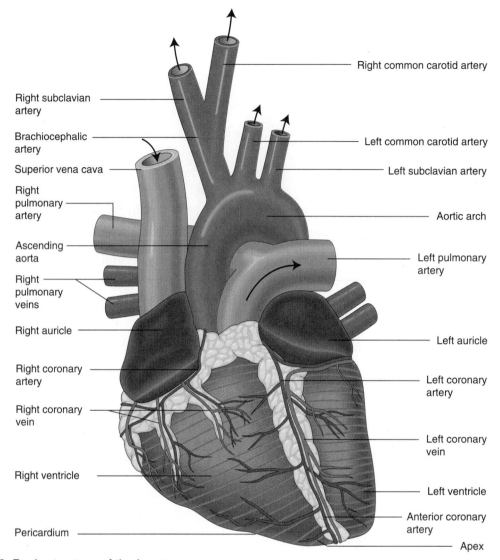

Figure 6-20 Basic structure of the heart.

One-way valves in the chambers of the heart keep the blood flowing in the right direction. The tricuspid valve is located between the right atrium and the right ventricle. It closes when the right ventricle contracts, allowing blood to flow to the lungs and preventing blood from flowing back into the right atrium. The pulmonary valve is located between the right ventricle and the pulmonary artery, a blood vessel that carries blood to the lungs. It closes when the right ventricle has finished contracting, preventing blood from flowing back into the right ventricle. The mitral valve is located between the left atrium and left ventricle. It closes when the left ventricle is contracting, allowing blood to flow into the aorta (for transport to the body) and preventing blood from flowing back into the left atrium. The aortic valve is located between the left ventricle and the aorta, the largest artery in

the body. It closes when the left ventricle is finished contracting, allowing blood to flow into the aorta and preventing blood from flowing back into the left ventricle.

Heartbeat Cycle

Although they are separated by the septum, the right and left sides of the heart work together in a cyclic manner. The cycle consists of a brief period of rest, called diastole, followed by a period of ventricular contraction, called systole (see figure 6-21). At the start of the cycle, the atria contract and push blood into the ventricles. The atria then relax, and blood returning from the body enters the right atrium, while blood returning from the lungs enters the left atrium. As the atria are filling, systole begins, and the ventricles contract. The right ventricle

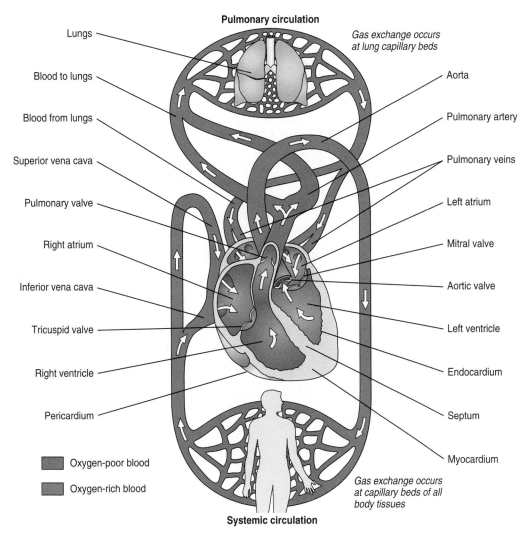

Pulmonary circulation

Lungs

*Gas exchange occurs
at lung capillary beds*

Blood to lungs

Aorta

Blood from lungs

Pulmonary artery

Superior vena cava

Pulmonary veins

Pulmonary valve

Left atrium

Right atrium

Mitral valve

Inferior vena cava

Aortic valve

Tricuspid valve

Left ventricle

Right ventricle

Endocardium

Pericardium

Septum

Myocardium

Oxygen-poor blood

Oxygen-rich blood

*Gas exchange occurs
at capillary beds of all
body tissues*

Systemic circulation

Figure 6-21 The pattern of circulation in the cardiovascular system.

pushes blood into the pulmonary artery, sending the blood to the lungs for oxygen. The left ventricle pushes blood into the aorta, sending the blood to all other parts of the body. The blood in the right side of the heart is low in oxygen and high in carbon dioxide. When this blood arrives in the lungs, the carbon dioxide is released into the lungs, and oxygen is taken into the blood. This oxygenated blood is then carried to the left side of the heart by the pulmonary veins. This blood in the left side of the heart, being high in oxygen and low in carbon dioxide, is ready for transport to the body cells.

Conductive Pathway

Electrical impulses originating in the heart cause the cyclic contraction of the muscles (see figure 6-22). A group of nerve cells located in the right atrium and called the *sinoatrial (SA) node,* or the

"pacemaker," sends out an electrical impulse, which spreads out over the muscles in the atria. The atrial muscles then contract and push blood into the ventricles. After the electrical impulse passes through the atria, it reaches the *atrioventricular (AV) node,* a group of nerve cells located between the atria and ventricles. The AV node sends the electrical impulse through the bundle of His, nerve fibers in the septum. The bundle of His divides into a right bundle branch and a left bundle branch, which carry the impulse down through the ventricles. The bundle branches further subdivide into the Purkinje fibers, a network of nerve fibers throughout the ventricles. In this way, the electrical impulse reaches all of the muscle tissue in the ventricles, and the ventricles contract. This electrical conduction pattern occurs approximately every 0.8 seconds. The movement of the electrical impulse can be recorded on an electrocardiogram (ECG or EKG) and used to detect abnormal activity or disease.

Superior vena cava

Right pulmonary artery

Right pulmonary veins

Sinoatrial (S-A) node (pacemaker)

Pulmonary semilunar valve

Right atrium

Atrioventricular (A-V) node

Tricuspid valve

Right ventricle

Inferior vena cava

Arch of aorta

Ascending aorta

Left pulmonary artery

Left pulmonary veins

Left atrium

Aortic semilunar valve

Bicuspid (mitral) valve

Atrioventricular bundle (bundle of His)

Left ventricle

Papillary muscle

Myocardium

Interventricular septum

Purkinje fibers

Apex

Descending aorta

Endocardium

Figure 6-22 Electrical conduction pathways in the heart.

BLOOD VESSELS

When the blood leaves the heart, it is carried throughout the body in blood vessels. The heart and blood vessels form a closed system for the flow of blood. There are three main types of blood vessels: arteries, capillaries, and veins.

Arteries (see figure 6-23) carry blood away from the heart. The aorta is the largest artery in the body; it receives the blood from the left ventricle of the heart. The aorta immediately begins branching into smaller arteries. The smallest branches of arteries are called *arterioles*. They join with capillaries. Arteries are more muscular and elastic than are the other blood vessels because they receive the blood as it is pumped from the heart.

Capillaries connect arterioles with *venules,* the smallest veins. Capillaries have thin walls contain-

ing only one layer of cells. These thin walls allow oxygen and nutrients to pass through to the cells and allow carbon dioxide and metabolic products from the cells to enter the capillaries.

Veins (see figure 6-24) are blood vessels that carry blood back to the heart. Venules, the smallest branches of veins, connect with the capillaries. The venules join together and, becoming larger, form veins. The veins continue to join together until they form the two largest veins: the superior vena cava and the inferior vena cava. The superior vena cava brings the blood from the upper part of the body, and the inferior vena cava brings the blood from the lower part of the body. Both vena cavae drain into the right atrium of the heart. Veins are thinner and have less muscle tissue than do arteries. Most veins contain valves, which keep the blood from flowing in a backward direction (see figure 6-25).

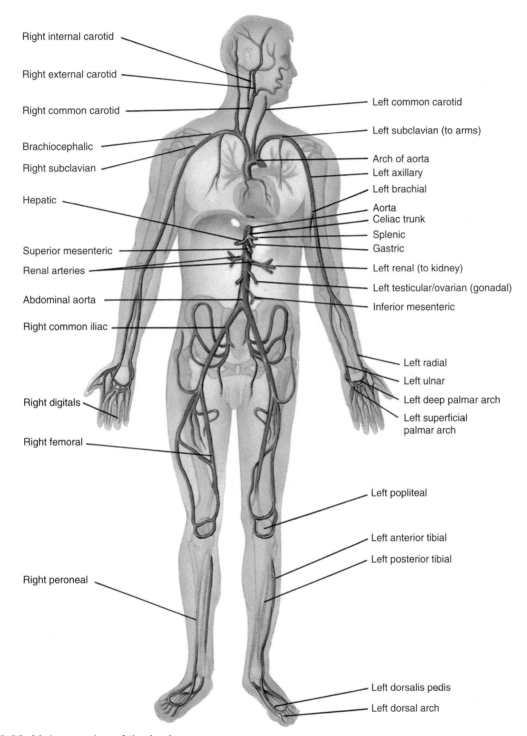

Right internal carotid

Right external carotid

Right common carotid

Brachiocephalic

Right subclavian

Hepatic

Superior mesenteric

Renal arteries

Abdominal aorta

Right common iliac

Right digitals

Right femoral

Right peroneal

Left common carotid

Left subclavian (to arms)

Arch of aorta

Left axillary

Left brachial

Aorta

Celiac trunk

Splenic

Gastric

Left renal (to kidney)

Left testicular/ovarian (gonadal)

Inferior mesenteric

Left radial

Left ulnar

Left deep palmar arch

Left superficial palmar arch

Left popliteal

Left anterior tibial

Left posterior tibial

Left dorsalis pedis

Left dorsal arch

Figure 6-23 Major arteries of the body.

BLOOD COMPOSITION

The **blood** that flows through the circulatory system is often called a tissue because it contains many kinds of cells. There are approximately four to six quarts of blood in the average adult. This blood continuously circulates throughout the body. It transports oxygen from the lungs to the body cells; carbon dioxide from the body cells to the lungs; nutrients from the digestive tract to the body cells; metabolic and waste products from the body cells to the organs of excretion; heat produced by

Figure 6-24 Major veins of the body.

various body parts; and hormones produced by endocrine glands to the body organs.

Blood is made of the fluid called plasma and solid elements called *blood cells* (see figure 6-26). Plasma is approximately 90 percent water, with many dissolved, or suspended, substances. Among these substances are blood proteins such as fibrinogen and prothrombin (both necessary for clotting); nutrients such as carbohydrates and proteins; mineral salts or electrolytes such as potassium, cal-

cium, and sodium; gases such as carbon dioxide and oxygen; metabolic and waste products; hormones, and enzymes.

Blood Cells

There are three main kinds of blood cells: erythrocytes, leukocytes, and thrombocytes.

The erythrocytes, or red blood cells, are produced in the red bone marrow at a rate of approxi-

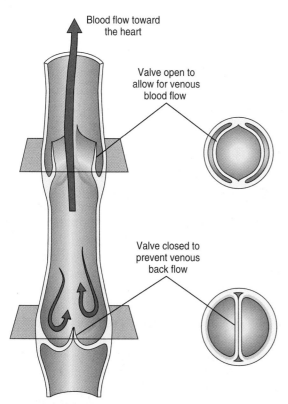

Blood flow toward the heart

Valve open to allow for venous blood flow

Valve closed to prevent venous back flow

Figure 6-25 Most veins contain valves to prevent the backflow of blood.

mately one million per minute. They live approximately 120 days. There are 4.5 to 5.5 million erythrocytes per cubic millimeter (approximately one drop) of blood, or approximately twenty-five trillion in the body. The mature form circulating in the blood lacks a nucleus and is shaped like a disc with a thinner central area. The erythrocytes contain **hemoglobin,** a complex protein composed of the protein molecule called *globin* and the iron compound called *heme.* Hemoglobin carries both oxygen and carbon dioxide. When carrying oxygen, hemoglobin gives blood its characteristic red color. When blood contains a lot of oxygen, it is bright red; when blood contains less oxygen and more carbon dioxide, it is a much darker red with a bluish cast.

Leukocytes, or white blood cells, are not as numerous as are erythrocytes. A normal count is 5,000 to 10,000 leukocytes per cubic millimeter of blood. There are several different types of leukocytes, each of which varies in shape and type of nucleus. Leukocytes can pass through capillary walls and enter body tissue. Their main function is to fight infection. Some do this by engulfing, ingesting, and destroying pathogens, or germs, by a process called *phagocytosis.*

Plasma (55% of total volume)

Formed elements (45% of total volume)

Test tube containing whole blood

Erythrocytes

Thrombocytes (platelets)

Neutrophil

Monocyte

Eosinophil

Lymphocyte

Basophil

Leukocytes

Figure 6-26 The major components of blood.

Thrombocytes, also called *platelets,* are usually described as fragments or pieces of cells because they lack nuclei and vary in shape and size. They contain an enzyme required for the clotting process, which stops bleeding. A normal thrombocyte count is 250,000 to 400,000 per cubic millimeter of blood.

DISEASES AND ABNORMAL CONDITIONS

Anemia is an inadequate number of red blood cells, hemoglobin, or both. Symptoms include pallor (paleness), fatigue, dyspnea (difficult breathing), and rapid heart rate. Hemorrhage can cause rapid blood loss, and result in acute-blood-loss anemia. Blood transfusions are used to correct this form of anemia. Iron deficiency anemia results when there is an inadequate amount of iron to form hemoglobin in erythrocytes. Iron supplements and increased iron intake in the diet from green leafy vegetables and other foods can correct this condition. Aplastic anemia is caused by injury to or destruction of the bone marrow, resulting in poor or no formation of red blood cells. Unless the damage can be reversed, it is frequently fatal. Pernicious anemia results in the formation of abnormally large and an inadequate number of erythrocytes. The cause is a lack of intrinsic factor, which prohibits adequate absorption of vitamin B12. Replacing the intrinsic factor and administering vitamin B12 injections can control and correct this condition. Sickle cell anemia is a chronic, inherited anemia. It results in the production of abnormal, crescent-shaped erythrocytes that carry less oxygen, break easily, and block blood vessels. Sickle cell anemia occurs almost exclusively among African Americans. Treatment methods include transfusions of packed cells and supportive therapy during crisis. Genetic counseling can lead to prevention of the disease if carriers make informed decisions and do not have children.

An *aneurysm* is a ballooning out of, or saclike formation on, an artery wall. Disease, congenital defects, and injuries leading to weakened arterial wall structure can cause this defect. Although some aneurysms cause pain and pressure, others generate no symptoms. Common sites are the cerebral, aortic, and abdominal arteries. If an aneurysm ruptures, hemorrhage, which can cause death, occurs.

Treatment usually involves surgically removing the damaged area of blood vessel and replacing it with a plastic graft or another blood vessel.

Arteriosclerosis is a hardening or thickening of the arterial walls, resulting in a loss of elasticity and contractility. It commonly occurs as a result of aging. Arteriosclerosis causes high blood pressure, or hypertension, and can lead to an aneurysm or cerebral hemorrhage.

Atherosclerosis occurs when fatty plaques (frequently cholesterol) are deposited on the walls of the arteries. This narrows the arterial opening, which reduces or eliminates blood flow. If plaques break loose, they can circulate through the bloodstream as *emboli.* A low-cholesterol diet and exercise are used to prevent atherosclerosis.

Congestive heart failure (CHF) is a condition that occurs when the heart muscles do not beat adequately to supply the blood needs of the body. It may involve either the right side or the left side of the heart. Symptoms include edema (swelling); dypsnea; pallor or cyanosis; distention of the neck veins; a weak, rapid pulse; and a cough accompanied by pink, frothy sputum. Cardiac drugs, diuretics (to remove retained body fluids), elastic support hose, oxygen therapy, bedrest, and/or a low-sodium diet are used as treatment methods.

An *embolus* is a foreign substance circulating in the bloodstream. It can be air, a blood clot, bacterial clumps, a fat globule, or other similar substances. When an embolus enters an artery or capillary too small for passage, blockage of the blood vessel occurs.

Hemophilia is an inherited disease that occurs almost exclusively in males but can be carried by females. Due to the lack of a plasma protein required for the clotting process, the blood is unable to clot. A minor cut can lead to prolonged bleeding, and a minor bump can cause internal bleeding. Treatment involves transfusing whole blood, or plasma, and administering the missing protein factor.

Hypertension is high blood pressure. A systolic pressure above 140 and a diastolic pressure above 90 millimeters of mercury is usually regarded as hypertension. Although there is no cure, hypertension can usually be controlled with antihypertensive drugs, diuretics (to remove retained body fluids), limited stress, avoidance of tobacco, and/or a low-sodium diet.

Leukemia is a malignant disease of the bone marrow or lymph tissue. It results in a high number of immature white blood cells. There are different types of leukemia, some acute and some chronic.

Symptoms include fever, pallor, swelling of lymphoid tissues, fatigue, anemia, bleeding gums, excessive bruising, and joint pain. Treatment methods vary with the type of leukemia but can include chemotherapy, radiation, and/or bone marrow transplant.

A *myocardial infarction,* or heart attack, occurs when a blockage in the coronary arteries cuts off the supply of blood to the heart. The affected heart tissue dies and is known as an *infarct.* Death can occur immediately. Symptoms include severe crushing pain that radiates to the arm, neck, and jaw; pressure in the chest; perspiration and cold, clammy skin; dypsnea; and a change in blood pressure. If the heart stops, cardiopulmonary resuscitation should be started immediately. Early treatment methods include complete bed rest, pain medications, oxygen therapy, anticoagulants, and control of arrhythmias (abnormal heart rhythms). Long-term care includes control of blood pressure; a diet low in cholesterol and saturated fat; avoidance of tobacco and stress; regular exercise; and weight control.

Phlebitis is an inflammation of a vein, frequently in the leg. If a thrombus, or clot, forms, the condition is termed *thrombophlebitis.* Symptoms include pain, edema, redness, and discoloration at the site. Treatment methods include anticoagulants; pain medication; elevation of the affected area; antiembolism or support hose; and, if necessary, surgery to remove the clot.

Varicose veins are dilated, swollen veins that have lost elasticity and cause stasis, or decreased blood flow. They frequently occur in the legs and result from pregnancy, prolonged sitting or standing, and hereditary factors. Treatment methods include exercise; antiembolism or support hose; and avoidance of prolonged sitting or standing and tight-fitting or restrictive clothing. In severe cases, surgery can be performed to remove the vein.

STUDENT *Go to the workbook and complete the assignment sheet for 6:6, Circulatory System.*

6:7 Lymphatic System

Objectives

After completing this section, you should be able to:

◆ Explain the function of lymphatic vessels
◆ List at least two functions of lymph nodes
◆ Identify the two lymphatic ducts and the areas of the body that each drains
◆ List at least three functions of the spleen
◆ Describe the function of the thymus
◆ Describe at least three diseases of the lymphatic system
◆ Define, pronounce, and spell all of the key terms

KEY TERMS

cisterna chyli
lacteals
lymph
  (limf´)

lymph nodes
lymphatic capillaries
  (lim-fat´-ik)
lymphatic vessels

right lymphatic duct
spleen
thoracic duct
  (tho-rass´-ik)

thymus
tonsils

6:7 INFORMATION

The lymphatic system consists of lymph, lymph vessels, lymph nodes, and lymphatic tissue. This system works in conjunction with the circulatory system to remove wastes and excess fluids from the tissues (see figure 6-27).

Lymph is a thin, watery fluid composed of intercellular, or interstitial, fluid, which forms when plasma diffuses into tissue spaces. It is composed of water, digested nutrients, salts, hormones, oxygen, carbon dioxide, lymphocytes, and metabolic

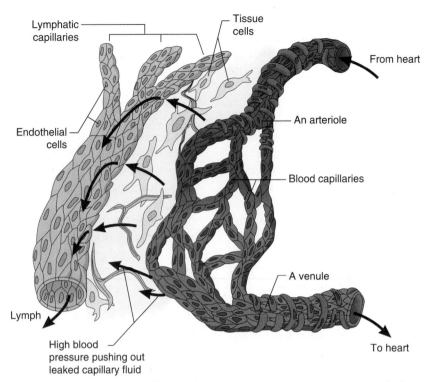

Figure 6-27 The lymphatic system works with the circulatory system to remove metabolic waste and excess fluid from the tissues.

wastes such as urea. When this fluid enters the lymphatic system, it is known as lymph.

Lymphatic vessels are located throughout the body. Small, open-ended lymph vessels act like drainpipes and are called **lymphatic capillaries.** The lymphatic capillaries pick up lymph at tissues throughout the body. The capillaries then join together to form larger lymphatic vessels, which pass through the lymph nodes. Contractions of skeletal muscles against the lymph vessels cause the lymph to flow through the vessels. Lymphatic vessels also have valves that keep the lymph flowing in only one direction. In the area of the small intestine, specialized lymphatic capillaries, called **lacteals,** pick up digested fats or lipids. When lymph is mixed with the lipids it is called *chyle.* The lacteals transport the chyle to the bloodstream.

Lymph nodes, popularly called "glands," are located all over the body, usually in groups or clusters. They are small, round masses ranging in size from that of a pinhead to that of an almond. Lymph vessels bring lymph to the nodes. The nodes filter the lymph and remove impurities such as carbon, cancer cells, pathogens (disease-producing organisms), and dead blood cells. In addition, the lymphatic tissue in the nodes produces lymphocytes (a type of leukocyte, or white blood cell) and antibod-

ies (substances used to combat infection). The purified lymph, with lymphocytes and antibodies added, leaves the lymph node by a single lymphatic vessel.

As lymphatic vessels leave the lymph nodes, they continue to join together to form larger lymph vessels (see figure 6-28). Eventually, these vessels drain into one of two lymphatic ducts: the right lymphatic duct or the thoracic duct. The **right lymphatic duct** is the short tube that receives all of the purified lymph from the right side of the head and neck, the right chest, and the right arm. It empties into the right subclavian vein, returning the purified lymph to the blood. The **thoracic duct,** a much larger tube, drains the lymph from the rest of the body. It empties into the left subclavian vein. At the start of the thoracic duct, the enlarged pouchlike structure called the **cisterna chyli** serves as a storage area for purified lymph before this lymph returns to the bloodstream.

In addition to being found in the lymph nodes, lymphatic tissue is located throughout the body. The tonsils, spleen, and thymus are examples of lymphatic tissue.

The **tonsils** are masses of lymphatic tissue that filter interstitial fluid. There are three pairs of tonsils: the *palatine tonsils,* located on each side of the soft palate; the *pharyngeal tonsils* (also called adenoids) located in the nasopharynx (the upper part of the throat); and the *lingual tonsils,* located on the back of the tongue.

The spleen is an organ located beneath the left side of the diaphragm and in back of the upper part of the stomach. It produces leukocytes and antibodies; destroys old erythrocytes (red blood cells); stores erythrocytes; destroys thrombocytes (platelets); and filters metabolites and wastes from body tissues.

The thymus is a mass of lymph tissue located in the center of the upper chest. It atrophies (wastes away) after puberty and is replaced by fat and connective tissue. During early life, it produces antibodies and manufactures lymphocytes to fight infection. Its function is taken over by the lymph nodes.

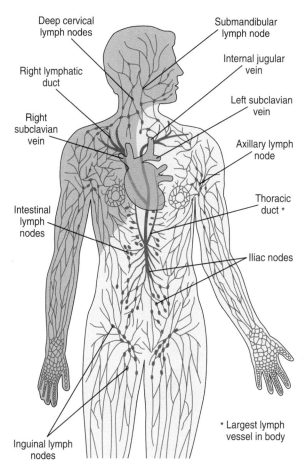

Figure 6-28 Main components of the lymphatic system.

DISEASES

Adenitis is an inflammation or infection of the lymph nodes. It occurs when large quantities of harmful substances, such as pathogens or cancer cells, enter the lymph nodes and infect the tissue. Symptoms include fever and swollen, painful nodes. If the infection is not treated, an abscess may form in the node. Usually treatment methods are antibiotics and warm, moist compresses. If an abscess forms, it is sometimes necessary to incise and drain the node.

Hodgkin's disease is a chronic, malignant disease of the lymph nodes. Symptoms include painless swelling of the lymph nodes, fever, night sweats, weight loss, fatigue, and pruritus (itching). Chemotherapy and radiation are usually effective forms of treatment.

Lymphangitis is an inflammation of lymphatic vessels, usually resulting from an infection in an extremity. Symptoms include a characteristic red streak extending up an arm or leg from the source of infection; fever; chills; and tenderness or pain. Treatment methods include antibiotics, rest, elevation of the affected part, and/or warm, moist compresses.

Splenomegaly is an enlargement of the spleen. It can result from an abnormal accumulation of red blood cells; mononucleosis; and cirrhosis of the liver. The main symptoms are swelling and abdominal pain. If the spleen ruptures, intraperitoneal hemorrhage and shock can lead to death. In severe cases, where the underlying cause cannot be treated, a splenectomy (surgical removal of the spleen) is performed.

Tonsillitis is an inflammation or infection of the tonsils. It usually involves the pharyngeal (adenoid) and palatine tonsils. Symptoms include throat pain; dysphagia (difficulty swallowing); fever; white or yellow spots of exudate on the tonsils; and swollen lymph nodes near the mandible. Antibiotics, warm throat irrigations, rest, and analgesics for pain are the main forms of treatment. Chronic, frequent infections or hypertrophy (enlargement) that causes obstruction are indications for a tonsillectomy, or surgical removal of the tonsils.

STUDENT   *Go to the workbook and complete the assignment sheet for 6:7, Lymphatic System.*

6:8 Nervous System

Objectives

After completing this section, you should be able to:

◆ Identify the four main parts of a neuron
◆ Name the two main divisions of the nervous system
◆ Describe the function of each of the five main parts of the brain
◆ Explain three functions of the spinal cord
◆ Name the three meninges
◆ Describe the circulation and function of cerebrospinal fluid
◆ Contrast the actions of the sympathetic and parasympathetic nervous systems
◆ Describe at least five diseases of the nervous system
◆ Define, pronounce, and spell all of the key terms

KEY TERMS

autonomic nervous
    system
brain
central nervous
    system
cerebellum
    (seh"-reh-bell´-um)
cerebrospinal fluid
    (seh-ree"-broh-spy´-
    nal fluid)
cerebrum
    (seh-ree´-brum)
diencephalon
hypothalamus
medulla oblongata
    (meh-due´-la
    ob-lawn-got´-ah)
meninges(singular:
    meninx)
    (meh-nin´-jeez)
midbrain
nerves
neuron
    (nur´-on)
parasympathetic
    (par"-ah-sim"-pah-
    thet´-ik)
peripheral nervous
    system
    (peh-rif´-eh-ral)
pons
    (ponz)
spinal cord
sympathetic
thalamus
ventricles

6:8 INFORMATION

The **nervous** system is a complex, highly organized system that coordinates all of the many activities of the body. This system enables the body to respond and adapt to changes that occur both inside and outside the body.

The basic structural unit of the nervous system is the **neuron,** or nerve cell (see figure 6-29). It consists of a cell body containing a nucleus; nerve

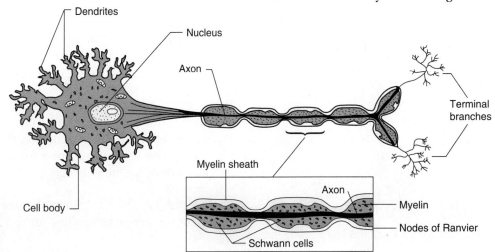

Figure 6-29 A neuron, the basic structural unit of the nervous system.

fibers, called *dendrites* (which carry impulses toward the cell body); and a single nerve fiber, called an *axon* (which carries impulses away from the cell body). Many axons have a lipid (fat) covering called a *myelin sheath,* which increases the rate of impulse transmission and insulates and maintains the axon. The axon of one neuron lies close to the dendrites of many other neurons. The spaces between them are known as *synapses.* Impulses coming from one axon "jump" the synapse to get to the dendrite of another neuron, which will carry the impulse in the right direction. In this way, impulses can follow many different routes.

Nerves are a combination of many nerve fibers located outside the brain and spinal cord. Afferent, or sensory, nerves carry messages from all parts of the body to the brain and spinal cord. Efferent, or motor, nerves carry messages from the brain and spinal cord to the muscles and glands. Connecting, or mixed, nerves carry both sensory and motor messages.

There are two main divisions to the nervous system: the central nervous system and the peripheral nervous system. The central nervous system consists of the brain and spinal cord. The peripheral nervous system consists of the nerves. A separate division of the peripheral nervous system is the autonomic nervous system. This system controls involuntary body functions.

CENTRAL NERVOUS SYSTEM

The brain is a mass of nerve tissue well protected by membranes and the cranium, or skull (see figure 6-30). The main sections include:

◆ Cerebrum—the largest and highest section of the brain. The outer part is arranged in folds, called *convolutions,* and separated into lobes. The lobes include the frontal, parietal, temporal, and occipital, named from the skull bones that surround them. The cerebrum is responsible for reasoning, thought, memory, speech, sensation, sight, hearing, and voluntary body movement.

◆ Cerebellum—the section below the back of the cerebrum. It is responsible for muscle coordination; balance and posture; and muscle tone.

◆ Diencephalon—the section located between the cerebrum and midbrain. It contains two structures; the thalamus and hypothalamus. The

Figure 6-30 The brain and spinal cord.

thalamus acts as a relay center and directs sensory impulses to the cerebrum. The hypothalamus regulates and controls the autonomic nervous system, temperature, appetite, water balance, sleep, and blood vessel constriction and dilation. The hypothalamus is also involved in emotions such as anger, fear, pleasure, pain, and affection.

◆ **Midbrain**—the section located below the cerebrum at the top of the brain stem. It is responsible for conducting impulses between brain parts and for certain eye and auditory reflexes.

◆ **Pons**—the section located below the midbrain and in the brain stem. It is responsible for conducting messages to other parts of the brain and for certain reflex actions including chewing, tasting, and saliva production.

◆ **Medulla oblongata**—the lowest part of the brain stem. It connects with the spinal cord and is responsible for regulating heartbeat, respiration, swallowing, coughing, and blood pressure.

The **spinal cord** continues down from the medulla oblongata and ends at the first or second lumbar vertebrae (see figure 6-31). It is surrounded and protected by the vertebrae. The spinal cord is responsible for many reflex actions and for carrying sensory (afferent) messages up to the brain and motor (efferent) messages from the brain to the nerves that go to the muscles and glands.

The **meninges** are three membranes that cover and protect the brain and spinal cord. The *dura mater* is the thick, tough, outer layer. The middle layer is delicate and weblike and called the *arachnoid membrane*. The innermost layer, the *pia mater*, is closely attached to the brain and spinal cord and contains blood vessels that nourish the nerve tissue.

The brain has four **ventricles,** hollow spaces that connect with each other and with the space under the arachnoid membrane (the subarachnoid space). The ventricles are filled with the fluid called **cerebrospinal fluid.** This fluid circulates continually between the ventricles and through the subarachnoid space. It serves as a shock absorber to protect the brain and spinal cord. It also carries nutrients to some parts of the brain and spinal cord and helps remove metabolic products and wastes. The fluid is produced in the ventricles of the brain by the special structures called *choroid plexuses.* After circulating, it is absorbed into the blood vessels of the dura mater and returned to the bloodstream through special structures called *arachnoid villi.*

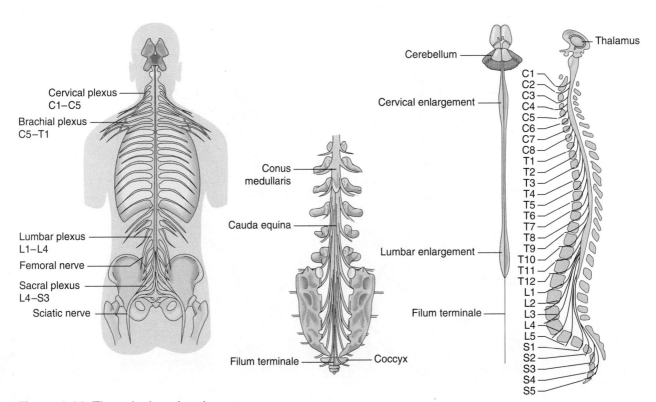

Figure 6-31 The spinal cord and nerves.

PERIPHERAL NERVOUS SYSTEM

The peripheral nervous system consists of the somatic and the autonomic nervous systems. The somatic nervous system consists of twelve pairs of cranial nerves and their branches, and thirty-one pairs of spinal nerves and their branches. Some of the cranial nerves are responsible for special senses such as sight, hearing, taste, and smell. Others receive general sensations such as touch, pressure, pain, and temperature and send out impulses for involuntary and voluntary muscle control. The spinal nerves carry messages to and from the spinal cord and are mixed nerves, both sensory (afferent) and motor (efferent).

Autonomic Nervous System

The autonomic nervous system is an important part of the peripheral nervous system. It helps maintain a balance in the involuntary functions of the body and allows the body to react in times of emergency. There are two divisions to the autonomic nervous system: the sympathetic and parasympathetic nervous systems. These two systems usually work together to maintain a balanced state, or *homeostasis,* in the body and to control involuntary body functions at proper rates. In times of emergency, the sympathetic nervous system prepares the body to act by increasing heart rate, respiration, and blood pressure, and slowing activity in the digestive tract. This is known as the *fight or flight response.* After the emergency, the parasympathetic nervous system counteracts the actions of the sympathetic system by slowing heart rate, decreasing respiration, lowering blood pressure, and increasing activity in the digestive tract.

DISEASES

Cerebral palsy is a disturbance in voluntary muscle action and is caused by brain damage. Lack of oxygen to the brain, birth injuries, prenatal rubella (German measles), and infections can all cause cerebral palsy. Of the three forms—spastic, athetoid, and atactic—spastic is the most common. Symptoms include exaggerated reflexes, tense muscles, contracture development, seizures, speech impairment, spasms, tremors and, in some cases, mental retardation. Although there is no cure, physical, occupational, and speech therapy are important aspects of treatment. Muscle relaxants, anticonvulsive drugs, casts, braces, and/or orthopedic surgery (for severe contractures) are also used.

A *cerebrovascular accident (CVA),* also called a *stroke* or *apoplexy,* occurs when the blood flow to the brain is impaired, resulting in a lack of oxygen and a destruction of brain tissue. It can be caused by cerebral hemorrhage resulting from hypertension, an aneurysm, or a weak blood vessel; or by an occlusion, or blockage, caused by atherosclerosis or a thrombus (blood clot). Symptoms vary depending on the area and amount of brain tissue damaged. Some common symptoms of an acute CVA include loss of consciousness; weakness or paralysis on one side of the body (hemiplegia); dizziness; dysphagia; visual disturbances; mental confusion; aphasia (speech and language impairment); and incontinence. Treatment depends on symptoms and is directed toward helping the person recover from or adapt to the symptoms that are present. Physical, occupational, and speech therapy are the main forms of treatment.

Encephalitis is an inflammation of the brain and is caused by a virus, bacteria, or chemical agent. The virus is frequently contracted from a mosquito bite, because mosquitos can carry the encephalitis virus. Symptoms vary but may include fever; extreme weakness or lethargy; visual disturbances; headaches; vomiting; stiff neck and back; disorientation; seizures; and coma. Treatment methods are supportive and include antiviral drugs; maintenance of fluid and electrolyte balance; antiseizure medication; and monitoring of respiratory and kidney function.

Epilepsy, or seizure syndrome, is a brain disorder associated with abnormal electrical impulses in the neurons of the brain. Although causes can include brain injury; birth trauma; tumors; toxins such as lead or carbon monoxide; and infections, many cases of epilepsy are idiopathic (spontaneous, or primary). Absence, or petit mal, seizures are milder and characterized by a loss of consciousness lasting several seconds. They are common in children and frequently disappear by late adolescence. Partial, or Jacksonian, seizures cause uncontrolled muscle movements on one extremity or side of the body. Generalized tonic-clonic, or grand mal, are the most severe seizures. They are characterized by a loss of consciousness lasting several minutes; convulsions accompanied by violent shaking and thrashing movements; hypersalivation causing foaming at the mouth; and loss of body functions. Anticonvulsant drugs are very effective in controlling epilepsy.

Hydrocephalus is an excessive accumulation of cerebrospinal fluid in the ventricles and, in some cases, the subarachnoid space of the brain. Symptoms include an abnormally enlarged head, prominent forehead, irritability, distended scalp veins, and, when pressure prevents proper development of the brain, retardation. The condition is treated by the surgical implantation of a shunt (tube) between the ventricles and the veins, heart, or abdominal peritoneal cavity to provide for drainage of the excess fluid.

Meningitis is an inflammation of the meninges of the brain and/or spinal cord and is caused by a bacteria or virus. Symptoms include high fever; headaches; back and neck pain and stiffness; nausea and vomiting, delirium; convulsions; and, if untreated, coma and death. Treatment methods include antibiotics, anticonvulsants, and/or medications for pain and cerebral edema.

Multiple sclerosis (MS) is a chronic, progressive, disabling condition resulting from a degeneration of the myelin sheath in the central nervous system. It usually occurs between the ages of twenty and forty. The cause is unknown. The disease progresses at different rates and has periods of remission. Early symptoms include visual disturbances, weakness, fatigue, poor coordination, and tingling and numbness. As the disease progresses, tremors, muscle spasticity, paralysis, speech impairment, emotional swings, and incontinence occur. There is no cure. Treatment methods such as physical therapy, muscle relaxants, steroids, and psychological counseling are used to maintain functional ability as long as possible.

Neuralgia is nerve pain. It is caused by inflammation, pressure, toxins, and other disease.

Treatment is directed toward eliminating the cause of the pain.

Paralysis usually results from a brain or spinal cord injury that destroys neurons and results in a loss of function and sensation below the level of injury. *Hemiplegia* is paralysis on one side of the body and is caused by a tumor, injury, or CVA. *Paraplegia* is paralysis in the lower extremities or lower part of the body and is caused by a spinal cord injury. *Quadriplegia i*s paralysis of the arms, legs, and body below the spinal cord injury. There is currently no cure, although much research is being directed toward repairing spinal cord damage. Treatment methods are supportive and include physical and occupational therapy.

Parkinson's disease is a chronic, progressive condition involving degeneration of brain cells, usually in persons over fifty years of age. Symptoms include tremors; stiffness; muscular rigidity; a forward leaning position; a shuffling gait; difficulty in stopping while walking; loss of facial expression; drooling; mood swings and frequent depression; and behavioral changes. Although there is no cure, a drug called Levodopa is used to relieve the symptoms. In some cases, surgery can be performed to selectively destroy a small area of the brain and control involuntary movements. Physical therapy is also used to limit muscular rigidity.

Shingles, or herpes zoster, is an acute inflammation of nerve cells and is caused by the herpes virus, which also causes chicken pox. It characteristically occurs in the thoracic area on one side of the body and follows the path of the affected nerves. Fluid-filled vesicles appear on the skin, accompanied by severe pain, redness, itching, fever, and abnormal skin sensations. Treatment is directed toward relieving pain and itching until the inflammation subsides, usually in one to four weeks.

STUDENT *Go to the workbook and complete the assignment sheet for 6:8, Nervous System.*

6:9 Special Senses

Objectives

After completing this section, you should be able to:

◆ Identify five special senses

◆ Label the major parts on a diagram of the eye

◆ Trace the pathway of light rays as they pass through the eye

◆ Label the major parts on a diagram of the ear

◆ Trace the pathway of sound waves as they pass through the ear

◆ Explain how the ear helps maintain balance and equilibrium

◆ State the locations of the four main taste receptors

◆ List at least four general senses located throughout the body

◆ Describe at least six diseases of the eye and ear

◆ Define, pronounce, and spell all of the key terms

KEY TERMS

aqueous humor
(a´-kwee″-us hue-more)
auditory canal
auricle
(or´-eh-kul″)
choroid coat
(koh´-royd)
cochlea
(co´-klee-ah)
conjunctiva
(kon-junk″-tye´-vah)
cornea
eustachian tube
(you-stay´-she-en)
iris
lacrimal glands
(lack´-rih″-mal)
lens

organ of Corti
ossicles
(os´-ick-uls)
pinna
(pin´-nah)
pupil
refracts
retina
(ret´-in-ah)
sclera
(sklee´-rah)
semicircular canals
tympanic membrane
(tim-pan´-ik)
vestibule
(ves´-tih-bewl)
vitreous humor
(vit´-ree-us hue´-more)

6:9 INFORMATION

Special senses allow the human body to react to the environment by providing for sight, hearing, taste, smell, and balance maintenance. These senses are possible because the body has structures that receive sensations, nerves that carry sensory messages to the brain, and a brain that interprets and responds to sensory messages.

THE EYE

The eye is the organ that controls the special sense of sight. It receives light rays and transmits impulses from the rays to the optic nerve, which carries the impulses to the brain, where they are interpreted as vision, or sight.

The eye (see figure 6-32A) is well protected. It is partially enclosed in a bony socket of the skull. Eyelids and eyelashes help keep out dirt and pathogens. Lacrimal glands in the eye produce tears, which constantly moisten and cleanse the eye. A mucous membrane, called the conjunctiva, lines the eyelids and covers the front of the eye to provide additional protection.

There are three main layers to the eye (see figure 6-32B). The outermost layer is the tough connective tissue called the sclera. It is frequently referred to as the "white" of the eye. The sclera maintains the shape of the eye. Extrinsic muscles, responsible for moving the eye within the socket, are attached to the outside of the sclera. The cornea is a circular, transparent part of the front of the sclera. It allows light rays to enter the eye. The middle layer of the eye, the choroid coat, is interlaced with many blood vessels, which nourish the eyes. The innermost layer of the eye is the retina. It is made of many layers of nerve cells, which transmit the light impulses to the optic nerve. Two such special cells are *cones* and *rods*. Cones are sensitive to color and are used mainly for vision when it is light. Most of the cones are located in a depression

Figure 6-32(A) External view of the eye; **(B)** structures of the eye.

located on the back surface of the retina and called the *fovea centralis;* this is the area of sharpest vision. Rods are used for vision when it is dark or dim.

The **iris** is the colored portion of the eye. The opening in the center of the iris is called the **pupil.** The iris contains two muscles, which control the size of the pupil and regulate the amount of light entering the eye.

Other special structures are also located in the eye. The **lens** is a circular structure located behind the pupil and suspended in position by ligaments. It **refracts** (bends) light rays so the rays focus on the retina. The **aqueous humor** is a clear, watery fluid that fills the space between the cornea and iris. It helps maintain the forward curvature of the eyeball and refracts light rays. The **vitreous humor** is the jellylike substance that fills the area behind the lens. It helps maintain the shape of the eyeball and also refracts light rays. A series of muscles located in the eye provide for eye movement.

When light rays enter the eye, they pass through a series of parts that refract the rays so that the rays focus on the retina. These parts are the cornea, the aqueous humor, the pupil, the lens, and the vitreous humor. In the retina, the light rays (image) are picked up by the rods and cones, changed into nerve impulses, and transmitted by the optic nerve to the occipital lobe of the cerebrum, where sight is interpreted. If the rays are not refracted correctly by the various parts, vision can be distorted or blurred.

Diseases

Amblyopia, or lazy eye, commonly occurs in early childhood. It results in poor vision in one eye and is caused by the dominance of the other eye. Treatment methods include covering the good eye to stimulate development of the "lazy" eye, exercises to strengthen the weak eye, corrective lenses, and/or surgery. If the condition is not treated before eight to nine years of age, blindness of the affected eye may occur.

Astigmatism is blurred vision caused by abnormal shape or curvature of the cornea. Corrective lenses (glasses or contact lenses) correct the condition.

A *cataract* occurs when the normally clear lens becomes cloudy, or opaque. This occurs gradually, usually as a result of aging. Symptoms include blurred vision, halos around lights, gradual vision loss, and, in later stages, a milky-white pupil. Sight is restored by the surgical removal of the lens. An implanted intraocular lens or prescription glasses or contact lenses correct the vision and compensate for the removed lens.

Conjunctivitis, or pink eye, is a contagious inflammation of the conjunctiva an is usually caused by a bacteria or virus. Symptoms include redness, swelling, pain, and, at times, pus formation in the eye. Antibiotics, frequently in the form of an eye ointment, are used to treat conjunctivitis.

Glaucoma is a condition of increased intraocular (within the eye) pressure caused by an excess amount of aqueous humor. It is common after age forty and is a leading cause of blindness. A tonometer (instrument that measures intraocular pressure) is usually used during regular eye examinations to check for this condition. Symptoms include loss of peripheral (side) vision, halos around lights, limited night vision, and mild aching. Glaucoma is usually controlled with medications that decrease the pressure. In severe cases, surgery is performed to create an opening for the flow of the aqueous humor.

Hyperopia is farsightedness. It occurs when the light rays are not refracted sharply enough, and the image focuses behind the retina. Vision is corrected by the use of convex lenses.

Myopia is nearsightedness. It occurs when the light rays are refracted too sharply, and the image focuses in front of the retina. Vision is corrected by the use of concave lenses.

Presbyopia is farsightedness caused by a loss of lens elasticity. It results from the normal aging process and is treated by the use of corrective lenses or "reading" glasses.

Strabismus is when the eyes do not move or focus together. The eyes may move inward (cross-eyed) or outward, or up or down. Treatment methods include eye exercises, covering the good eye, corrective lenses, and/or surgery on the muscles that move the eye.

THE EAR

The ear is the organ that controls the special senses of hearing and balance. It transmits impulses from sound waves to the auditory nerve (vestibulocochlear), which carries the impulses to the brain for interpretation as hearing. The ear is divided into three main sections: the outer ear, the middle ear, and the inner ear (see figure 6-33).

The outer ear contains the visible part of the ear, called the pinna, or auricle. The pinna is elastic cartilage covered by skin. It leads to a canal, or tube, called the *external auditory meatus*, or auditory canal. Special glands in this canal produce *cerumen*, a wax that protects the ear. Sound waves travel through the auditory canal until they reach the eardrum, or tympanic membrane. The tympanic membrane separates the outer ear from the middle ear. It vibrates when sound waves hit it and transmits the sound waves to the middle ear.

The middle ear is a small space, or cavity, in the temporal bone. It contains three small bones (ossicles): the malleus, the incus, and the stapes. The bones are connected and transmit sound waves from the tympanic membrane to the inner ear. The middle ear is connected to the pharynx, or throat, by a tube called the eustachian tube. This tube allows air to enter the middle ear and helps equalize air pressure on both sides of the tympanic membrane.

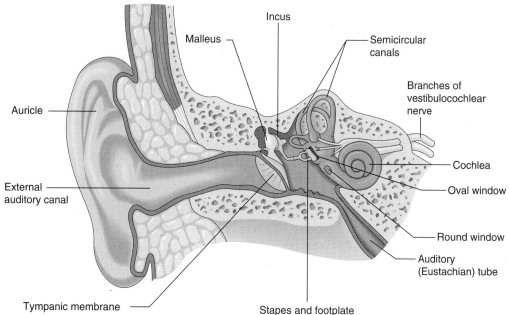

Figure 6-33 Structures of the ear.

The inner ear is the most complex portion of the ear. It is separated from the middle ear by a membrane called the *oval window.* The first section is the vestibule, which acts as the entrance to the two other parts of the inner ear. The cochlea, shaped like a snail's shell, contains delicate, hairlike cells, which compose the organ of Corti, a receptor of sound waves. The organ of Corti transmits the impulses from sound waves to the auditory nerve. This nerve carries the impulses to the temporal lobe of the cerebrum, where they are interpreted as hearing. Semicircular canals are also located in the inner ear. These canals contain a liquid that moves with head and body movements. Impulses sent from the semicircular canals to the brain constitute our sense of balance and equilibrium.

Diseases

Hearing loss is classified as either conductive or sensory. Conductive hearing loss or deafness is when sound waves are not conducted to the inner ear. Possible causes include a wax (cerumen) plug, a foreign body obstruction, otosclerosis, an infection, or a ruptured tympanic membrane. Treatment is directed toward eliminating the cause. Surgery and the use of hearing aids are common forms of treatment. Sensory hearing loss or deafness is when there is damage to the inner ear or auditory nerve. This type of hearing loss usually cannot be corrected.

Meniere's disease results from a collection of fluid in the labyrinth of the inner ear and a degeneration of the hair cells in the cochlea and vestibule. Symptoms include severe vertigo (dizziness); tinnitus (ringing in the ears); nausea and vomiting; loss of balance; and a tendency to fall. Forms of treatment include drugs to reduce the fluid, draining the fluid, and antihistamines. In severe, chronic cases, surgery to destroy the cochlea may be performed; however, this causes permanent deafness.

Otitis externa is an inflammation of the external auditory canal. It is caused by a pathogenic organism such as a bacteria or virus. Swimmer's ear is one form. It is caused by swimming in contaminated water. Inserting bobby pins, fingernails, or cotton swabs into the ear can also cause this condition. Treatment methods include antibiotics; warm, moist compresses; and/or pain medications.

Otitis media is an inflammation or infection of the middle ear and is caused by a bacteria or virus. It frequently follows a sore throat because organisms from the throat can enter the middle ear through the eustachian tube. Symptoms include severe pain; fever; vertigo (dizziness); nausea and vomiting; and fluid buildup in the middle ear. Treatment usually consists of administering antibiotics and pain medications. At times, a myringotomy (incision of the tympanic membrane) is performed, and tubes are inserted to relieve pressure and allow fluid to drain.

Otosclerosis is when the stapes becomes immobile causing conductive hearing loss. Symptoms include gradual hearing loss, tinnitus, and, at times, vertigo. Surgical removal of the stapes and insertion of an artificial stapes corrects the condition.

OTHER SENSES

The sense of taste is made possible by the taste receptors, which are located on the tongue (see figure 6-34). There are four main tastes: sweet tastes and salty tastes at the tip of the tongue; sour tastes at the sides of the tongue; and bitter tastes at the back of the tongue.

The sense of smell is made possible by olfactory receptors, which are located in the upper part of the nasal cavity. Impulses from these receptors are carried to the brain by the olfactory nerve. The sense of smell is closely related to the sense of taste. This is clearly illustrated by the fact that when you have a head cold and your sense of smell is impaired, food does not taste as good.

General sense receptors for pressure, heat, cold, touch, and pain are located throughout the body. Messages from these receptors allow the human body to respond to its environment and help it react to conditions that can cause injury.

STUDENT *Go to the workbook and complete the assignment sheet for 6:9, Special Senses.*

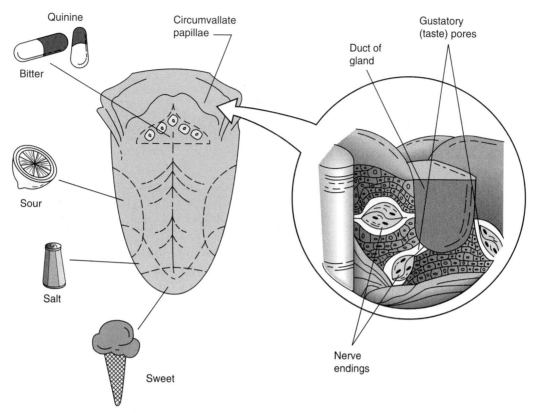

Figure 6-34 Locations of taste buds.

6:10 Respiratory System

Objectives

After completing this section, you should be able to:

◆ Label a diagram of the respiratory system

◆ List five functions of the nasal cavity

◆ Identify the three sections of the pharynx

◆ Explain how the larynx helps create sound and speech

◆ Describe the function of the epiglottis

◆ Compare the processes of inspiration and expiration, including the muscle action that occurs during each process

◆ Describe at least five diseases of the respiratory system

◆ Define, pronounce, and spell all of the key terms

KEY TERMS

alveoli
  (ahl-vee´-oh˝-lie)
bronchi
  (bron´-kie)
bronchioles
  (bron´-key˝-ohlz)
cilia
  (sil´-lee-ah)
epiglottis
  (ep-ih-glot´-tiss)
expiration
inspiration
larynx
  (lar´-inks)

lungs
nasal cavities
nasal septum
nose
pharynx
  (far´-inks)
respiration
sinuses
trachea
  (tray´-key˝-ah)
ventilation

6:10 INFORMATION

The **respiratory** system consists of the lungs and air passages. This system is responsible for taking in oxygen, a gas needed by all body cells, and removing carbon dioxide, a gas that is a metabolic waste product produced by the cells. Because the body has only a four- to six-minute supply of oxygen, the respiratory system must work continuously to prevent death.

The parts of the respiratory system are the nose, pharynx, larynx, trachea, bronchi, alveoli, and lungs (see figure 6-35).

The **nose** has two openings, called *nostrils* or *nares,* through which air enters. A wall of cartilage, called the **nasal septum,** divides the nose into two hollow spaces, called **nasal cavities.** The nasal cavities are lined with a mucous membrane and have a rich blood supply. As air enters the cavities, it is warmed, filtered, and moistened. Mucus, produced by the mucous membranes, helps trap pathogens and dirt. Tiny, hairlike structures, called **cilia,** help move the mucous layer that lines the airways pushing trapped particles toward the esophagus, where they can be swallowed. The olfactory receptors for the sense of smell are also located in the nose. The lacrimal ducts drain tears from the eye into the nose to provide additional moisture for the air.

Sinuses are cavities in the skull that surround the nasal area. They are connected to the nasal cavity by short ducts. The sinuses are lined with a mucous membrane, which warms and moistens air. The sinuses also provide resonance for the voice.

The **pharynx,** or throat, lies directly behind the nasal cavities. As air leaves the nose, it enters the

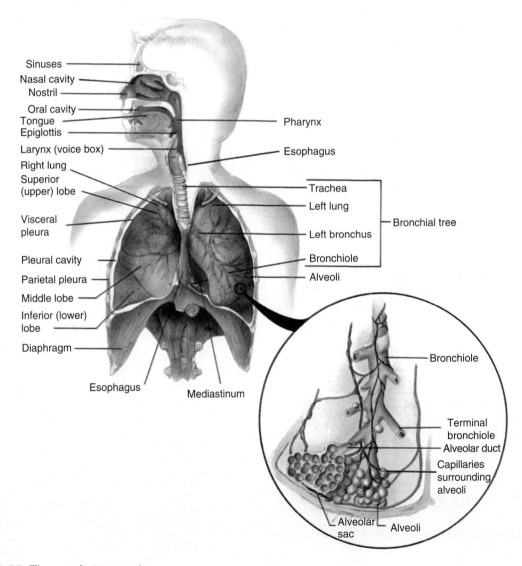

Figure 6-35 The respiratory system.

pharynx. The pharynx is divided into three sections. The nasopharynx is the upper portion, located behind the nasal cavities. The pharyngeal tonsils, or adenoids (lymphatic tissue), and the eustachian tube (tube to middle ear) openings are located in this section. The oropharynx is the middle section, located behind the oral cavity (mouth). This section receives both air from the nasopharynx and food and air from the mouth. The laryngopharynx is the bottom section of the pharynx. The esophagus, which carries food to the stomach, and the trachea, which carries air to and from the lungs, branch off the laryngopharynx.

The larynx, or voice box, lies between the pharynx and trachea. It has nine layers of cartilage. The largest, the thyroid cartilage, is commonly called the *Adam's apple.* The larynx contains two folds, called *vocal cords.* The opening between the vocal cords is called the *glottis.* As air leaves the lungs, the vocal cords vibrate and produce sound or speech. The epiglottis, a special leaflike piece of cartilage, closes the opening into the larynx during swallowing. This prevents food and liquids from entering the respiratory tract.

The trachea (windpipe) is a tube extending from the larynx to the center of the chest. It carries air between the pharynx and the bronchi. A series of C-shaped cartilages (which are open on the dorsal, or back, surfaces) help keep the trachea open.

The trachea divides into two bronchi near the center of the chest. Each bronchus enters a lung and carries air from the trachea to the lung. In the lungs, the bronchi continue to divide into smaller and smaller bronchi until, finally, they divide into the smallest branches, called bronchioles. The smallest bronchioles end in air sacs, called *alveoli.*

The alveoli resemble a bunch of grapes. They are made of one layer of squamous epithelial tissue and contain a rich network of blood capillaries. The capillaries allow oxygen and carbon dioxide to be exchanged between the blood and the lungs.

The divisions of the bronchi and the alveoli are found in organs called lungs. The right lung has three sections or lobes: the superior, the middle, and the inferior. The left lung has only two lobes: the superior and the inferior. The left lung is smaller because the heart is located toward the left side of the chest. Each lung is enclosed in a membrane, or sac, called the *pleura.* Both of the lungs, along with the heart and major blood vessels, are located in the thoracic cavity.

Ventilation is the process of breathing. It involves two phases: inspiration and expiration.

Inspiration (inhalation) is the process of breathing in air. The diaphragm (dome-shaped muscle between the thoracic and abdominal cavities) and the intercostal muscles (between the ribs) contract and enlarge the thoracic cavity to create a vacuum. Air rushes in through the airways to the alveoli, where the exchange of gases takes place. This process is known as respiration. When the diaphragm and intercostal muscles relax, the process of expiration (exhalation) occurs. Air is forced out of the lungs and air passages. The process of respiration is controlled by the respiratory center in the medulla oblongata of the brain. An increased amount of carbon dioxide in the blood causes the center to increase the rate of respiration. Although this process is usually involuntary, a person can control the rate of breathing by breathing faster or slower.

There are two main stages of respiration: external respiration and internal respiration (see figure 6-36). External respiration is the exchange of oxygen and carbon dioxide between the lungs and bloodstream. Oxygen, breathed in through the respiratory system, enters the alveoli. Since the oxygen concentration in the alveoli is higher than the oxygen concentration in the blood capillaries, oxygen leaves the alveoli and enters the capillaries and the bloodstream. Carbon dioxide, a metabolic waste product, is carried in the bloodstream. Since the carbon dioxide concentration in the capillaries is higher than the carbon dioxide concentration in the alveoli, carbon dioxide leaves the capillaries and enters the alveoli, where it is expelled from the body during exhalation. Internal respiration is the exchange of carbon dioxide and oxygen between the cells and the bloodstream. Oxygen is carried to the cells by the blood. Since the oxygen concentration is higher in the blood than in the body cells, oxygen leaves the blood capillaries and enters the body cells. The cells then use the oxygen and nutrients to produce energy, water, and carbon dioxide. This process is called *cellular respiration.* Since the carbon dioxide concentration is higher in cells than in the bloodstream, carbon dioxide leaves the cells and enters the bloodstream to be transported back to the lungs, where external respiration takes place.

DISEASES

Asthma is a respiratory disorder usually caused by a sensitivity to an allergen such as dust, pollen, an animal, or a food. Stress, overexertion, and infec-

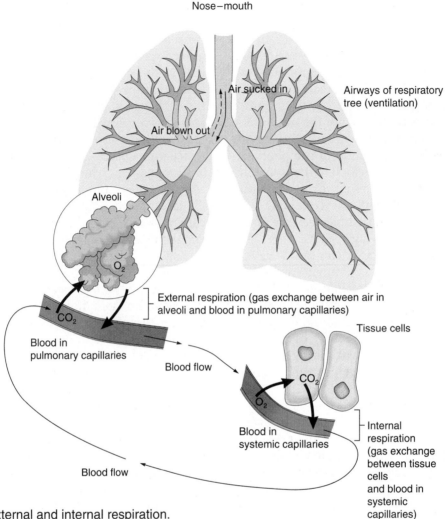

Figure 6-36 External and internal respiration.

tion can also cause an asthma attack, during which bronchospasms narrow the openings of the bronchioles, mucus production increases, and edema develops in the mucosal lining. Symptoms of an asthma attack include dyspnea (difficult breathing), wheezing, coughing accompanied by expectoration of sputum, and tightness in the chest. Treatment methods include bronchodilators (to enlarge the bronchioles), epinephrine, and oxygen therapy. Identification and elimination of or disensitization to allergens are important in preventing asthma attacks.

Bronchitis is an inflammation of the bronchi and bronchial tubes. Acute bronchitis is usually caused by infection and is characterized by a productive cough, dyspnea, chest pain, and fever. It is treated with antibiotics and expectorants (to remove excessive mucus). Chronic bronchitis results from frequent attacks of acute bronchitis and long-

term exposure to pollutants or smoking. It is characterized by chronic inflammation, damaged cilia, and enlarged mucous glands. Symptoms include excessive mucus resulting in a productive cough, wheezing, dyspnea, chest pain, and prolonged air expiration. Although there is no cure, antibiotics, bronchodilators, and/or respiratory therapy are used in treatment.

Chronic obstructive pulmonary disease (COPD) is a term used to describe any chronic lung disease that results in obstruction of the airways. Disorders such as asthma, chronic bronchitis, emphysema, and tuberculosis lead to COPD. Smoking is the primary cause, but allergies and chronic respiratory infections are also factors.

Emphysema is a noninfectious, chronic respiratory condition that occurs when the walls of the alveoli deteriorate and lose their elasticity. Carbon dioxide remains trapped in the alveoli, and there is poor exchange of gases. The most common causes are heavy smoking and prolonged exposure to air pollutants. Symptoms include dyspnea, a feeling of suffocation, pain, barrel chest, chronic cough, cyanosis, rapid respirations accompanied by prolonged expirations, and eventual respiratory failure and death. Although there is no cure, treatment methods include bronchodilators, prompt treatment of respiratory infections, oxygen therapy, respiratory therapy, and avoidance of smoking.

Epistaxis, or a nosebleed, occurs when capillaries in the nose become congested and bleed. It can be caused by an injury or blow to the nose; hypertension; chronic infection; anticoagulant drugs; and blood diseases such as hemophilia and leukemia. Compressing the nostrils toward the septum; elevating the head and tilting it slightly forward; and applying cold compresses will usually control epistaxis, although it is sometimes necessary to insert nasal packs or cauterize (burn and destroy) the bleeding vessels. Treatment of any underlying cause, such as hypertension, is important in preventing epistaxis.

Influenza, or flu, is a highly contagious, viral infection of the upper respiratory system. Onset is sudden, and symptoms include chills, fever, a cough, sore throat, runny nose, muscle pain, and fatigue. Treatment methods include bed rest, fluids, and analgesics (for pain and fever). Antibiotics are not effective against the viruses causing influenza, but they are sometimes given to prevent secondary infections such as pneumonia.

Laryngitis is an inflammation of the larynx and vocal cords. It frequently occurs in conjunction with other respiratory infections. Symptoms include hoarseness or loss of voice; sore throat; and dysphagia (difficult swallowing). Treatment methods include rest, limited voice use, fluids, and medication, if an infection is present.

Pleurisy is an inflammation of the pleura, or membranes, of the lungs. It usually occurs in conjunction with pneumonia or other lung infections. Symptoms include sharp, stabbing pain while breathing; crepitation (grating sounds in the lungs); dyspnea; and fever. Treatment methods include rest and medications to relieve pain and inflammation. If fluid collects in the pleural space, a thoracentesis (withdrawal of fluid through a needle) is performed to remove the fluid and prevent compression of the lungs.

Pneumonia is an inflammation or infection of the lungs characterized by exudate (a buildup of fluid) in the alveoli. It is usually caused by bacteria, viruses, or chemicals. Symptoms include chills, fever, chest pain, productive cough, dyspnea, and fatigue. Treatment methods include bed rest, fluids, antibiotics (if indicated), respiratory therapy, and/or pain medication.

Rhinitis is an inflammation of the nasal mucous membrane, resulting in a runny nose, soreness, and congestion. Common causes are infections and allergens. Treatment consists of administering fluids and medications to relieve congestion. Rhinitis is usually self limiting.

Sinusitis is an inflammation of the mucous membrane lining the sinuses. One or more sinuses may be affected. Sinusitis is usually caused by a bacteria or virus. Symptoms include headache or pressure; thick nasal discharge; congestion; and loss of voice resonance. Treatment methods include analgesics (for pain), medications to loosen secretions, and moist inhalations. Surgery is used in cases of chronic sinusitis to open the cavities and encourage drainage.

Tuberculosis (TB) is an infectious lung disease caused by the bacteria *Mycobacterium tuberculosis.* At times, white blood cells surround the invading TB organisms and wall them off creating nodules, called *tubercles,* in the lungs. The TB organisms remain dormant in the tubercles but can cause an active case of tuberculosis later, if body resistance is lowered. Symptoms of an active case of TB include fatigue, fever, night sweats, weight loss, hemoptysis (coughing up blood-tinged sputum), and chest pain. Treatment includes administering drugs for one or more years to destroy the bacteria. Good nutrition and rest are also important. In recent years, a new strain of the TB bacteria resistant to drug therapy has created concern that tuberculosis will become a widespread infectious disease.

An *upper respiratory infection (URI),* or common cold, is an inflammation of the mucous membrane lining the upper respiratory tract. Caused by viruses, URIs are highly contagious. Symptoms include fever, runny nose, watery eyes, congestion, sore throat, and hacking cough. There is no cure, and symptoms usually last approximately one week. Analgesics (for pain and fever), rest, increased fluid intake, and antihistamines (to relieve congestion) are used to treat the symptoms.

STUDENT   *Go to the workbook and complete the assignment sheet for 6:10, Respiratory System.*

6:11 Digestive System

Objectives

After completing this section, you should be able to:

◆ Label the major organs on a diagram of the digestive system
◆ Identify at least three organs that are located in the mouth and aid in the initial breakdown of food
◆ Cite two functions of the salivary glands
◆ Describe how the gastric juices act on food in the stomach
◆ Explain how food is absorbed into the body by the villi in the small intestine
◆ List at least three functions of the large intestine
◆ List at least four functions of the liver
◆ Explain how the pancreas helps digest foods
◆ Describe at least five diseases of the digestive system
◆ Define, pronounce, and spell all of the key terms

KEY TERMS

alimentary canal
   (ahl-ih-men´-tar″-ee)
anus
colon
   (coh´-lun)
duodenum
   (dew-oh-deh´-num)
esophagus
   (ee″-sof´-eh-gus)
gallbladder
hard palate
ileum
   (ill´-ee″-um)
jejunum
   (jeh-jew´-num)
large intestine
liver

mouth
pancreas
   (pan´-cree″-as)
peristalsis
   (pair″-ih-stall″-sis)
pharynx
   (far´-inks)
rectum
salivary glands
small intestine
soft palate
stomach
teeth
tongue
vermiform appendix
villi
   (vil´-lie)

6:11 INFORMATION

The digestive system, also known as the *gastrointestinal system,* is responsible for the physical and chemical breakdown of food so that it can be taken into the bloodstream and used by body cells and tissues. The system consists of the alimentary canal and accessory organs (see figure 6-37). The alimentary canal is a long, muscular tube that begins at the mouth and includes the mouth (oral cavity), pharynx, esophagus, stomach, small intestine, large intestine, and anus. The accessory organs are the salivary glands, tongue, teeth, liver, gallbladder, and pancreas.

The mouth (see figure 6-38) receives food as it enters the body. While food is in the mouth, it is tasted, broken down physically by the teeth; lubricated and partially digested by saliva; and swallowed. The teeth are special structures in the mouth that physically break down food by chewing and grinding. This process is called *mastication.* The tongue is a muscular organ that contains special receptors, called *taste buds.* The taste buds allow a person to taste sweet, salt, sour, and bitter sensations. The tongue also aids in chewing and swallowing food. The hard palate is the bony structure that forms the roof of the mouth and separates the mouth from the nasal cavities. Behind the hard palate is the soft palate, which separates the mouth from the nasopharynx. Three pairs of salivary glands, the parotid, sublingual, and submandibular, produce a liquid called *saliva.* Saliva lubricates the mouth during speech and chewing and moistens food so that it can be swallowed easily. Saliva also contains the enzyme (substance that speeds up a chemical reaction) called *salivary amylase,* formerly known as *ptyalin.* Salivary amylase begins the chemical breakdown of carbohydrates, or starches, into sugars that can be taken into the body.

After the food is chewed and mixed with saliva, it is called a *bolus.* When the bolus is swallowed, it enters the pharynx (throat). The pharynx is a tube

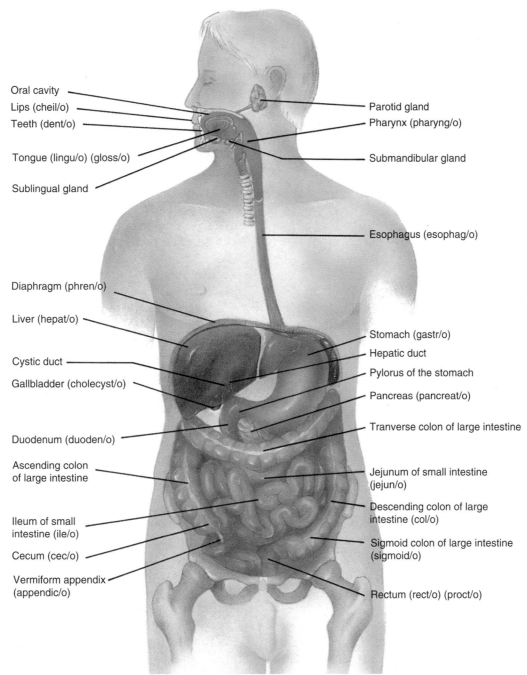

Oral cavity
Lips (cheil/o)
Teeth (dent/o)
Tongue (lingu/o) (gloss/o)
Sublingual gland

Parotid gland
Pharynx (pharyng/o)
Submandibular gland

Esophagus (esophag/o)

Diaphragm (phren/o)
Liver (hepat/o)
Cystic duct
Gallbladder (cholecyst/o)
Duodenum (duoden/o)
Ascending colon of large intestine
Ileum of small intestine (ile/o)
Cecum (cec/o)
Vermiform appendix (appendic/o)

Stomach (gastr/o)
Hepatic duct
Pylorus of the stomach
Pancreas (pancreat/o)
Tranverse colon of large intestine
Jejunum of small intestine (jejun/o)
Descending colon of large intestine (col/o)
Sigmoid colon of large intestine (sigmoid/o)
Rectum (rect/o) (proct/o)

Figure 6-37 The digestive system.

that carries both air and food. It carries the air to the trachea, or windpipe, and food to the esophagus. When a bolus is being swallowed, muscle action causes the epiglottis to close over the larynx preventing the bolus from entering the respiratory tract and causing it to enter the esophagus.

The **esophagus** is the muscular tube dorsal to (behind) the trachea. This tube receives the bolus from the pharynx and carries the bolus to the stomach. The esophagus, like the remaining part of the alimentary canal, relies on a rhythmic, wavelike, involuntary movement of its muscles, called **peristalsis,** to move the food in a forward direction.

The **stomach** is an enlarged part of the alimentary canal. It receives the food from the esophagus. The mucous membrane lining of the stomach contains folds, called *rugae*. These disappear as the stomach fills with food and expands. The cardiac sphincter, a circular muscle between the esophagus and stomach, closes after food enters the stomach

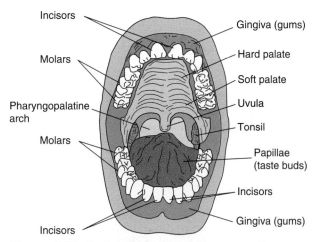

Incisors

Molars

Pharyngopalatine arch

Molars

Incisors

Gingiva (gums)

Hard palate

Soft palate

Uvula

Tonsil

Papillae (taste buds)

Incisors

Gingiva (gums)

Figure 6-38 Parts of the oral cavity, or mouth.

and prevents food from going back up into the esophagus. The pyloric sphincter, a circular muscle between the stomach and small intestine, keeps food in the stomach until the food is ready to enter the small intestine. Food usually remains in the stomach for approximately one to four hours. During this time, food is converted into a semifluid material, called *chyme,* by gastric juices produced by glands in the stomach. The gastric juices contain hydrochloric acid and enzymes. Hydrochloric acid kills bacteria, facilitates iron absorption, and activates the enzyme pepsin. The enzymes in gastric juices include lipase, which starts the chemical breakdown of fats, and pepsin, which starts protein digestion. In infants, the enzyme rennin is also secreted to aid in the digestion of milk. Rennin is not present in adults.

When the food, in the form of chyme, leaves the stomach, it enters the small intestine. The small intestine is a coiled section of the alimentary canal. It is approximately twenty feet in length and one inch in diameter, and is divided into three sections: the duodenum, the jejunum, and the ileum. The duodenum is the first nine to ten inches of the small intestine. Bile (from the gallbladder and liver) and pancreatic juice (from the pancreas) enter this section through ducts, or tubes. The jejunum is approximately eight feet in length and forms the middle section of the small intestine. The ileum is the final twelve feet of the small intestine, and it connects with the large intestine at the cecum. The circular muscle called the *ileocecal valve* separates the ileum and cecum and prevents food from returning to the ileum. While food is in the small intestine, the process of digestion is completed, and the products of digestion are absorbed into the

bloodstream for use by the body cells. Intestinal juices, produced by the small intestine, contain the enzymes maltase, sucrase, and lactase, which break down sugars into simpler forms. The intestinal juices also contain enzymes known as *peptidases,* which complete the digestion of proteins. Bile, from the liver and gallbladder, emulsifies (physically breaks down) fats. Enzymes from the pancreatic juice complete the process of digestion. These enzymes include pancreatic amylase (which acts on sugars); trypsin and chymotrypsin (which act on proteins); and lipase (which acts on fats). After food has been digested, it is absorbed into the bloodstream. The walls of the small intestine are lined with fingerlike projections called villi (see figure 6-39). The villi contain blood capillaries and lacteals. The blood capillaries absorb the digested nutrients and carry them to the liver, where they are either stored or released into general circulation for use by the body cells. The lacteals absorb most of the digested fats and carry them to the lymphatic system, which releases them into the circulatory system. When food has completed its passage through the small intestine, only wastes, indigestible materials, and excess water remain.

The large intestine is the final section of the alimentary canal. It is approximately five feet in length and two inches in diameter. Functions include absorption of water and any remaining nutrients; storage of indigestible materials before they are eliminated from the body; synthesis (formation) and absorption of some B-complex vitamins and vitamin K by bacteria present in the intestine; and transportation of waste products out of the alimentary canal. The large intestine is divided into a series of connected sections. The cecum is the first section and is connected to the ileum of the small intestine. It contains a small projection, called the vermiform appendix. The next section, the colon, has several divisions. The *ascending colon* continues up on the right side of the body from the cecum to the lower part of the liver. The *transverse colon* extends across the abdomen, below the liver and stomach and above the small intestine. The *descending colon* extends down the left side of the body. It connects with the *sigmoid colon,* an S-shaped section that joins with the rectum. The rectum is the final six to eight inches of the large intestine and is a storage area for indigestibles and wastes. It has a narrow canal, called the *anal canal,* which opens at a hole, called the anus. Fecal material, or stool, the final waste product of the digestive process, is expelled through this opening.

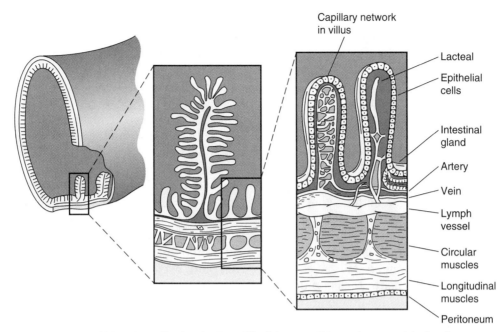

Figure 6-39 Lymphatic and blood capillaries in the villi of the small intestine provide for the absorption of the products of digestion.

The **liver** (see figure 6-40), is the largest gland in the body and is an accessory organ to the digestive system. It is located under the diaphragm and in the upper right quadrant of the abdomen. The liver secretes bile, which is used to emulsify fats in the digestive tract. Bile also makes fats water soluble, which is necessary for absorption. The liver stores sugar in the form of glycogen. The glycogen is converted to glucose and released into the bloodstream when additional blood sugar is needed. The liver also stores iron and certain vitamins. It produces heparin, which prevents clotting of the blood; blood proteins such as fibrinogen and prothrombin, which aid in clotting of the blood; and cholesterol. Finally, the liver detoxifies (renders less harmful) substances such as alcohol and pesticides, and destroys bacteria that have been taken into the blood from the intestine.

The **gallbladder** is a small, muscular sac located under the liver and attached to it by connective tissue. It stores and concentrates bile, which it receives from the liver. When the bile is needed to emulsify fats in the digestive tract, the gallbladder contracts and pushes the bile through the common bile duct and into the duodenum.

The **pancreas** is a fish-shaped organ located behind the stomach. It produces pancreatic juices, which contain enzymes to digest food. These juices enter the duodenum through the pancreatic duct. The enzymes in the juices include pancreatic amy-lase (to break down sugars); trypsin and chymotrypsin (to break down proteins); and lipase (to act on fats). The pancreas also produces insulin, which is secreted into the bloodstream. Insulin regulates the metabolism, or burning, of carbohydrates to convert glucose (blood sugar) to energy.

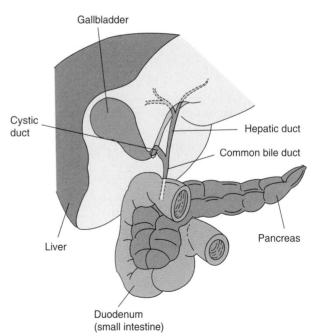

Figure 6-40 The liver, gallbladder, and pancreas

DISEASES

Appendicitis is an acute inflammation of the appendix, usually resulting from an obstruction and infection. Symptoms include generalized abdominal pain that later localizes at the lower right quadrant; nausea and vomiting; mild fever; and elevated white blood cell count. If the appendix ruptures, the infectious material will spill into the peritoneal cavity and cause peritonitis, a serious condition. Appendicitis is treated by an appendectomy (surgical removal of the appendix).

Cholecystitis is an inflammation of the gallbladder. When gallstones form from crystallized cholesterol, bile salts, and bile pigments, the condition is known as *cholelithiasis.* Symptoms frequently occur after eating fatty foods and include indigestion; nausea and vomiting; and pain that starts under the rib cage and radiates to the right shoulder. If a gallstone blocks the bile ducts, the gallbladder can rupture and cause peritonitis. Treatment methods include low-fat diet, lithotripsy (shock waves that are used to shatter the gallstones), and/or a cholecystectomy (surgical removal of the gallbladder).

Cirrhosis is a chronic destruction of liver cells accompanied by the formation of fibrous connective and scar tissue. Causes include hepatitis, bile duct disease, chemical toxins, and malnutrition associated with alcoholism. Symptoms vary and become more severe as the disease progresses. Some common symptoms are liver enlargement; anemia; indigestion; nausea and vomiting, nosebleeds; jaundice (yellow discoloration); and ascites (an accumulation of fluid in the abdominal peritoneal cavity). When the liver fails, disorientation, hallucinations, hepatic coma, and death occur. Treatment is directed toward preventing further damage to the liver. Alcohol avoidance, proper nutrition, vitamin supplements, rest, infection prevention, and appropriate exercise are encouraged.

Constipation is when fecal material remains in the colon too long, causing excessive reabsorption of water. The feces or stool becomes hard, dry, and difficult to eliminate. Causes include poor bowel habits, chronic laxative use leading to a "lazy" bowel, a diet low in fiber, and certain digestive diseases. The condition is usually corrected by a high-fiber diet, adequate fluids, and exercise. Although laxatives are sometimes used to stimulate defecation, frequent laxative use may be habit forming and lead to chronic constipation.

Diarrhea is a condition characterized by frequent watery stools. Causes include infection, stress, diet, an irritated colon, and toxic substances. Diarrhea can be extremely dangerous in infants and small children due to the excessive fluid loss. Treatment is directed toward eliminating the cause, providing adequate fluid intake, and modifying the diet.

Diverticulitis is an inflammation of the diverticula, pouches (or sacs) that form in the intestine as the mucosal lining pushes through the surrounding muscle. When fecal material and bacteria become trapped in the diverticula, inflammation occurs. This can result in an abscess or rupture leading to peritonitis. Symptoms vary depending on the amount of inflammation but may include abdominal pain; irregular bowel movements; flatus (gas); constipation or diarrhea; abdominal distention (swelling); low-grade fever; nausea, and vomiting. Treatment methods include antibiotics, stool-softening medications, pain medications, and, in severe cases, surgery to remove the affected section of colon.

Gastroenteritis is an inflammation of the mucous membrane that lines the stomach and intestinal tract. Causes include food poisoning, infection, and toxins. Symptoms include abdominal cramping, nausea, vomiting, fever, and diarrhea. Usual treatment methods are rest and increased fluid intake. In severe cases, antibiotics, intravenous fluids, and medications to slow peristalsis may be used.

Hemorrhoids are painful, dilated or varicose veins of the rectum and/or anus. They may be caused by straining to defecate, constipation, pressure during pregnancy, insufficient fluid intake, laxative abuse, and prolonged sitting or standing. Symptoms include pain, itching, and bleeding. Treatment methods include a high-fiber diet; increased fluid intake; stool softeners; sitz baths or warm, moist compresses; and, in some cases, a hemorrhoidectomy (surgical removal of the hemorrhoids).

Hepatitis is a viral inflammation of the liver. Type A, or infectious hepatitis, is highly contagious and is transmitted in food or water contaminated by the feces of an infected person. Type B, or serum hepatitis, is transmitted by blood and serum. It is more serious than type A and can lead to chronic hepatitis or to cirrhosis of the liver. Symptoms include fever, anorexia (lack of appetite), nausea, vomiting, fatigue, dark-colored urine, clay-colored stool, enlarged liver, and jaundice. Treatment methods include rest and a diet high in protein and calories and low in fat.

A *hernia,* or rupture, occurs when an internal organ pushes through a weakened area or natural opening in a body wall. A hiatal hernia is when the stomach protrudes through the diaphragm and into the chest cavity through the opening for the esophagus. Symptoms include heartburn, stomach distention, chest pain, and difficult swallowing. Treatment methods include a bland diet, small frequent meals, staying upright after eating, and surgical repair. An inguinal hernia is when a section of the small intestine protrudes through the inguinal rings of the lower abdominal wall. If the hernia cannot be reduced (pushed back in place), a herniorrhaphy (surgical repair) is performed.

Peritonitis, an inflammation of the abdominal peritoneal cavity, usually occurs when a rupture in the intestine allows the intestine contents to enter the peritoneal cavity. A ruptured appendix or gallbladder can cause this condition. Symptoms include abdominal pain and distention; fever; nausea; and vomiting. Treatment methods include antibiotics and, if necessary, surgical repair of the damaged intestine.

An *ulcer* is an open sore on the lining of the digestive tract. Peptic ulcers include gastric (stomach) ulcers and duodenal ulcers. Symptoms include burning pain, indigestion, hematemesis (bloody vomitus), and melena (dark, tarry stool). Usual treatment methods are antacids, a bland diet, decreased stress, and avoidance of irritants such as alcohol, fried foods, tobacco, and caffeine. In severe cases, surgery is performed to remove the affected area.

Ulcerative colitis is a severe inflammation of the colon accompanied by the formation of ulcers and abscesses. It is thought to be caused by stress, food allergy, or an autoimmune reaction. The main symptom is diarrhea containing blood, pus, and mucus. Other symptoms include weight loss, weakness, abdominal pain, anemia, and anorexia. Periods of remission and exaccerbation are common. Treatment is directed toward controlling inflammation, reducing stress with mild sedation, maintaining proper nutrition, and avoiding substances that aggravate the condition. In some cases, surgical removal of the affected colon and creation of a colostomy (an artificial opening in the colon that allows fecal material to be excreted through the abdominal wall) is necessary.

STUDENT *Go to the workbook and complete the assignment sheet for 6:11, Digestive System.*

6:12 Urinary System

Objectives

After completing this section, you should be able to:

◆ Label a diagram of the urinary system
◆ Explain the action of the following parts of a nephron: glomerulus, Bowman's capsule, convoluted tubule, and collecting tubule
◆ State the functions of the ureter, bladder, and urethra
◆ Explain why the urethra is different in males and females
◆ Interpret at least five terms used to describe conditions affecting urination
◆ Describe at least three diseases of the urinary system
◆ Define, pronounce, and spell all of the key terms

KEY TERMS

bladder
Bowman's capsule
cortex
(core´-tex)
glomerulus
(glow"-mare´-you-luss)
kidneys
medulla
(meh-due´-la)
nephrons
(nef´-ronz)

ureters
(you´-reh"-turz)
urethra
(you"-wreath´-rah)
urinary meatus
(you´-rih-nah-ree" me-ate´-as)
urine

INFORMATION

The urinary system, also known as the excretory system, is responsible for both removing certain wastes and excess water from the body and maintaining the body's acid-base balance. The parts of the urinary system are two kidneys, two ureters, one bladder, and one urethra (see figure 6-41).

The kidneys (see figure 6-42A) are two bean-shaped organs located on either side of the vertebral column, behind the upper part of the abdominal cavity, and separated from this cavity by the peritoneum. The kidneys are protected by the ribs and a heavy cushion of fat. Connective tissue helps hold the kidneys in position. Each kidney is enclosed in a mass of fatty tissue, called an *adipose capsule*, and covered externally by a tough, fibrous tissue, called the *renal fascia*, or *fibrous capsule*.

Each kidney is divided into two main sections: the cortex and the medulla. The cortex is the outer section of the kidney. It contains most of the nephrons, which aid in the production of urine. The medulla is the inner section of the kidney. It contains most of the collecting tubules, which carry the urine from the nephrons through the kidney.

Nephrons (figure 6-42B) are microscopic filtering units located in the kidneys. There are more than one million nephrons per kidney. Each nephron consists of a glomerulus, a Bowman's capsule, a proximal convoluted tubule, a distal convoluted tubule, and a collecting duct (tubule). The renal artery carries blood to the kidney. Branches of the renal artery pass through the medulla to the cortex, where the blood enters the first part of the nephron, the glomerulus (a cluster of capillaries). As blood passes through the glomerulus, water, salt, sugar, metabolic products, and other substances are filtered out of the blood. Red blood cells and proteins are not filtered out. The filtered blood leaves the glomerulus and eventually makes its way to the renal vein, which carries it away from the kidney. The substances filtered out in the glomeru-

Figure 6-41 The urinary system.

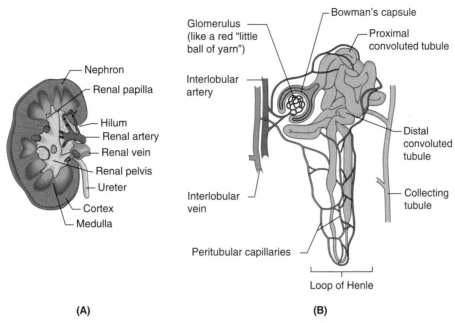

Figure 6-42 (A) A cross section of the kidney; **(B)** a nephron unit.

lus enter the next section of the nephron, the **Bowman's capsule.** The Bowman's capsule is a C-shaped structure that surrounds the glomerulus and is the start of the convoluted tubule. It picks up the materials filtered from the blood in the glomerulus and passes them into the convoluted tubule. As these materials pass through the various sections of the tubule, substances needed by the body are reabsorbed and returned to the blood capillaries. By the time the filtered materials pass through the tubule, most of the water, sugar, and salts have been reabsorbed. Excess sugar and salts; some water; and wastes (including urea, uric acid, and creatinine) remain in the tubule and become known as the concentrated liquid called *urine.* The urine then enters collecting ducts, or tubules, located in the medulla. These collecting ducts empty into the renal basin (renal pelvis), which is the first section of the ureter.

The **ureters** are two muscular tubes approximately ten to twelve inches in length. One extends from the renal pelvis of each kidney to the bladder. Peristalsis (a rhythmic, wavelike motion of muscle) moves the urine through the ureter from the kidney to the bladder.

The **bladder** is a hollow, muscular sac that lies behind the symphysis pubis and at the midline of the pelvic cavity. It has a mucous membrane lining arranged in a series of folds, called *rugae.* The rugae disappear as the bladder expands to fill with urine. Three layers of visceral (smooth) muscle form the walls of the bladder, which receive the

urine from the ureters and store the urine until it is eliminated from the body. Although the urge to void (urinate, or micturate) occurs when the bladder contains approximately 250 cubic centimeters (1 cup) of urine, the bladder can hold much more. A series of circular sphincter muscles controls the opening to the bladder to prevent emptying. When the bladder is full, receptors in the bladder wall send out a reflex action, which opens these muscles. Infants cannot control this reflex action. As children age, however, they learn to control the reflex.

The **urethra** is the tube that carries the urine from the bladder to the outside. The external opening is called the **urinary meatus.** The urethra is different in females and males. In females, it is a tube approximately one and one-half inches in length that opens in front of the vagina and carries only urine to the outside. In males, the urethra is approximately eight inches in length and passes through the prostate gland and out through the penis. It carries both urine (from the urinary system) and semen (from the reproductive system), although not at the same time.

Urine is the liquid waste product produced by the urinary system. It is approximately 95 percent water. Waste products dissolved in this liquid are urea, uric acid, creatinine, mineral salts, and various pigments. Excess useful products, such as sugar, can also be found in the urine, but their presence usually indicates disease. Approximately 1,500 to 2,000 cubic centimeters (1 1/2 to 2 quarts) of urine are produced daily from the approximately 150 quarts of liquid that is filtered through the kidneys.

Terms used to describe conditions affecting urination include:

polyuria: excessive urination
oliguria: below normal amounts of urination
anuria: absence of urination
hematuria: blood in the urine
nocturia: urination at night
dysuria: painful urination
retention: inability to empty the bladder
incontinence: involuntary urination

DISEASES

Cystitis is an inflammation of the bladder, usually caused by pathogens entering the urinary meatus. It is more common in females due to the shortness of the urethra. Symptoms include frequent urination, dysuria, a burning sensation during urination, hematuria, bladder spasm, and fever. Treatment methods are antibiotics and increased fluid intake.

Glomerulonephritis, or nephritis, is an inflammation of the glomerulus of the kidney. Acute glomerulonephritis usually follows a streptococcal infection such as strep throat, scarlet fever, or rheumatic fever. Symptoms include chills, fever, fatigue, edema, oliguria, hematuria, and albuminuria (protein in the urine). Treatment methods include rest; restriction of salt; maintenance of fluid and electrolyte balance; and, at times, antibiotics. With treatment, kidney function is usually restored, and the prognosis is good. Repeated attacks can cause a chronic condition. Chronic glomerulonephritis is a progressive disease that causes scarring and sclerosing of the glomeruli. Early symptoms include hematuria, albuminuria, and hypertension. As the disease progresses and additional glomeruli are destroyed, edema, fatigue, anemia, hypertension, congestive heart failure, and, finally, renal failure and death occur. Treatment is directed at treating the symptoms, and treatment methods include a low-sodium diet; antihypertensive drugs; maintenance of fluids and electrolytes; and dialysis (removal of the waste products from the blood by a hemodialysis machine). When both kidneys are severely damaged, a kidney transplant can be performed.

Pyelonephritis is an inflammation of the kidney tissue and renal pelvis (upper end of the ureter), usually caused by pyogenic (pus-forming) bacteria. Symptoms include chills, fever, back pain, dysuria, hematuria, and pyuria (pus in the urine). Treatment methods are antibiotics and increased fluid intake.

A *renal calculus,* or urinary calculus, is a kidney stone. A calculus is formed when salts in the urine precipitate (settle out of solution). Some small calculi may be eliminated in the urine, but larger stones often become lodged in the renal pelvis or ureter. Symptoms include sudden, intense pain (renal colic); hematuria; and, in some cases, urinary retention. Initial treatment consists of increasing fluids, providing pain medication, and straining all urine through gauze or filter paper to determine whether stones are being eliminated. Lithotripsy is a procedure where laser beams or sound waves are used to crush the stones so that they can be eliminated through the urine. In some cases, surgery is required to remove the calculi.

Renal failure is when the kidneys stop functioning. Acute renal failure can be caused by hemorrhage, shock, injury, poisoning, nephritis, or dehydration. Symptoms include oliguria or anuria; headache; an ammonia odor to the breath; edema; cardiac arrhythmia; and uremia. Prompt treatment involving dialysis, restricted fluid intake, and correction of the condition causing renal failure results in a good prognosis. Chronic renal failure results from the progressive loss of kidney function. It can be caused by chronic glomerulonephritis, hypertension, toxins, and endocrine disease. Waste products accumulate in the blood and affect many body systems. Symptoms include nausea; vomiting; diarrhea; decreased mental ability; convulsions; muscle irritability; an ammonia odor to the breath and perspiration; and, in later stages, coma and death. Treatment methods are dialysis; diet modifications and restrictions; careful skin and mouth care; and control of fluid intake. A kidney transplant is the only cure.

Uremia is a toxic condition that occurs when the kidneys fail and urinary waste products are present in the bloodstream. It can result from any condition that affects the proper functioning of the kidneys, such as renal failure, chronic glomerulonephritis, and hypotension. Symptoms include headache; nausea; vomiting; an ammonia odor to the breath; oliguria or anuria; mental confusion; coma; and, eventually, death. Treatment consists of a restricted diet and dialysis until a kidney transplant can be performed.

Urethritis is an inflammation of the urethra, usually caused by bacteria (such as gonococcus), viruses, or chemicals (such as bubble bath solutions). Symptoms include frequent and painful urination; redness and itching at the urinary meatus; and a purulant (pus) discharge. Treatment methods include sitz baths or warm, moist compresses; antibiotics; and/or increased fluid intake.

STUDENT *Go to the workbook and complete the assignment sheet for 6:12, Urinary System.*

6:13 Endocrine System

Objectives

After completing this section, you should be able to:

◆ Label a diagram of the main endocrine glands
◆ Describe how hormones influence various body functions
◆ Describe at least five diseases of the endocrine glands
◆ Define, pronounce, and spell all of the key terms

KEY TERMS

adrenal glands
  (ah"-dree´-nal)
endocrine
  (en´-doh"-krin)
hormones
ovaries
pancreas
  (pan-kree-as)
parathyroid glands

pineal body
  (pin´-knee"-ahl)
pituitary gland
  (pih"-too´-ih-tar-ee)
placenta
testes
  (tess´-tees)
thymus
thyroid gland

6:13 INFORMATION

The endocrine system consists of a group of ductless (without tubes) glands that secrete substances directly into the bloodstream. These substances are called *hormones*. The endocrine system consists of the pituitary gland, thyroid gland, parathyroid gland, adrenal glands, pancreas, ovaries, testes, thymus, pineal body, and placenta (see figure 6-43).

Hormones, the substances produced and secreted by the endocrine glands, are frequently called "chemical messengers." They are transported throughout the body by the bloodstream and perform many functions including stimulating exocrine glands (glands with ducts, or tubes) to produce secretions; stimulating other endocrine glands; regulating growth and development; regulating metabolism; maintaining fluid and chemical balance; and controlling various sex processes. Table 6-2 lists the main hormones produced by each endocrine gland and the actions they perform.

PITUITARY GLAND

The pituitary gland is often called the "master gland" of the body because it produces many hormones that affect other glands. It is located under the brain and in the stella turcica, a small, bony depression of the sphenoid bone. It is divided into two sections, or lobes: the anterior lobe and the posterior lobe. Each lobe secretes certain hormones, as shown in table 6-2.

Diseases

Acromegaly results from an oversecretion of somatotropin (growth hormone) in an adult and is usually caused by a tumor of the pituitary. Bones of the hands, feet, and face enlarge and create a grotesque appearance. The skin and tongue thicken, and slurred speech develops. Surgical removal and/or radiation of the tumor is the usual treatment.

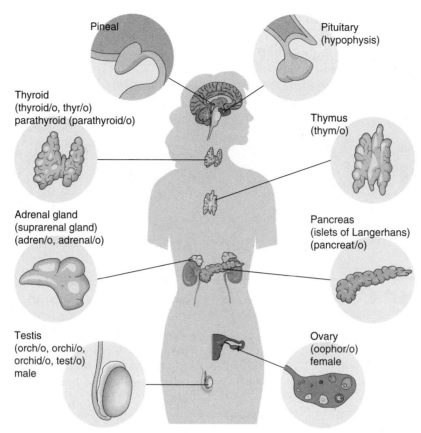

Figure 6-43 The endocrine system.

TABLE 6-2 **Hormones Produced by the Endocrine Glands and Their Actions**

GLAND	HORMONE	ACTION
Pituitary		
Anterior lobe	ACTH—adrenocorticotrophic	Stimulates growth and secretion of the cortex of the adrenal gland
	TSH—thyrotropin	Stimulates growth and secretion of the thyroid gland
	GH—somatotropin	Growth hormone, accelerates body growth
	FSH—follicle stimulating	Stimulates growth and hormone production in the ovarian follicles of female, production of sperm in males
	LH—Luteinizing (female) OR	Causes ovulation and secretion of estrogen in females, production of sperm and testosterone in males
	ICSH—Interstitial cell-stimulating (male)	Stimulates testes to secrete testosterone
	LTH—Lactogenic or prolactin	Stimulates secretion of milk
	Melanocyte stimulating (MSH)	Stimulates production and dispersion of melanin pigment in the skin
Posterior lobe	ADH—Vasopressin	Antidiuretic, promotes reabsorption of water in kidneys
	Oxytocin (pitocin)	Cause contraction of uterus during childbirth, stimulates milk flow

TABLE 6-2 **Hormones of Endocrine Glands** *(continued)*

GLAND	HORMONE	ACTION
Thyroid		
	Thyroxine and triiodothyronine	Increase metabolic rate, stimulate physical and mental growth
	Calcitocin	Accelerates absorption of calcium by the bones and lowers blood calcium level
Parathyroid		
	Parathormone (PTH)	Regulates amount of calcium of blood
Adrenal		
Cortex	Mineralocorticoids Aldosterone	Regulate the reabsorption of sodium in the kidney and the elimination of potassium
	Glucocorticoids Cortisol-hydrocortisone Corticosterone Cortisone	Aid in metabolism of proteins, fats, and carbohydrates; provide resistance to stress; and depress immune responses (anti-inflammatory)
	Gonadocorticoids Estrogens Androgens	Act as sex hormones Stimulate female sexual characteristics Stimulate male sexual characteristics
Medulla	Epinephrine (adrenaline)	Activates sympathetic nervous system, acts in stress
	Norepinephrine	Activates body in stress situations
Pancreas		
	Insulin	Used in metabolism of glucose (sugar) by promoting entry of glucose into cells
	Glucagon	Maintains blood level of glucose
Ovaries		
	Estrogen	Promotes growth and development of sex organs in female
	Progesterone	Maintains lining of uterus
Testes		
	Testosterone	Stimulates growth and development of sex organs in the male
Thymus		
	Thymosin	Stimulates production of antibodies in early life
Pineal		
	Melatonin	May delay puberty by inhibiting gonadotropic (sex) hormones
	Adrenoglomerulotropin	May stimulate adrenal cortex to secrete aldosterone
	Serotonin	May prevent vasoconstriction of blood vessels in the brain
Placenta	Estrogen	Stimulates growth of reproductive organs
	Chorionic gonadotropin	Causes corpus luteum of ovary to continue secretions
	Progesterone	Maintains lining of uterus to provide fetal nutrition

Giantism results from an oversecretion of somatotropin before puberty. It causes excessive growth of long bones, extreme tallness, decreased sexual development, and, at times, retarded mental development. If a tumor is involved, surgical removal or radiation is the treatment.

Diabetes insipidus is caused by decreased secretion of antidiuretic hormone (ADH). A low level of ADH prevents water from being reabsorbed in the kidneys. Symptoms include polyuria (excessive urination), polydipsia (excessive thirst), dehydration, weakness, constipation, and dry skin. The condition is corrected by administering ADH.

Dwarfism results from an undersecretion of somatotropin and can be caused by a tumor, infection, genetic factors, or injury. It is characterized by small body size, short extremities, and lack of sexual development. Mental development is normal. If the condition is diagnosed early, it can be treated with injections of somatotropic hormone for five or more years until long bone growth is complete.

THYROID GLAND

The **thyroid gland** synthesizes hormones that regulate the body's metabolism and control the level of calcium in the blood. It is located in front of the upper part of the trachea (windpipe) in the neck. It has two lobes, one on either side of the larynx (voice box), connected by the isthmus, a small piece of tissue. In order to produce its hormones, the thyroid gland requires iodine, which is obtained from certain foods (see table 6-2).

Diseases

A *goiter* is an enlargement of the thyroid gland. Causes can include a hyperactive thyroid, an iodine deficiency, an oversecretion of thyroid stimulating hormone on the part of the pituitary gland, or a tumor. Symptoms include thyroid enlargement, dysphagia (difficult swallowing), a cough, and a choking sensation. Treatment is directed toward eliminating the cause. For example, iodine is given if a deficiency exists. Surgery may be performed to remove very large goiters.

Hyperthyroidism is an overactivity of the thyroid gland, which causes increased production of thyroid hormones and increased basal metabolic rate (BMR). Symptoms include extreme nervousness, tremors, irritability, rapid pulse, weight loss, goiter formation, and hypertension. Treatment consists of either radiation to destroy part of the thyroid or a thyroidectomy (surgical removal of the thyroid).

Grave's disease is a severe form of hyperthyroidism more common in women than men. Symptoms include a strained and tense facial expression; exophthalmia (protuding eyeballs); goiter; nervous irritability; emotional instability; tachycardia; a tremendous appetite accompanied by weight loss; and diarrhea. Treatment methods include medication to inhibit the synthesis of thyroxine, radioactive iodine to destroy thyroid tissue, and/or a thyroidectomy.

Hypothyroidism is an underactivity of the thyroid gland and a deficiency of thyroid hormones. Two main forms exist: *cretinism* and *myxedema*. Cretinism develops in infancy or early childhood and results in a lack of mental and physical growth, leading to mental retardation and an abnormal, dwarfed stature. If diagnosed early, oral thyroid hormone can be given to minimize mental and physical damage. Myxedema occurs in later childhood or adulthood. Symptoms include coarse, dry skin; slow mental function; fatigue; weakness; intolerance of cold; weight gain; edema; puffy eyes; and a slow pulse. Treatment consists of administering oral thyroid hormone to restore normal metabolism.

PARATHYROID GLANDS

The **parathyroid glands** are four small glands located behind and attached to the thyroid gland. Their hormone regulates the amount of calcium in the blood (see table 6-2). Although most of the body's calcium is in the bones, the calcium circulating in the blood is very important for blood clotting, the tone of heart muscle, and muscle contraction. Since there is a constant exchange of calcium and phosphate between the bones and blood, the parathyroid hormone plays an important function in maintaining the proper level of circulating calcium.

Diseases

Hyperparathyroidism is an overactivity of the parathyroid gland, resulting in an overproduction of parathormone. This results in hypercalcemia (increased calcium in the blood), which leads to renal calculi (kidney stones) formation, lethargy, gastrointestinal disturbances, and calcium deposits on the walls of blood vessels and organs. Because the calcium is drawn from the bones, they become weak, deformed, and likely to fracture. This condition is often caused by an adenoma (glandular tumor), and removal of the tumor usually results in normal parathyroid function.

Hypoparathyroidism is an underactivity of the parathyroid gland, which causes a low level of calcium in the blood. Symptoms include tetany (a sustained muscular contraction), hyperirritability of the nervous system, and convulsive twitching. Death can occur if the larynx and respiratory muscles are involved. The condition is easily treated with calcium, vitamin D (which increases the absorption of calcium from the digestive tract), and parathormone.

ADRENAL GLANDS

The **adrenal glands** are frequently called the "suprarenal" glands because one is located above each kidney. Each gland has two parts: the outer portion or cortex, and the inner portion, or medulla. The adrenal cortex secretes many steroid hormones, which are classified into three groups: mineralocorticoids, glucocorticoids, and gonadocorticoids. The groups and the main hormones in each group are listed in table 6-2. The adrenal medulla secretes two main hormones: epinephrine and norepinephrine. These hormones are sympathominmetic, meaning that they mimic the sympathetic nervous system and cause the fight or flight response.

Diseases

Addison's disease is caused by decreased secretion of aldosterone on the part of the adrenal cortex. This interferes with the reabsorption of sodium and water and causes an increased level of potassium in the blood. Symptoms include dehydration, hypotension (low blood pressure), mental lethargy, weight loss, muscle weakness, excessive pigmentation leading to a "bronzing" (yellow-brown color) of the skin, hypoglycemia (low blood sugar), and edema. Treatment methods include steroid hormones, controlled intake of sodium, and fluid regulation to combat dehydration.

Cushing's syndrome results from an oversecretion of glucocorticoids on the part of the adrenal cortex. It can be caused by either a tumor of the adrenal cortex or excess production of ACTH on the part of the pituitary gland. Symptoms include hyperglycemia (high blood sugar), hypertension, muscle weakness, poor wound healing, a tendency to bruise easily, a "moon" face, and obesity. If a tumor is causing the disease, treatment is removal of the tumor. If the glands are removed, hormonal therapy is required to replace the missing hormones.

PANCREAS

The **pancreas** is a fish-shaped organ located behind the stomach. It is both an exocrine gland and an endocrine gland. As an exocrine gland, it secretes pancreatic juices, which are carried to the small intestine by the pancreatic duct to aid in the digestion of food. Special B, or beta, cells located throughout the pancreas in patches of tissue called *islets of Langerhans* produce the hormone insulin, which is needed for the cells to absorb sugar from the blood. Alpha, or A, cells produce the hormone glucagon, which increases the glucose level in blood.

Disease

Diabetes mellitus is a chronic disease caused by decreased secretion of insulin. The metabolism of carbohydrates, proteins, and fats is affected. There are two main types of diabetes mellitus named according to the age of onset and need for insulin. Insulin-dependent diabetes mellitus (IDDM), or type I, usually occurs early in life, is more severe, and requires insulin. Noninsulin-dependent diabetes mellitus (NIDDM), or type II, is the mature-onset form of diabetes mellitus. It frequently occurs in obese adults and is controlled with diet and/or oral hypoglycemic (lower-blood-sugar) medications. The main symptoms include hyperglycemia (high blood sugar), polyuria (excessive urination), polydipsia (thirst), polyphagia (hunger), glycosuria (sugar in the urine), weight loss, fatigue, slow healing of skin infections, and vision changes. If the condition is not treated, diabetic coma and death may occur. Treatment methods are a carefully regulated diet to control the blood sugar level, regulated exercise, and oral hypoglycemic drugs or insulin injections.

OTHER ENDOCRINE GLANDS

The ovaries are the gonads, or sex glands, of the female. They are located in the pelvic cavity, one on each side of the uterus. They secrete hormones that regulate menstruation and secondary sexual characteristics (see table 6-2).

The testes are the gonads of the male. They are located in the scrotal sac and are suspended outside the body. They produce hormones that regulate sexual characteristics of the male (see table 6-2).

The thymus is a mass of tissue located in the upper part of the chest and under the sternum. It contains lymphoid tissue. The thymus is active in early life, activating cells in the immune system, but atrophies (wastes away) during puberty,

when it becomes a small mass of connective tissue and fat. It produces one hormone, thymosin (see table 6-2).

The pineal body is a small structure attached to the roof of the third ventricle in the brain. Knowledge regarding the physiology of this gland is limited. Three main hormones secreted by this gland are listed in table 6-2.

The placenta is a temporary endocrine gland produced during pregnancy. It acts as a link between the mother and infant, provides nutrition for the developing infant, and promotes lactation (the production of milk in the breasts). It is expelled after the birth of the child (when it is called *afterbirth*). Three hormones secreted by this gland are listed in table 6-2.

STUDENT *Go to the workbook and complete the assignment sheet for 6:13, Endocrine System.*

6:14 Reproductive System

Objectives

After completing this section, you should be able to:

◆ Label a diagram of the male reproductive system
◆ Trace the pathway of sperm from where they are produced to where they are expelled from the body
◆ Identify at least three organs of the male reproductive system that secrete fluids added to semen
◆ Label a diagram of the female reproductive system
◆ Describe how an ovum is released from an ovary
◆ Explain the action of the endometrium
◆ Describe at least six diseases of the reproductive systems
◆ Define, pronounce, and spell all of the key terms

KEY TERMS

Bartholin's glands
  (Bar´-tha-lens)
breasts
Cowper's glands
  (Cow´-purrs)
ejaculatory ducts
  (ee-jack´-you-lah-tore"-ee)
endometrium
  (en"-doe-me´-tree-um)
epididymis
  (eh"-pih-did´-ih-muss)

fallopian tubes
  (fah-low´-pea"-an)
fertilization
  (fur"-til-ih-zay´-shun)
labia majora
  (lay´-bee"-ah mah"-jore´-ah)
labia minora
  (lay´-bee"-ah ma-nore´-ah)
ovaries
penis

perineum
   (pear″-ih-knee′-um)
prostate gland
scrotum
   (skrow′-tum)
seminal vesicles
   (sem′-ih-null ves′-ik-ullz)
testes
   (tes′-tees)
urethra

uterus
vagina
   (vah-jie′-nah)
vas deferens
   (vass deaf′-eh-rens)
vestibule
vulva
   (vull′-vah)

6:14 INFORMATION

The function of the reproductive system is to produce new life. Although the anatomical parts differ in males and females, the reproductive systems of both have the same types of organs: gonads (sex glands); ducts (tubes) to carry the sex cells and secretions; and accessory organs.

MALE REPRODUCTIVE SYSTEM

The male reproductive system consists of the testes, epididymis, vas deferens, seminal vesicles, ejaculatory ducts, urethra, prostate gland, Cowper's glands, and penis (see figure 6-44).

The male gonads are the testes. The two testes are located in the scrotum, a sac suspended between the thighs. The testes produce the male sex cell called the *sperm,* or *spermatozoa*. Because the scrotum is located outside the body, the temperature in the scrotum is lower than that inside the body. This lower temperature is essential for the production of sperm. The testes also produce male hormones. The main hormone is testosterone, which aids in the maturation of the sperm and also is responsible for the secondary male sex characteristics such as body hair, facial hair, large muscles, and a deep voice.

After the sperm develop in tubes in the testes, they enter the epididymis. The epididymis is a

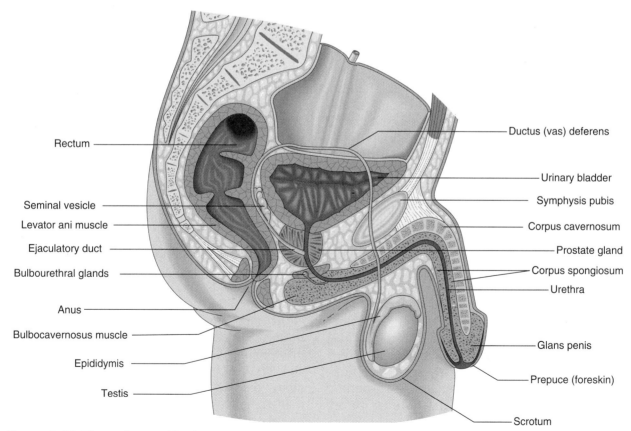

Figure 6-44 The male reproductive system.

tightly coiled tube approximately twenty feet in length and located in the scrotum and above the testes. It stores the sperm while they mature and become motile (able to move by themselves). It also produces a fluid that becomes part of the semen (fluid released during ejaculation). The epididymis connects with the next tube, the vas deferens.

The **vas deferens,** also called the *ductus deferens,* receives the sperm and fluid from the epididymis. On each side, a vas deferens joins with the epididymis and extends up into the abdominal cavity, where it curves behind the urinary bladder and joins with a seminal vesicle. Each vas deferens acts as both a passageway and a temporary storage area for sperm. The vas deferens are also the tubes that are cut during a vasectomy (procedure to produce sterility in the male).

The **seminal vesicles** are two small tubes located behind the bladder and near the junction of the vas deferens and the ejaculatory ducts. They contain a glandular lining. This lining produces a thick, yellow fluid that is rich in sugar and other substances and provides nourishment for the sperm. This fluid composes a large part of the semen.

The **ejaculatory ducts** are two short tubes formed by the union of the vas deferens and the seminal vesicles. They carry the sperm and fluids known collectively as *semen* through the prostate gland and into the urethra.

The **prostate gland** is a doughnut-shaped gland located below the urinary bladder and on either side of the urethra. It produces an alkaline secretion that both increases sperm motility and neutralizes the acidity in the vagina, providing a more favorable environment for the sperm. The muscular tissue in the prostate contracts during ejaculation (expulsion of the semen from the body) to aid in the expulsion of the semen into the urethra. When the prostate contracts, it also closes off the urethra, preventing urine passage through the urethra.

Cowper's (or bulbourethral) **glands,** are two small glands located below the prostate and connected by small tubes to the urethra. They secrete a mucouslike fluid, which serves as a lubricant for intercourse, and an alkaline fluid, which decreases the acidity of the urine residue in the urethra, providing a more favorable environment for the sperm.

The **urethra** is the tube that extends from the urinary bladder, through the penis, and to the outside of the body. It carries urine, from the urinary bladder, and semen, from the reproductive tubes.

The **penis** is the external male reproductive organ and is located in front of the scrotum. At the distal end is an enlarged structure, called the *glans penis.* The glans penis is covered with a prepuce (foreskin), which is sometimes removed surgically in a procedure called a *circumcision.* The penis is made of spongy, erectile tissue. During sexual arousal, the spaces in this tissue fill with blood, causing the penis to become erect. The penis functions as the male organ of copulation, or intercourse; deposits the semen in the vagina; and provides for the elimination of urine from the bladder and through the urethra.

Diseases

Epididymitis is an inflammation of the epididymis, usually caused by a pathogenic organism such as gonococcus, streptococcus, or staphyloccus. Symptoms include intense pain in the testes, swelling, and fever. Treatment methods include antibiotics, cold applications, and pain medication.

Orchitis is an inflammation of the testes, usually caused by mumps, pathogens, or injury. It can lead to atrophy of the testes and cause sterility. Symptoms include swelling of the scrotum, pain, and fever. Treatment methods include antibiotics and pain medication.

Prostatic hypertrophy, or hyperplasia, is an enlargement of the prostate gland. Common in men over age fifty, prostatic hypertrophy can be a benign condition, caused by inflammation, a tumor, or a change in hormonal activity, or a malignant (cancerous) condition. Symptoms include difficulty in starting to urinate, frequent urination, nocturia (voiding at night), dribbling, urinary infections, and, when the urethra is blocked, urinary retention. Initial treatment methods include fluid restriction, antibiotics (for infections), and prostatic massage. When hypertrophy causes urinary retention, a prostatectomy (surgical removal of all or part of the prostate) is necessary. A transurethral resection (TUR), removal of part of the prostate, is performed by inserting a scope into the urethra and resecting, or removing, the enlarged area. A prostatectomy can also be done by a perineal, or suprapubic (above the pubis bone), incision. If the condition is malignant, a prostatectomy, orchidectomy (removal of the testes), radiation, and estrogen therapy are the main treatments.

FEMALE REPRODUCTIVE SYSTEM

The female reproductive system consists of the ovaries, fallopian tubes, uterus, vagina, Bartholin's glands, vulva, and breasts (see figure 6-45).

The ovaries are the female gonads (see figure 6-46). They are small, almond-shaped glands located in the pelvic cavity and attached to the uterus by ligaments. The ovaries contain thousands of small sacs, called *follicles.* Each follicle contains an immature ovum, or female sex cell. When an ovum matures, the follicle enlarges and then ruptures to release the mature ovum. This process, called *ovulation,* usually occurs once every twenty-eight days. The ovaries also produce hormones that aid in the development of the reproductive organs and produce secondary sexual characteristics.

The fallopian tubes are two tubes, each approximately five inches in length and attached to the upper part of the uterus. The lateral ends of these tubes are located above the ovaries but are not directly connected to the ovaries. These ends have fingerlike projections, called *fimbriae.* The fimbriae help move the ovum, which is released by the ovary, into the fallopian tube. Each fallopian tube serves as a passageway for the ovum as the ovum moves from the ovary to the uterus. The muscle layers of the tube move the ovum by peristalsis. Cilia, hairlike structures on the lining of the tubes, also keep the ovum moving toward the uterus. Fertilization, the union of the ovum and a sperm to create a new life, usually takes place in the fallopian tubes.

The uterus is a hollow, muscular, pear-shaped organ located behind the urinary bladder and in front of the rectum. It is divided into three parts: the fundus (the top section, where the fallopian tubes attach); the body, or corpus (the middle section); and the cervix (the narrow, bottom section, which

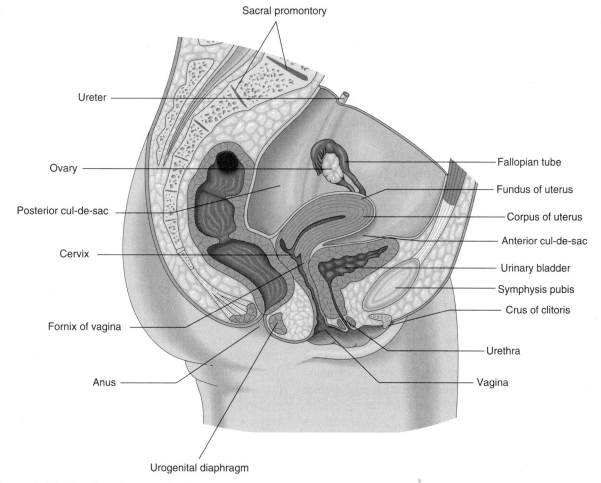

Figure 6-45 The female reproductive system.

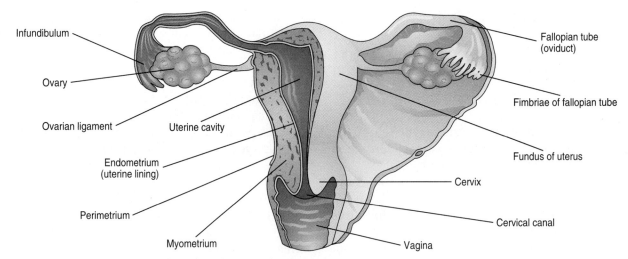

Figure 6-46 Anterior view of the female reproductive system.

attaches to the vagina). The uterus is the organ of menstruation; allows for the development and growth of the fetus; and contracts to aid in expulsion of the fetus during birth. The uterus has three layers. The inner layer is called the **endometrium**. This layer of specialized epithelium provides for implantation of a fertilized ovum and aids in the development of the fetus. If fertilization does not occur, the endometrium deteriorates and causes the bleeding known as *menstruation*. The middle layer of the uterus is a muscle layer. It allows for the expansion of the uterus during pregnancy and contracts to expel the fetus during birth. The outer layer is a serous membrane.

The **vagina** is a muscular tube that connects the cervix of the uterus to the outside of the body. It serves as a passageway for the menstrual flow; receives the sperm and semen from the male; is the female organ of copulation; and acts as the birth canal during delivery of the infant. The vagina is lined with a mucous membrane arranged in folds called rugae. The rugae allow the vagina to enlarge during childbirth and intercourse.

Bartholin's glands, also called *vestibular glands,* are two small glands located one on each side of the vaginal opening. They secrete mucous for lubrication during intercourse.

The **vulva** is the collective name for the structures that form the external female genital area (see figure 6-47). The mons veneris is the triangular pad of fat that is covered with hair and lies over the pubic area. The **labia majora** are the two large folds of fatty tissue that are covered with hair on their outer surfaces; they enclose and protect the vagina. The **labia minora** are the two smaller folds of tissue that are located within the labia majora. The area of

the vulva located inside the labia minora is called the **vestibule**. It contains the openings to the urethra and the vagina. An area of erectile tissue, called the *clitoris,* is located at the junction of the labia minora. It produces sexual arousal when stimulated directly or indirectly during intercourse. The **perineum** is defined as the area between the vagina and anus in the female, although it can be used to describe the entire pelvic floor in both the male and female.

The **breasts,** or mammary glands, contain lobes separated into sections by connective and fatty tissue. Milk ducts located in the tissue exit on the surface at the nipples. The main function of the glands is to secrete milk (lactate) after childbirth.

DISEASES

Breast tumors can be benign or malignant. Symptoms include a lump or mass in the breast tissue, a change in breast size, and a discharge from the nipple. Breast self-examination (BSE) can often detect tumors early. Mammography and ultrasonography are also used to detect tumors. Treatment methods include a lumpectomy (removal of the tumor), a simple mastectomy (surgical removal of the breast), or a radical mastectomy (surgical removal of the tissue, underlying muscles, and axillary lymph nodes). If the tumor is malignant, chemotherapy and/or radiation are usually used in addition to surgery.

Cancer of the cervix and/or uterus is common in females. Cervical cancer can be detected early by a

Pap smear. Symptoms of cervical cancer include abnormal vaginal discharge and bleeding. Symptoms of uterine cancer include an enlarged uterus, a watery discharge, and abnormal bleeding. Treatment methods include a hysterectomy (surgical removal of the uterus and cervix) or panhysterectomy (surgical removal of the uterus, ovaries, and fallopian tubes); chemotherapy; and/or radiation.

Endometriosis is the growth of endometrial tissue outside the uterus. The tissue can be transferred from the uterus by the fallopian tubes, blood, or lymph, or during surgery. It usually becomes embedded in a structure in the pelvic area, such as the ovaries or the peritoneal tissues, and constantly grows and sheds. Symptoms include pelvic pain, abnormal bleeding, and dysmenorrhea (painful menstruation). Treatment methods vary with the age of the patient and the degree of abnormal growth but can include hormonal therapy, pain medications, and/or surgical removal of affected organs.

Pelvic inflammatory disease (PID) is an inflammation of the cervix, the endometrium of the uterus, fallopian tubes, and, at times, the ovaries. It is usually caused by pathogenic organisms such as bacteria, viruses, and fungi. Symptoms include pain in the lower abdomen, fever, and a purulent (pus) vaginal discharge. Treatment methods include antibiotics, increased fluid intake, rest, and/or pain medication.

Premenstrual syndrome (PMS) is actually a group of symptoms that appear three to fourteen days before menstruation. A large percentage of women experience some degree of PMS. The cause is unknown but may be related to a hormonal or biochemical imbalance; poor nutrition; or stress. Symptoms vary and may include nervousness, irritability, depression, headache, edema, backache, constipation, abdominal bloating, temporary weight gain, and breast tenderness and enlargement. Treatment is geared mainly toward relieving symptoms, and methods include diet modification, exercise, stress reduction, and/or medications to relieve the emotional symptoms.

SEXUALLY TRANSMITTED DISEASES

Sexually transmitted diseases (STDs), or venereal diseases, affect both males and females. The incidence of these diseases has increased greatly in recent years, especially among young people. If not treated, STDs can cause serious chronic conditions and, in some cases, sterility or death.

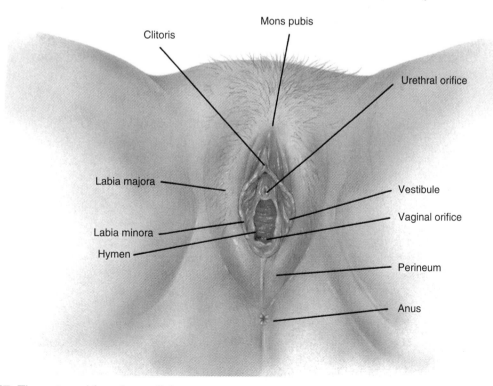

Figure 6-47 The external female genital area.

Acquired immune deficiency syndrome (AIDS) is caused by a virus called the *human immuno-deficiency virus (HIV)*. This virus attacks the body's immune system, rendering the immune system unable to fight off certain infections and diseases, and, eventually, causing death. The virus is spread through sexual secretions or blood, and from an infected mother to her infant during pregnancy or childbirth.

The HIV virus does not live long outside the body and is not transmitted by casual, nonsexual contact. Individuals infected with HIV can remain free of any symptoms for years after infection. During this asymptomatic period, the infected individual can transmit the virus to any other individual with whom they exchange sexual secretions, blood, or blood products. After this initial asymptomatic period, many individuals develop AIDS-related complex (ARC). Symptoms of ARC include a positive blood test for antibodies to the HIV virus, lack of infection resistance, appetite loss, weight loss, recurrent fever, night sweats, skin rashes, diarrhea, fatigue, and swollen lymph nodes. When opportunistic diseases appear, AIDS is diagnosed. Two of the most common opportunistic diseases include the rare type of pneumonia called *Pneumocystis carinii* and the slow-growing cancer called Kaposi's sarcoma (see figure 6-48).

At present, there is no cure for AIDS, although much research is being directed toward developing a vaccine to prevent and drugs to cure AIDS. One drug currently in use is Zidovudine (formerly AZT). Although several other experimental drugs are currently being tested, many patients cannot tolerate the side effects and bone marrow toxicity of these drugs. Some of the drugs do reduce the symptoms and prolong life. Prevention is the best method in dealing with AIDS. Universal precautions should be followed while handling blood, body secretions, and sexual secretions. High-risk sexual activities should be avoided. A condom and an effective spermicide should be used to form a protective barrier during intercourse. The use of drugs and sharing of intravenous (IV) needles should be avoided. Females infected with HIV should avoid pregnancy. *Everyone* must concern themselves with eliminating the transmission of AIDS.

Chlamydia is one of the most frequently occurring STDs and is caused by several strains of the chlamydia organism, a specialized bacteria that lives as an intracellular parasite. Symptoms are similar to those of gonorrhea. Males experience burning when urinating and a mucoid discharge. Females

Figure 6-48 A common opportunistic disease that occurs in AIDS patients is Kaposi's sarcoma. *(Courtesy of The Centers of Disease Control, Atlanta, GA).*

are frequently asymptomatic, although some may have a vaginal discharge. The disease frequently causes pelvic inflammatory disease and sterility in females, if not treated. Chlamydia can be treated with tetracycline or erythromycin antibiotics.

Gonorrhea is caused by the gonococcus bacteria. Symptoms in males include a greenish-yellow discharge, burning when urinating, sore throat, and swollen glands. Females are frequently asymptomatic but may experience dysuria, pain in the lower abdomen, and vaginal discharge. An infected woman can transmit the gonococcus organism to her infant's eyes during childbirth, causing blindness. To prevent this, a drop of silver nitrate or antibiotic is routinely placed in the eyes of newborn babies. Gonorrhea is treated with large doses of penicillin or tetracycline antibiotics.

Herpes is a viral disease caused by the herpes simplex virus type II. Symptoms include a burning sensation, fluid-filled vesicles (blisterlike sores) that rupture and form painful ulcers, and painful urination. After the sores heal, the virus becomes dormant. Many people have repeated attacks, but the attacks are milder. There is no cure, and treatment is directed toward promoting healing and easing discomfort.

Pubic lice are parasites that are usually transmitted sexually, although they can be spread by contact with clothing, bed linen, or other items containing the lice. Symptoms include an intense itching and redness of the perineal area. Medications that kill the lice are used as treatment.

To prevent a recurrence, it is essential to wash all clothing and bed linen to destroy any lice or nits (eggs).

Syphilis is caused by a spirochete bacteria. The symptoms occur in stages. During the primary stage, a painless chancre, or sore, appears, usually on the penis of the male and in the vulva or on the cervix of the female. This chancre heals within several weeks. During the second stage, which occurs if the chancre is not treated, the organism enters the bloodstream and causes a nonitching rash, a sore throat, a fever, and swollen glands. These symptoms also disappear within several weeks. The third stage occurs years later after the spirochete has damaged vital organs. Damage to the heart and blood vessels causes cardiovascular disease; damage to the spinal cord causes a characteristic gait and paralysis; and brain damage causes mental disorders, deafness, and blindness. At this stage, damage is irreversible, and death occurs. Early diagnosis and treatment with antibiotics can cure syphilis during the first two stages.

Trichomonas vaginalis is caused by a parasitic protozoa. The main symptom is a large amount of white or yellow, foul-smelling discharge. Males are frequently asymptomatic. The oral medication Flagyl is used to treat this disease; both sexual partners must be treated to prevent reinfection.

STUDENT *Go to the workbook and complete the assignment sheet for 6:14, Reproductive System.*

tegumentary system, or skin, provides a protective covering for the body. The skeletal and muscular systems provide structure and movement. The circulatory system transports oxygen and nutrients to all body cells, and carries carbon dioxide and metabolic materials away from the cells. The lymphatic system assists the circulatory system in removing wastes and excess fluid from the cells and tissues. The nervous system coordinates the many activities that occur in the body and allows the body to respond and adapt to changes. Special senses provided by organs such as the eyes and ears also allow the body to react to the environment. The respiratory system takes in oxygen for use by the body and eliminates carbon dioxide, a waste product produced by body cells. The digestive system is responsible for the physical and chemical breakdown of food so it can be used by body cells. The urinary system removes certain wastes and excess water from the body. The endocrine system, composed of a group of glands, controls many body functions. The reproductive system allows the human body to create new life.

All of the systems are interrelated, working as a unit to maintain a constant balance within the human body. When disease occurs, this balance frequently is disturbed. Some of the major diseases and disorders of each system were also discussed in this unit.

UNIT **6** SUMMARY

A health care worker must understand normal functioning of the human body in order to understand disease processes. A study of anatomy, the form and structure of an organism, and physiology, the processes of living organisms, adds to this understanding.

The basic structural unit of the human body is the cell. Cells join together to form tissues. Tissues join together to form organs, which work together to form body systems.

Systems work together to provide for proper functioning of the human body. The in-

UNIT 6 SUGGESTED REFERENCES

Borgstadt, Marcia. *Understanding and Caring for Human Diseases.* Albany, NY: Delmar Publishers, 1997.

Burke, Shirley R. *Human Anatomy and Physiology in Health and Disease.* 3rd ed. Albany, NY: Delmar Publishers, 1992.

Colbert, Bruce, et al. *An Integrated Approach to Health Sciences: Anatomy and Physiology, Math, Physics, and Chemistry.* Albany, NY: Delmar Publishers, 1997.

Creager, Joan C. *Human Anatomy and Physiology.* 2nd ed. Dubuque, IA: Wm. C. Brown Publishers, 1991.

Des Jardins, Terry R. *Cardiopulmonary Anatomy and Physiology: Essentials for Respiratory Care.* 2nd ed. Albany, NY: Delmar Publishers, 1993.

Fong, Elizabeth, and Ann Senisi-Scott. *Body Structures and Functions.* 8th ed. Albany, NY: Delmar Publishers, 1993.

Fox, Stuart I. *Perspectives on Human Biology.* Dubuque, IA: Wm. C. Brown Publishers, 1991.

Hampton, John K. *The Biology of Human Aging.* Dubuque, IA: Wm. C. Brown Publishers, 1991.

Keir, Lucille, Connie Krebs, and Barbara A. Wise. *Medical Assisting: Administrative and Clinical Comptetencies.* 3rd ed. Albany, NY: Delmar Publishers, 1993.

Mader, Sylvia. *Understanding Human Anatomy and Physiology.* Dubuque, IA: Wm. C. Brown Publishers, 1991.

Memmler, Ruth Lundeen, and Dena L. Wood. *The Human Body in Health and Disease.* 7th ed. Philadelphia, PA: J. B. Lippincott, 1992.

Mulvihill, Mary Lou. *Human Disease: A Systematic Approach.* 4th ed. Norwalk, CT: Appleton-Lange, 1994.

Rice, Jane. *Medical Terminology with Human Anatomy.* 3rd ed. Norwalk, CT: Appleton-Lange, 1994.

Seeley, Rod, Trent Stephens, and Philip Tate. *Essentials of Anatomy and Physiology.* 3rd ed. St. Louis, MO: Mosby, 1996.

Short, Marjorie J., and Deborah Goldstein. *Head, Neck, and Dental Anatomy.* 2nd ed. Albany, NY: Delmar Publishers, 1994.

Tate, Phil, and Rod Seeley. *Understanding the Human Body.* St. Louis, MO: Mosby, 1994.

Thibodeau, Gary, and Kevin Patton. *Anatomy and Physiology.* 2nd ed. St. Louis, MO: C. V. Mosby, 1993.

UNIT 7

Human Growth and Development

UNIT OBJECTIVES

After completing this unit of study, you should be able to:

- Identify at least two physical, mental, emotional, and social developments that occur during each of the seven main life stages
- Explain the main causes and the treatments for eating disorders, chemical abuse, and suicide
- Recognize ways that life stages affect an individual's needs
- Describe the five stages of grieving that occur in the dying patient and the role of the health care worker during each stage
- List at least two purposes of hospice care
- Justify what is meant by the "right to die"
- Create examples for each of the five basic groups of needs in Maslow's Hierarchy of Needs
- Name the two main methods people use to meet or satisfy needs
- Describe a situation that shows the use of each of the following defense mechanisms: rationalization, projection, displacement, compensation, daydreaming, repression, and denial
- List the three main factors of the communication process
- Identify at least four factors that can interfere with the communication process
- Explain the importance of listening, nonverbal behavior, reporting, and recording in the communication process
- Justify the importance of recognizing cultural diversity
- Define, pronounce, and spell all of the key terms

KEY TERMS

acceptance
adolescence
affection
Alzheimer's disease
   (Altz´-high-merz)
anger
anorexia nervosa
   (an-oh-rex´-see-ah ner-voh´-sah)
arteriosclerosis
   (ar-tear"-ee-oh-skleh-row´-sis)
bargaining
bulimarexia
   (byou-lee"-mah-rex´-ee-ah)
bulimia
   (byou-lee´-me-ah)
chemical abuse
communication
compensation
   (cahm"-pen-say´-shun)
cultural diversity
daydreaming

defense mechanisms
denial
depression
displacement
early adulthood
early childhood
emotional
esteem
hospice
   (hoss´-pis)
infancy
late adulthood
late childhood
life stages
listening
mental
middle adulthood
motivated
needs
nonverbal
physical

physiological needs
   (fizz"-ee-oh-lodg´-ih-kal)
projection
puberty
   (pew´-burr"-tee)
rationalization
   (rash"-en-nal-ih-zay´-shun)
repression
right to die
safety
satisfaction
self-actualization
sexuality
social
suicide
tension
terminal illness
verbal
withdrawal

INTRODUCTION

Human growth and development is a process that begins at birth and does not end until death. During all stages of growth and development, individuals have needs that must be met. A health care worker must be aware of the various life stages and of individual needs in order to provide quality health care (see figure 7-1).

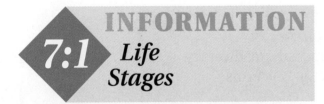

INFORMATION
7:1 Life Stages

Even though individuals differ greatly, each person passes through certain stages of growth and development from birth to death. These stages are frequently called **life stages**. A common method of classifying life stages is as follows:

- Infancy—birth to 1 year
- Early childhood—1 to 6 years
- Late childhood—6 to 12 years
- Adolescence—12 to 20 years
- Early adulthood—20 to 40 years
- Middle adulthood—40 to 65 years
- Late adulthood—65 years and up

As individuals pass through these life stages, four main types of growth and development occur: physical, mental, emotional, and social. **Physical** refers to body growth and includes height and weight changes, muscle and nerve development, and changes in body organs. **Mental** refers to development of the mind and includes learning how to solve problems, make judgments, and deal with situations. **Emotional** refers to feelings and includes dealing with love, hate, joy, fear, excitement, and other similar feelings. **Social** refers to interactions and relationships with other people.

Each stage of growth and development has its own characteristics and has specific developmental

Figure 7-1 An understanding of life stages is important for the health care worker, who may provide care to individuals of all ages; from the very young (left) to the elderly (above).

tasks that an individual must master. These tasks progress from the simple to the more complex. For example, an individual first learns to sit, then stand, then walk, and then, finally, run. Each stage establishes the foundation for the next stage. In this way, growth and development proceeds in an orderly pattern. It is important to remember, however, that the rate of progress varies among individuals. Some children master speech early, others master it later. Similarly, an individual may experience a sudden growth spurt and then maintain the same height for a period of time.

Each life stage creates certain needs in individuals. Likewise, other factors can affect life stages and needs. An individual's sex, race, and heredity (factors inherited from parents, such as hair color and body structure) can influence needs. Injury or illness usually has a negative effect and can change needs or impair development.

INFANCY

Physical Development

The most dramatic and rapid changes in growth and development occur during the first year of life. A newborn baby usually weighs approximately 6 to 8

pounds (2.7 to 3.6 kg) and measures 18 to 22 inches (46 to 55 cm) (see figure 7-2). By the end of the first year of life, weight has usually tripled, to 21 to 24 pounds (9.5 to 11 kg), and height has increased to approximately 29 to 30 inches (74 to 76 cm).

Muscular system and nervous system developments are also dramatic. The muscular and nervous systems are very immature at birth. Certain reflex actions present at birth allow the infant to

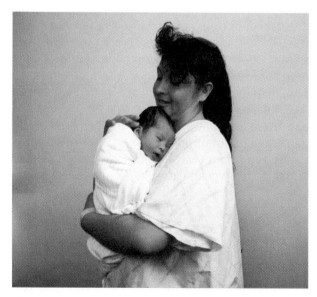

Figure 7-2 A newborn baby usually weighs approximately 6 to 8 pounds and measures 18 to 22 inches in length.

respond to the environment. These include the Moro, or startle, reflex to a loud noise or sudden movement; the rooting reflex, in which a slight touch on the cheek causes the mouth to open and the head to turn; the sucking reflex, caused by a slight touch on the lips; and the grasp reflex, in which infants can grasp an object placed in the hand. Muscle coordination develops in stages. At first, infants are able to lift the head slightly. By 2 months, they can usually roll from side to back. By 4 to 5 months, they can turn the body completely around, accept objects handed to them, grasp stationary objects, and, with support, hold the head up while sitting. By 6 to 7 months, infants can sit unsupported for several minutes, grasp moving objects, and crawl on the stomach. By 12 months, infants frequently can walk without assistance, grasp objects with the thumb and fingers, and throw small objects.

Other physical developments are also dramatic. Most infants are born without teeth, but usually have ten to twelve teeth by the end of the first year of life. At birth, vision is poor and may be limited to black and white, and eye movements are not coordinated. By 1 year of age, however, close vision is good, in color, and can readily focus on small objects. Sensory abilities such as those of smell, taste, sensitivity to hot and cold, and hearing, while good at birth, become more refined and exact.

Mental Development

Mental development is also rapid during the first year. Newborns respond to discomforts such as pain, cold, or hunger by crying. As their needs are met, they gradually become more aware of their surroundings and begin to recognize individuals associated with their care. As infants respond to stimuli in the environment, learning activities grow. At birth, they are unable to speak. By 6 months of age, however, infants understand some words and can make basic sounds; and by 12 months, infants understand many words and use many single words in their vocabularies.

Emotional Development

Emotional development is observed very early in life. Newborns show excitement. By 4 to 6 months of age, distress, delight, anger, disgust, and fear can often be seen. By 12 months of age, elation and affection for adults is evident. Events that occur in

Figure 7-3 By 4 months of age, infants recognize their caregivers and stare intently at others.

the first year of life when these emotions are first exhibited can have a strong influence on an individual's emotional behavior during adulthood.

Social Development

Social development progresses gradually from the self-centeredness concept of the newborn to the recognition of others in the environment. By 4 months of age, infants recognize their caregivers, smile readily, and stare intently at others (see figure 7-3). By 6 months of age, infants watch the activities of others, show signs of possessiveness, and may become shy or withdraw when in the presence of strangers. By 12 months of age, infants may still be shy with strangers, but they socialize freely with familiar people, and mimic and imitate gestures, facial expressions, and vocal sounds.

Infants are dependent on others for all needs. Food, cleanliness, and rest are essential for physical growth. Love and security are essential for emotional and social growth. Stimulation is essential for mental growth.

EARLY CHILDHOOD

Physical Development

During early childhood, from 1 to 6 years of age, physical growth is slower than during infancy. By age 6, the average weight is 45 pounds (20.4 kg), and the average height is 46 inches (116 cm). Skeletal and muscle development helps the child assume a more adult appearance. The legs and lower body tend to grow more rapidy than do the head, arms, and chest. Muscle coordination allows the child to run, climb, and move freely. As muscles of the fingers develop, the child learns to write, draw, and use a fork and knife. By age 2 or 3, most teeth have erupted, and the digestive system is mature enough to handle most adult foods. Between 2 and 4 years of age, most children learn bladder and bowel control.

Mental Development

Mental development advances rapidly during early childhood. Verbal growth progresses from the use of several words at age 1 to a vocabulary of 1,500 to 2,500 words at age 6. Two-year-olds have short attention spans but are interested in many different activities (see figure 7-4). They can remember details and begin to understand concepts. Four-year-olds ask frequent questions and usually recognize letters and some words. They begin to make decisions based on logic rather than on trial and error. By age 6, children are very verbal and want to learn how to read and write. Memory has developed to the point where the child can make decisions based on both past and present experiences.

Emotional Development

Emotional development also advances rapidly. At ages 1 to 2, children begin to develop self-awareness and to recognize the effect they have on other peo-

Figure 7-5 Two- to four-year-olds like routine, such as regular periods set aside for reading.

ple and things. Limits are usually established for safety, leading the 1- or 2-year-old to either accept or defy such limits. Children feel impatience and frustration as they try to do things beyond their abilities. Anger, often in the form of "temper tantrums," occurs when they cannot perform as desired. Children at this age also like routine (see figure 7-5), and become stubborn, angry, or frustrated when changes occur. From ages 4 to 6, children begin to gain more control over their emotions. They understand the concept of right and wrong, and because they have achieved more independence, they are not frustrated as much by their lack of ability. By age 6, most children also show less anxiety when faced with new experiences, because they have learned they can deal with new situations.

Social Development

Social development expands from a self-centered 1-year-old to a very sociable 6-year-old. In the early years, children are usually strongly attached to their parents (or to the individuals who provide their care), and they fear any separation. They begin to enjoy the company of others, but are still very possessive. Playing alongside other children is more common than playing with other children. Gradually, children learn to put "self" aside and begin to take more of an interest in others. They learn to trust other people and make more of an effort to please others by becoming more agreeable and social. Friends of their own age are usually important to 6-year-olds.

Figure 7-4 Two-year-olds are interested in many different activities, but they have short attention spans.

The needs of early childhood still include food, rest, shelter, protection, love, and security. In addition, children need routine, order, and consistency in their daily lives. They must be taught to be responsible and must learn how to conform to rules. This can be accomplished by making reasonable demands based on the child's ability to comply.

LATE CHILDHOOD

Physical Development

This life stage, which covers ages 6 to 12, is also called *preadolescence*. Physical development is slow but steady. Weight gain averages 5 to 7 pounds (2.3 to 3.2 kg) per year, and height usually increases approximately 2 to 3 inches (5 to 7.5 cm) per year. Muscle coordination is well developed, and children can engage in physical activities that require complex motor-sensory coordination. During this age, most of the primary teeth are lost, and permanent teeth erupt. The eyes are well developed, and visual acuity is at its best. During ages 10 to 12, sexual maturation may begin in some children.

Mental Development

Mental development increases rapidly because much of the child's life centers around school. Speech skills develop more completely, and reading and writing skills are learned. Children learn to use information to solve problems and the memory becomes more complex. They begin to understand more abstract concepts such as loyalty, honesty, values, and morals. Children use more active thinking and become more adept at making judgments (see figure 7-6).

Emotional Development

Emotional development continues to help the child achieve a greater independence and a more distinct personality. At age 6, children are often frightened and uncertain as they begin school. Reassuring parents and success in school help children gain self-confidence. Gradually, fears are replaced by the ability to cope. Emotions are slowly brought under control and dealt with in a more effective manner.

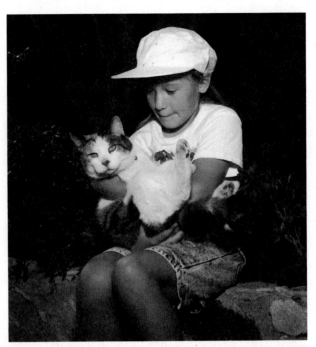

Figure 7-6 In late childhood (ages 6 to 12), children become more adept at making judgments.

By ages 10 to 12, sexual maturation and changes in body functions can lead to periods of depression followed by periods of joy. These emotional changes can cause children to be restless, anxious, and difficult to understand.

Social Development

Social changes are evident during these years. Seven-year-olds tend to like activities they can do by themselves and do not usually like group activities. However, they want the approval of others, especially their parents and friends. Children from ages 8 to 10 tend to be more group oriented, and they typically form groups with members of their own sex. They are more ready to accept the opinions of others and learn to conform to rules and standards of behavior followed by the group. Toward the end of this period, children tend to make friends more easily, and they begin to develop an increasing awareness of the opposite sex. As children spend more time with others their own age, their dependency on their parent(s) lessens, as does the time they spend with their parents.

Needs of children in this age group include the same basic needs of infancy and early childhood along with the need for reassurance, parental approval, and peer acceptance.

ADOLESCENCE

Physical Development

Adolescence, ages 12 to 20, is often a traumatic life stage. Physical changes occur most dramatically in the early period. A sudden "growth spurt" can cause rapid increases in weight and height. A weight gain of up to 25 pounds (11 kg) and a height increase of several inches can occur in a period of months. Muscle coordination does not advance as quickly. This can lead to awkwardness or clumsiness in motor coordination. This growth spurt usually occurs anywhere from ages 11 to 13 in girls and ages 13 to 15 in boys.

The most obvious physical changes in adolescents relate to the development of the sexual organs and the secondary sexual characteristics, frequently called puberty. Secretion of sex hormones leads to the onset of menstruation in girls and the production of sperm and semen in boys. Secondary sexual characteristics in females include growth of pubic hair, development of breasts and wider hips, and distribution of body fat leading to the female shape. The male develops a deeper voice; attains more muscle mass and broader shoulders; and grows pubic, facial, and body hair.

Mental Development

Since most of the foundations have already been established, mental development primarily involves an increase in knowledge and a sharpening of skills. Adolescents learn to make decisions and to accept responsibility for their actions. At times, this causes conflict because they are treated as both children and adults, or are told to "grow up" while being reminded that they are "still children."

Emotional Development

Emotional development is often stormy and in conflict. As adolescents try to establish their identities and independence, they are often uncertain and feel inadequate and insecure. They worry about their appearances, their abilities, and their relationships with others. They frequently respond more and more to peer group influences. At times, this leads to changes in attitude and behavior and conflict with

values previously established. Toward the end of adolescence, self-identity has been established. At this point, teenagers feel more comfortable with who they are and turn attention toward what they may become. They gain more control of their feelings and become more mature emotionally.

Social Development

Social development usually involves spending less time with family and more time with peer groups. As adolescents attempt to develop self-identity and independence, they seek security in groups of people their own age who have similar problems and conflicts (see figure 7-7). If these peer relationships help develop self-confidence through the approval of others, adolescents become more secure and satisfied. Toward the end of this life stage, adolescents develop a more mature attitude and begin to develop patterns of behavior that they associate with adult behavior or status.

In addition to basic needs, adolescents need reassurance, support, and understanding. Many problems that develop during this life stage can be traced to the conflict and feelings of inadequacy and insecurity that adolescents experience. Examples include eating disorders, drug and alcohol abuse, and suicide. Even though these types of problems also occur in earlier and later life stages, they are frequently associated with adolescence.

Eating disorders often develop from an excessive concern with appearance. Two common eating disorders are anorexia nervosa and bulimia. Anorexia nervosa, commonly called *anorexia*, is a psychological disorder in which a person drastically reduces food intake or refuses to eat at all. This

Figure 7-7 Adolescents use the peer group as a safety net as they try to establish their identities and independence. *(Courtesy of Suzanne Fronk).*

results in metabolic disturbances, excessive weight loss, weakness, and, if not treated, death. Bulimia is a psychological disorder in which a person alternately binges (eats excessively) and then fasts, or refuses to eat at all. When a person induces vomiting or uses laxatives to get rid of food that has been eaten, the condition is called bulimarexia. All three conditions are more common in females than males. Psychological or psychiatric help is usually needed to treat these conditions.

Chemical abuse is the use of substances such as alcohol or drugs and the development of a physical and/or mental dependence on these chemicals. Chemical abuse can occur in any life stage, but it frequently begins in adolescence. Reasons for using chemicals include anxiety or stress relief, peer pressure, escape from emotional or psychological problems, experimentation with feelings the chemicals produce, desire for "instant gratification," hereditary traits, and cultural influences. Chemical abuse can lead to physical and mental disorders and disease. Treatment is directed toward total rehabilitation that allows the chemical abuser to return to a productive and meaningful life.

Suicide, found in many life stages, is one of the leading causes of death in adolescents. Reasons for suicide include depression, grief over a loss or love affair, failure in school, inability to meet expectations, influence of suicidal friends, or lack of self-esteem. The impulsive nature of adolescents increases the possibility of suicide. Most individuals who are thinking of suicide give warning signs such as verbal statements like "I'd rather be dead" or "You'd be better off without me." Other warning signs include sudden changes in appetite and sleep habits, withdrawal and moodiness, excessive fatigue or agitation, alcohol or drug abuse, and loss of interest in hobbies and other aspects of life. These individuals are calling out for attention and help and usually respond to efforts of assistance. Their direct and indirect pleas should never be ignored. Support, understanding, and psychological or psychiatric counseling are used to prevent suicide.

EARLY ADULTHOOD

Physical Development

Early adulthood, ages 20 to 40, is frequently the most productive life stage. Physical development is basically complete, muscles are developed and strong, and motor coordination is at its peak. This is also the prime childbearing time and usually produces the healthiest babies (see figure 7-8). Both male and female sexual development is at its peak.

Mental Development

Mental development usually continues throughout this stage. Many young adults pursue additional education to establish and progress in their chosen careers. Frequently, formal education continues for many years. The young adult often also deals with independence, makes career choices, establishes a lifestyle, selects a marital partner, starts a family, and establishes values, all of which involve making many decisions and forming many judgments.

Emotional Development

Emotional development usually involves preserving the stability established during previous stages. Young adults are subjected to many emotional stresses related to career, marriage, family, and other similar situations. If emotional structure is strong, most young adults can cope with these worries. They find satisfaction in their achievements, take responsibility for their actions, and learn to accept criticism and to profit from mistakes.

Social Development

Social development frequently involves moving away from the peer group, and young adults instead tend to associate with others who have similar

Figure 7-8 Early adulthood is the prime childbearing time and usually produces the healthiest babies.

ambitions and interests, regardless of age. The young adult often becomes involved with a mate and forms a family. Young adults do not necessarily accept traditional sex roles, and frequently adopt nontraditional roles. For example, males fill positions as nurses and secretaries, and females enter administrative or construction positions. Such choices have caused and will continue to cause changes in the traditional patterns of society.

MIDDLE ADULTHOOD

Physical Development

Middle adulthood, ages 40 to 65, is frequently called middle age. Physical changes begin to occur during these years. The hair tends to gray and thin, the skin begins to wrinkle, muscle tone tends to decrease, hearing loss starts, visual acuity declines, and weight gain occurs. Females experience menopause, or the end of menstruation, along with decreased hormone production that causes physical and emotional changes. Males also experience a slowing of hormone production. This can lead to physical and psychological changes, a period frequently referred to as the *male climacteric.* However, except in cases of injury, disease, or surgery, males never lose the ability to produce sperm or to reproduce.

Mental Development

Mental ability can continue to increase during middle age, a fact that has been proven by the many individuals in this life stage who seek formal education. Middle adulthood is a period when individuals have acquired an understanding of life and have learned to cope with many different stresses. This allows them to be more confident in decision making and excellent at analyzing situations.

Emotional Development

Emotionally, middle age can be a period of contentment and satisfaction, or it can be a time of crisis. The emotional foundation of previous life stages and the situations that occur during middle age determine emotional status during this period. Job stability, financial success, the end of child rearing, and good health due to disease prevention can all

Figure 7-9 Job stability and enjoyment during middle adulthood contribute to emotional satisfaction.

contribute to emotional satisfaction (see figure 7-9). Stress, created by loss of job, fear of aging, loss of youth and vitality, illness, marital problems, or problems with children or aging parents, can contribute to emotional feelings of depression, insecurity, anxiety, and even anger. Therefore, emotional status varies in this age group and is largely determined by events that occur during this period.

Social Development

Social relationships also depend on many factors. Family relationships often see a decline as children begin lives of their own and parents die. Relationships between husband and wife can become stronger as they have more time together and opportunities to enjoy success. However, divorce rates are also high in this age group, as couples who have remained together "for the children's sake" now separate. Friendships are usually with people who have the same interests and lifestyles.

LATE ADULTHOOD

Physical Development

Late adulthood, age 65 and up, has many different terms associated with it. These include "elderly," "senior citizen," "golden ager," and "retired citizen."

Much attention has been directed toward this life stage in recent years because people are living longer, and the number of people in this age group is increasing daily.

Physical development is on the decline. All body systems are usually affected. The skin becomes dry, wrinkled, and thinner. Brown or yellow spots (frequently called "age spots") appear. The hair becomes thin and frequently loses its luster or shine. Bones become more brittle and porous and are more likely to fracture or break. Cartilage between the vertebrae thins and can lead to a stooping posture. Muscles lose tone and strength, which can lead to fatigue and poor coordination. A decline in the function of the nervous system leads to hearing loss, decreased visual acuity, and decreased tolerance for temperatures that are too hot or too cold. Memory loss can occur, and reasoning ability can diminish. The heart is less efficient, and circulation decreases. The kidney and bladder are less efficient. Breathing capacity decreases and causes shortness of breath. However, it is important to note that these changes usually occur slowly over a long period of time. Many individuals, because of better health and living conditions, do not show physical changes of aging until their seventies and even eighties.

Mental Development

Mental abilities vary among individuals. Although some 90-year-olds remain alert and well oriented, other elderly individuals show decreased mental capacities at much earlier ages. Short-term memory is usually first to decline. Many elderly individuals can clearly remember events that occurred 20 years ago, but do not remember yesterday's events. Diseases such as Alzheimer's disease can lead to irreversible loss of memory, deterioration of intellectual functions, speech and gait disturbances, and disorientation. Arteriosclerosis, a thickening and hardening of the walls of the arteries, can also decrease the blood supply to the brain and cause a decrease in mental abilities.

Emotional Development

Emotional stability also varies among individuals in this age group. Some elderly people cope well with the stresses presented by aging and remain happy and able to enjoy life. Others become lonely, frustrated, withdrawn, and depressed. Emotional adjustment is necessary throughout this cycle.

Retirement, death of a spouse and friends, physical disabilities, financial problems, loss of independence, and knowledge that life must end all can cause emotional distress. The adjustments that the individual makes during this life stage are similar to those made throughout life.

Social Development

Social adjustment also occurs during late adulthood. Retirement can lead to a loss of self-esteem, especially if work is strongly associated with self-identity: "I am a teacher," instead of "I am Sandra Jones." Less contact with coworkers and a more limited circle of friends usually occurs. Many elderly individuals engage in other activities and continue to make new social contacts (see figure 7-10). Others limit their social relationships. Death of a spouse and friends, and moving to a new environment can also cause changes in social relationships. Development of new social contacts is important at this time. Senior centers, golden age groups, churches, and many other organizations help provide the elderly with the opportunity to find new social roles.

Needs of this life stage are the same as those of all other life stages. In addition to basic needs, the elderly need a sense of belonging, self-esteem, financial security, social acceptance, and love.

STUDENT *Go to the workbook and complete the assignment sheet for 7:1, Life Stages.*

Figure 7-10 Social contacts and activities are important during late adulthood.

INFORMATION
7:2 *Death and Dying*

Death is often referred to as "the final stage of growth." It is experienced by everyone and cannot be avoided. In our society, the young tend to ignore its existence. It is usually the elderly, having lost spouses and/or friends, who begin to think of their own deaths.

When a patient is told that he or she has a **terminal illness,** a disease that cannot be cured and will result in death, the patient may react in different ways. Some patients react with fear and anxiety. They fear pain, abandonment, and loneliness. They fear the unknown. They become anxious about their loved ones and about unfinished work or dreams. Anxiety diminishes in patients who feel they have had full lives and who have strong religious beliefs regarding life after death. Some patients view death as a final peace. They know it will bring an end to loneliness, pain, and suffering.

Dr. Elizabeth Kübler-Ross has done extensive research on the process of death and dying and is known as a leading expert on this topic. Because of her research, most medical personnel now feel patients should be told of their approaching deaths. However, patients should be left with "some hope" and the knowledge that they will "not be left alone." It is important that all staff members who provide care to the dying patient know both the extent of information given to the patient and how the patient reacted.

Dr. Kübler-Ross has identified five stages of grieving that dying patients and their families/friends may experience in preparation for death. The stages may not occur in order, and they may overlap or be repeated several times. Some patients may not progress through all of the stages before death occurs. Other patients may be in several stages at the same time. The stages are denial, anger, bargaining, depression, and acceptance.

Denial is the "No, not me!" stage, which usually occurs when a person is first told of a terminal illness. It occurs when the person cannot accept the reality of death or when the person feels loved ones cannot accept the truth. The person may make statements such as "The doctor does not know what he is talking about" or "The tests have to be wrong." Some patients seek second medical opinions or request additional tests. Others refuse to discuss their situations and avoid any references to their illnesses. It is important for patients to discuss these feelings. The health care worker should listen to a patient and try to provide support without confirming or denying. Statements such as "It must be hard for you" or "You feel additional tests will help?" will allow the patient to express feelings and move on to the next stage.

Anger occurs when the patient is no longer able to deny death. Statements such as "Why me?" or "It's your fault" are common. Patients may strike out at anyone who comes in contact with them and become very hostile and bitter. They may blame themselves, their loved ones, or health care personnel for their illnesses. It is important for the health care worker to understand that this anger is not a personal attack; the anger is due to the situation the patient is experiencing. Providing understanding and support, listening, and making every attempt to respond to the patient's demands quickly and with kindness is essential during this stage. This stage continues until the anger is exhausted or the patient must attend to other concerns.

Bargaining occurs when patients accept death but want more time to live. Frequently, this is a period when patients turn to religion and spiritual beliefs. At this point, the will to live is strong, and patients fight hard to achieve goals set. They want to see their children graduate or get married; they want time to arrange care for their families; they want to hold new grandchildren; or other similar desires. Patients make promises to God to obtain more time. Health care workers must again be supportive and be good listeners. Whenever possible, they should help patients meet their goals.

Depression occurs when patients realize that death will come soon and they will no longer be with their families or be able to complete their goals. They may express these regrets, or they may withdraw and become quiet (see figure 7-11). They experience great sadness, and, at times, overwhelming despair. It is important for health care workers to let patients know that it is "OK" to be depressed. Providing quiet understanding, support, and/or a simple touch, and allowing patients to cry or express grief are important during this stage.

Acceptance is the final stage. Patients understand and accept the fact that they are going to die. Patients may complete unfinished business and try to help those around them deal with the oncoming death. Gradually, patients separate themselves from the world and other people. At the end, they

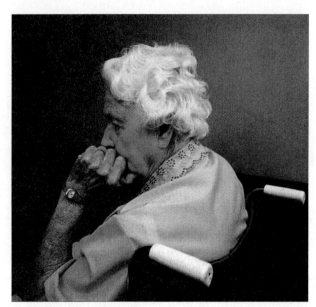

Figure 7-11 Depression can be a normal stage of grieving in a dying patient.

are at peace and can die with dignity. During this final stage, patients still need emotional support and the presence of others, even if it is just the touch of a hand (see figure 7-12).

Providing care to dying patients can be very difficult, but very rewarding. Providing supportive care when families and patients require it most can be one of the greatest satisfactions a health care worker can experience. In order to be able to provide this care, however, health care workers must first understand their own personal feelings about death and come to terms with these feelings. Feelings of fear, frustration, and uncertainty about death can cause workers to avoid dying patients or provide superficial, mechanical care. With experience, health care workers can find ways to deal with their feelings and learn to provide the supportive care needed by the dying.

Hospice care can play an important role in meeting the needs of the dying patient. Hospice care can be offered in hospitals, medical centers, and special facilities, but most frequently it is offered in the patient's home. The philosophy behind this care is to allow the patient to die with dignity and comfort. Pain is controlled so that the patient can remain active as long as possible. Psychological, spiritual, social, and financial counseling are provided for both the patient and family. In medical facilities, personal care of the patient is provided by the staff; in the home situation, this care is provided by home health aides and other health care profes-

sionals. Specially trained volunteers are an important part of many hospice programs. They make regular visits to the patient and family, stay with the patient while the family leaves the home for brief periods of time, and help provide the support and understanding that the patient and family need. When the time for death arrives, the patient is allowed to die with dignity and in peace.

The **right to die** is another issue that health care workers must understand. Because health care workers are ethically concerned with promoting life, allowing patients to die can cause conflict. However, a large number of surveys have shown that most people feel that an individual who has a terminal illness, with no hope of being cured, should be allowed to refuse measures that would prolong life. This is called the *right to die.* Most states have passed, or are now creating, laws that allow adults who have terminal illnesses to instruct their doctors, in writing, to withhold treatments that might prolong life. Most of the laws involve the use of a living will, discussed in Unit 4:4. Under these laws, specific actions to end life cannot be taken. However, the use of respirators, pacemakers, and other medical devices can be withheld, and the person can be allowed to die with dignity.

Health care workers deal with death and with dying patients because death is a part of life. By understanding the process of death and by thinking about the needs of dying patients, the health care worker will be able to provide the special care needed by these individuals.

STUDENT   *Go to the workbook and complete the assignment sheet for 7:2, Death and Dying.*

Figure 7-12 The support and presence of others is important to the dying person.

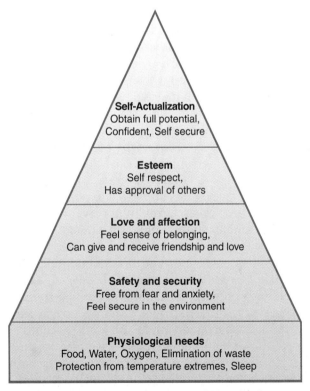

INFORMATION
7:3 *Human Needs*

Needs are frequently defined as "a lack of something that is required or desired." From the moment of birth to the moment of death, every human being has needs. Needs motivate the individual to behave or act so that these needs will be met, if at all possible.

Certain needs have priority over other needs. For example, at times a need for food may take priority over a need for social approval, or the approval of others. If individuals have been without food for a period of time, they will direct most of their actions toward obtaining food. Even though they want social approval and the respect of others, they may steal for food, knowing that stealing may cause a loss of social approval or respect.

MASLOW'S HIERARCHY OF NEEDS

Abraham Maslow, a noted psychologist, developed a hierarchy of needs (see figure 7-13). According to Maslow, the lower needs must be met before an individual can strive to meet the higher needs. Only when satisfaction has been obtained at one level is an individual motivated toward meeting needs at a higher level. The levels of needs include physiological needs, safety, affection, esteem, and self-actualization.

Physiological Needs

Physiological needs are often called "physical," "biological," or "basic" needs. These needs are required by every human being to sustain life. They include food, water, oxygen, elimination of waste materials, sleep, and protection from extreme temperatures. These needs must be met in order for life to continue. If any of these needs goes unmet, death will occur. Even among these needs, a priority exists. For example, because lack of oxygen will cause death in a matter of minutes, the need for oxygen has priority over the need for food. A patient with severe lung disease who is gasping for every breath will not be concerned with food intake. This individual's main concern will be to obtain enough oxygen to live through the next minute.

Other physiological needs include sensory and motor needs. If these needs are unmet, individuals may not die, but their body functions will be affected. Sensory needs include hearing, seeing, feeling, smelling, tasting, and mental stimulation. When these needs are met, they allow the individual to respond to the environment. If these needs are not met, the person may lose contact with the environment or with reality. An example is motor needs, which include the ability to move and respond to the individual's environment. If muscles are not stimulated, they will atrophy (waste away), and function will be lost.

Many of the physiological needs are automatically controlled by the body. The process of breathing is usually not part of the conscious thought process of the individual until something occurs to interfere with breathing. Another example is the functioning of the urinary bladder. The bladder fills automatically, and the individual only becomes aware of the bladder when it is full. If the individual does not respond and go to the restroom to empty the bladder, eventually control will be lost, and the bladder will empty itself.

Self-Actualization
Obtain full potential,
Confident, Self secure

Esteem
Self respect,
Has approval of others

Love and affection
Feel sense of belonging,
Can give and receive friendship and love

Safety and security
Free from fear and anxiety,
Feel secure in the environment

Physiological needs
Food, Water, Oxygen, Elimination of waste
Protection from temperature extremes, Sleep

Figure 7-13 Maslow's Hierarchy of Needs: the lower needs must be met before the individual can try to meet the higher needs.

Safety

Safety becomes important when physiological needs have been met. Safety needs include the need to be free from anxiety and fear and the need to feel secure in the environment. The need for order and routine is another example of an individual's effort to remain safe and secure. Individuals often prefer the familiar over the unknown. New environments, a change in routine, marital problems, job loss, injury, disease, and other similar events can threaten an individual's safety.

Love and Affection

The need for love and affection occupy the third level of Maslow's Hierarchy of Needs. When an individual feels safe and secure, and after all physiological needs have been met, the individual next strives for social acceptance, friendship, and to be loved. The need to belong, to relate to others, and to win approval of others motivates an individual's actions at this point. The individual may now attend a social function that was avoided when safety was more of a priority. Individuals who feel safe and secure are more willing to accept and adapt to change and more willing to face unknown situations. The need for love and affection is satisfied when friends are made, social contacts are established, acceptance by others is received, and the individual is able to both give and receive affection and love (see figure 7-14).

Maslow states that sexuality is both a part of the need for love and affection as well as a physiological need. Sexuality in this context is defined by people's feelings concerning their masculine/feminine natures, their abilities to give and receive love and affection, and, finally, their roles in reproduction of the species. It is important to note that in all three of these areas, sexuality involves a person's feelings and attitudes, not just the person's sexual relationships.

It is equally important to note that a person's sexuality extends throughout the life cycle. At conception, a person's sexual organs are determined. Following birth, a person is given a name, at least generally associated with the person's sex. Studies have shown that children receive treatment according to gender from early childhood and frequently are rewarded for behavior that is deemed "gender appropriate." With the onset of puberty, adolescents become more aware of their emerging sexuality and of the standards that society places on

Figure 7-14 Individuals of all ages need love and affection. *(Courtesy of Sandy Clark).*

them. During both childhood and adolescence, much of what is learned about sexuality comes from observing adult role models. As the adolescent grows into young adulthood, society encourages a reexamination of sexuality and the role it plays in helping to fulfill the need for love and affection. In adulthood, sexuality develops new meanings according to the roles that the adult takes on. Sexuality needs do not cease in late adulthood. Long-term care facilities are recognizing this fact by allowing married couples to each share a room, instead of separating people according to sex. Even after the death of a spouse, an individual may develop new relationships. Determining what role sexuality will play in a person's life is a dynamic process that allows people to meet their need for love and affection throughout their life.

Sexuality, in addition to being related to the satisfaction of needs, is also directly related to an individual's moral values. Issues such as the appropriateness of sex before marriage, the use of birth control, how to deal with pregnancy, and how to deal with sexually transmitted diseases all require individuals to evaluate their moral beliefs. These beliefs then serve as guidelines to help people reach decisions on their behaviors.

Some individuals use sexual relationships as substitutes for love and affection. Individuals who seek to meet their needs only in this fashion cannot successfully complete Maslow's third level.

Esteem

Maslow's fourth level includes the need for esteem. Esteem includes feeling important and worthwhile. When others show respect, approval, and appreciation, an individual begins to feel esteem and gains self-respect. The self-concept, or beliefs, values, and feelings people have about themselves, becomes positive. Individuals will engage in activities that bring achievement, success, and recognition in an effort to maintain their need for esteem. Failure in an activity can cause a loss of confidence and lack of esteem. When esteem needs are met, individuals gain confidence in themselves and begin to direct their actions toward becoming what they want to be.

Self-Actualization

Self-actualization, frequently called *self-realization*, is the final need in Maslow's hierarchy. All other needs must be met, at least in part, before self-actualization can occur. Self-actualization means that people have obtained their full potentials, or that they are what they want to be. People at this level are confident and willing to express their beliefs and stick to them. They feel so strongly about themselves that they are willing to reach out to others to provide assistance and support.

MEETING NEEDS

When needs are felt, individuals are motivated (stimulated) to act. If the action is successful and the need is met, satisfaction, or a feeling of pleasure or fulfillment, occurs. If the need is not met, tension, or frustration, an uncomfortable inner sensation or feeling, occurs. Several needs can be felt at the same time, so individuals must decide which needs are stronger. For example, if individuals need both food and sleep, they must decide which need is most important, because an individual cannot eat and sleep at the same time.

Individuals feel needs at different levels of intensity. The more intense a need, the greater the desire to meet or reduce the need. Also, when an individual first experiences a need, the individual may deal with it by trying different actions in a trial-and-error manner, a type of behavior frequently seen in very young children. As they grow older, children learn more effective means of meeting the need, and are able to satisfy the need easily.

METHODS OF SATISFYING HUMAN NEEDS

Needs can be satisfied by direct or indirect methods. Direct methods work at meeting the need and obtaining satisfaction. Indirect methods work at reducing the need or relieving the tension and frustration created by the unmet need.

Direct Methods

Direct methods include hard work, realistic goals, situation evaluation, and cooperation with others. All of these methods are directed toward meeting the need. Students who constantly fail tests but who want to pass a course have a need for success. They can work harder by listening more in class, asking questions on points they do not understand, and studying longer for the tests. They can set realistic goals that will allow them to find success. By working on one aspect of the course at a time, by concentrating on new material for the next test, by planning to study a little each night rather than studying only the night before a test, and by working on other things that will enable them to pass, they can establish goals they can achieve. They can evaluate the situation to determine why they are failing and to try to find other ways to pass the course. They may determine that they are always tired in class and that by getting more sleep, they will be able to learn the material. They can cooperate with others. By asking the teacher to provide extra assistance, by having parents or friends question them on the material, by asking a counselor to help them learn better study habits, or by having a tutor provide extra help, they may learn the material, pass the tests, and achieve satisfaction by meeting their need.

Indirect Methods

Indirect methods of dealing with needs usually reduce the need and help relieve the tension created by the unmet need. The need is still present, but its intensity decreases. Defense mechanisms are the main indirect methods used. Everyone uses defense mechanisms to some degree. Defense mechanisms provide methods for maintaining self-esteem and relieving discomfort. Some use of defense mechanisms is helpful because it allows individuals to cope with certain situations. However, defense mechanisms can be unhealthy if they are used all the time and individuals substitute them for more effective ways of dealing with situations. Being aware of the use of defense mechanisms and the reason for using them is a healthy use. This allows the individual to relieve tension while modifying habits, learning to accept reality, and striving to find more efficient ways to meet needs.

Examples of defense mechanisms include:

◆ **Rationalization**—This involves using a reasonable excuse or acceptable explanation for behavior in order to avoid the real reason or true motivation. For example, a patient who fears having laboratory tests performed may tell the health worker, "I can't take time off from my job," rather than admit fear.

◆ **Projection**—This involves placing the blame for one's own actions or inadequacies on someone else or on circumstances rather than accepting responsibility for the actions. Examples include, "The teacher failed me because she doesn't like me," rather than, "I failed because I didn't do the work"; and, "I'm late because the alarm clock didn't go off," rather than, "I forgot to set the alarm clock, and I overslept." When people use projection to blame others, they avoid having to admit that they have made mistakes.

◆ **Displacement**—This involves transferring feelings about one person to someone else. Displacement usually occurs because individuals cannot direct the feelings toward the person who is responsible. Many people fear directing hostile or negative feelings toward their bosses or supervisors because they fear job loss. They then direct this anger toward coworkers and/or family members. The classic example is the man who is mad at his boss. When the man gets home, he yells at his wife or children. In such a case, a constructive talk with the boss may solve the problem. If not, or if this is not possible, physical activity can help work off hostile or negative feelings.

◆ **Compensation**—This involves the substitution of one goal for another goal in order to achieve success. If a substitute goal meets needs, this can be a healthy defense mechanism. For example, Joan wanted to be a doctor, but she did not have enough money for a medical education. So she changed her educational plans and became a physician's assistant. Compensation was an ef-

ficient defense mechanism because she enjoyed her work and found satisfaction.

◆ **Daydreaming**—This is a dreamlike thought process that occurs when a person is awake. Daydreaming provides a means of escape when a person is not satisfied with reality. If it allows a person to establish goals for the future and leads to a course of action to accomplish those goals, it is a good defense mechanism. If daydreaming is a substitute for reality, and the dreams become more satisfying than actual life experiences, it can contribute to a poor adjustment to life. For example, if a person dreams about becoming a dental hygienist and takes courses and works toward this goal, daydreaming is effective. If the person dreams about the goal but is satisfied by the thoughts and takes no action, the person will not achieve the goal and is simply escaping from reality.

◆ **Repression**—This involves the transfer of unacceptable or painful ideas, feelings, and thoughts into the unconscious mind. An individual is not aware that this is occurring. When feelings or emotions become too painful or frightening for the mind to deal with, repression allows the individual to continue functioning and to "forget" the fear or feeling. Repressed feelings do not vanish, however. They can resurface in dreams or affect behavior. For example, a person is terrified of heights but does not know why. It is possible that a frightening experience regarding heights happened in early childhood and that the experience was repressed.

◆ **Denial**—This involves disbelief of an event or idea that is too frightening or shocking for a person to cope with. Often, an individual is not aware that denial is occurring. Denial frequently occurs when a terminal illness is diagnosed. The individual will say that the doctor is wrong and seek another opinion. When the individual is ready to deal with the event or idea, denial becomes acceptance.

◆ **Withdrawal**—There are two main ways withdrawal can occur: individuals can either cease to communicate or remove themselves physically from a situation. Withdrawal is sometimes a satisfactory means of avoiding conflict or an unhappy situation. For example, if you are forced to work with an individual who you dislike and who is constantly criticizing your work, you can withdraw by either avoiding any and all communication with this individual or quitting your job or asking for a transfer to another area. At times, interpersonal conflict cannot be avoided, however. In these cases, an open and honest communication with the individual may lead to improved understanding in the relationship.

It is important for health care workers to be aware of both their own and patients' needs. By recognizing needs and understanding the actions individuals take to meet needs, more efficient and higher quality care can be provided. Health care workers will be better able to understand their own behavior and the behavior of others.

STUDENT   *Go to the workbook and complete the assignment sheet for 7:3, Human Needs.*

INFORMATION
7:4 *Effective Communications*

C Communicating effectively with others is an important part of any health career. The health care worker must be able to relate to patients and their families, to coworkers, and to other professionals. An understanding of communication skills will assist the health care worker who is trying to relate effectively.

Communication is the exchange of information, thoughts, ideas, and feelings. It can occur through **verbal** means (spoken words), written communications, and **nonverbal** behavior such as facial expressions, body language, and touch.

COMMUNICATION PROCESS

The communication process involves several factors. The sender begins the process by creating a message, or material, that the sender wants to convey. The message is picked up by a receiver, the person for whom the message is intended. Without a sender, message, and receiver, communication cannot occur.

Even though the communication process seems simple, many factors can interfere with the completion of the process. The message must be clear, the sender must deliver the message effectively, the receiver must be able to hear or receive the message, the receiver must be able to understand the message, and interruptions or distractions must be kept to a minimum.

In order for a message to be clear, it must be in terms that both the sender and receiver understand. Health care workers learn and use terminology that is frequently not understood by those people who are not in health care. Even though these terms are familiar to the health care worker, they must be modified, defined, or substituted with other words when messages are conveyed to people not in health care. For example, if a health care worker needs a urine specimen, some patients can be told to urinate in a container. Others, such as very small children or individuals with limited education, may have to be told to "pee" or "do number one." Even a term such as *apical pulse* is not understood by many individuals. Instead of telling a patient, "I am going to take your apical pulse," say, "I am going to listen to your heart." It requires experience and constant practice to learn to create a message that can be clearly understood.

The sender must deliver the message in a clear and concise manner. Correct pronunciation and the use of good grammar are essential. The use of slang words or words with double meanings should be avoided. Meaningless phrases or terms such as "you know," "all that stuff," "um," and "OK," distract from the message and also must be avoided. In verbal communications, the tone and pitch of voice is important. A moderate level, neither too soft nor too loud, and good inflection, to avoid monotone, are essential. Think of the many different ways the sentence "I really like this job" can be said and the different meanings that can be interpreted depending on the tone and pitch of the voice. The proper rate, or speed, of delivering a message is also important. If a message is delivered too quickly, the receiver may not have enough time to hear all parts of the message. In written communications, the message should be spelled correctly, contain correct grammar and punctuation, and be concise but thorough.

The receiver must be able to hear and receive the message. Patients who are heavily medicated or are weak may nod their heads as if messages are heard, when, in reality, the patients are not receiving the information. They may hear it, but it is not being interpreted and understood because of their physical states. Patients with hearing or visual impairments or patients with limited English-speaking abilities are other examples of individuals who may not be able to easily receive messages (see figure 7-15). Repeating the message, changing the form of the message, and getting others to interpret or clarify the message are some ways to help the receiver receive and respond to the message.

Receivers may hear messages, but they may not understand them. Using unfamiliar terminology can cause this breakdown in communication. Many people do not want to admit that they do not understand terms because they think others will think they are dumb. The health care worker should ask questions or repeat information in different terms if it appears that the patient does not understand the information. The receiver's attitude and prejudices can also interfere with understanding. If a patient feels that health care workers do not know what they are talking about, the patient will not accept the information presented. Receivers must have some confidence and belief in the sender before they will accept and understand a message. It is important that health care workers are willing to say, "I don't know, but I will try to find out that information for you" when they are asked a question about which they do not have correct

knowledge. It is also important for health care workers to be aware of their own prejudices and attitudes when they are receiving messages from patients. If health care workers feel that certain patients are lazy, ignorant, or uncooperative, they will not respond correctly to messages sent by these patients. Health care workers must be aware of these feelings and work to overcome them so they can accept patients as they are.

Interruptions or distractions can interfere with any communication. Trying to talk with others while answering the phone or writing a message can decrease the effectiveness of spoken and/or written communication. Loud noises, or distractions in the form of bright light or uncomfortable temperature can interrupt communication. When two people are talking outside in freezing temperatures, for example, the conversation will be limited due to the discomfort from the cold. A small child jumping around or climbing up and down off a mother's lap will distract the mother as she is getting instructions from a health care worker. A loud television or radio interferes with verbal messages, because receivers may pay more attention to the radio or television than to the person speaking to them. It is important to eliminate or at least limit distractions if meaningful communication is to take place.

LISTENING

Listening is another essential part of effective communication. Listening means paying attention to and making an effort to hear what the other person is saying. Good listening skills require constant practice. The listener must convey a sincere interest and concern in what the speaker is saying. The listener must be alert and maintain eye contact with the speaker. An open mind free of prejudice and personal views allows the listener to hear the ideas being presented. The listener should observe the speaker closely for actions that may contradict what the speaker is saying. For example, if a patient says, "I'm not worried about this surgery," but is very restless and seems nervous, the patient's body movements may indicate fear that is being denied by words.

Reflecting statements back to the speaker lets the speaker know that statements are being heard. It also allows the speaker to clarify a message and express further feelings. For example, in the previous case, the health care worker could reflect the

Figure 7-15 In communicating with a person who has a hearing impairment, face the individual and speak slowly and distinctly.

patient's statement by saying, "You're not at all worried about this surgery?" The patient may respond by saying, "Well, not really. It's just that I worry about my family if something should happen to me." Good listening allowed the patient to express fears and opened the way to more effective communication. In this same case, the entire pattern of communication could have been blocked if the health care worker had instead responded, "That's good."

NONVERBAL COMMUNICATION

Nonverbal communication involves the use of facial expressions, body language, and touch to convey messages or ideas. If a person is smiling and sitting in a very relaxed position while saying, "I am very angry about this entire situation," two different messages are being conveyed. A smile, a frown, a wink, a shrug of the shoulders, a bored expression, a tapping of fingers or feet, and other similar body gestures or actions all convey messages to the receiver. It is important for health care workers to be aware of both their own and patients' nonverbal behaviors because these are an important part of any communication process. A touch of the hand, a pat on the back, a firm handshake, and a hug can convey more interest and caring than words could ever do. When verbal and nonverbal messages agree, the receiver is more likely to understand the message being sent.

BARRIERS TO COMMUNICATION

A communication barrier is something that gets in the way of clear communication. Three common barriers are physical disabilities, psychological attitudes and prejudice, and cultural diversity.

Physical disabilities may include deafness or hearing loss, blindness or impaired vision, and aphasia or speech disabilities. People who are deaf or hearing impaired have difficulty receiving messages. To improve communication, it is essential to use body language such as gestures and signs, speak clearly in short sentences, face the individual to improve the potential for lip reading, write mes-

sages if necessary, and make sure that any hearing aids have good batteries and are inserted correctly. People who are blind or visually impaired may be able to hear what is being said, but they will not see body language, gestures, or facial expressions. To improve communication, use a soft tone of voice, describe events that are occurring, announce your presence as you enter a room, explain sounds or noises, and use touch when appropriate. Individuals with aphasia or speech impairments can have difficulty with not only the spoken word but also written communications. They may know what they want to say but have difficulty remembering the correct words, may not be able to pronounce certain words, or may have slurred and distorted speech. Patience is essential while working with these individuals. Allow them to try to speak, encourage them to take their time, repeat messages to be sure they are correct, encourage them to use gestures or point to objects, provide writing materials if they can write messages, or use pictures with key messages to communicate.

Psychological barriers to communication are often caused by prejudice, attitudes, and personality. Our judgments of others are too often based on appearance, lifestyle, and social or economic status. Stereotypes such as "dumb blonde," "lazy bum," or "fat slob" cause us to make snap judgments about an individual and affect the communication process. Health care workers must learn to put prejudice aside and show respect to all individuals. A homeless person brought in from the street deserves the same quality of health care as the president of the United States. It is important to respect each person as an individual and to remember that each person has the right to good care and considerate treatment. At times, this can be extremely difficult, and patience and practice are essential. When individuals have negative attitudes or constantly complain or criticize your work, it can be difficult to show them respect. The health care worker must learn to see beyond the surface attitude to the human being underneath. Frequently, fear is the cause of anger or a negative attitude. Allow patients to express their fears or anger, encourage them to talk about their feelings, avoid arguing, remain calm, talk in a soft and nonthreatening tone of voice, and provide quality care. If other health care workers seem to be able to communicate more effectively with patients, watch these workers to learn how they handle difficult or angry patients. This is often the most effective means of learning good communication skills.

Cultural diversity is another possible communication barrier. Culture consists of the values, beliefs, attitudes, and customs shared by a group of people and passed from one generation to the next. It is often defined as a set of rules, because culture allows an individual to interpret the environment and actions of others and behave appropriately. Each cultural group has beliefs and practices regarding health and illness. An individual will respond to health care treatment according to his or her own cultural beliefs. One cultural group believes that health is a state of spiritual and physical harmony between body, mind, and spirit in harmony with nature. This is controlled by the forces of *yin* (female, negative energy such as darkness, cold, weakness, and death) and *yang* (male, positive energy such as light, heat, regeneration, and strength). An imbalance in these forces causes discomfort and illness. Treatment is directed toward balancing these forces. For example, if the body is "cold," an individual should eat "hot" foods and/or herbs to correct the imbalance. Another cultural group believes that illness is due to demons and evil spirits. White magic, voodoo, talismans, and bangles (silver bracelets) are used as treatments. A common concept among several cultural groups is that health is the result of good luck or is a reward from God for good behavior, while illness is the result of bad luck or is a punishment from God. These individuals often strive to practice their religions more faithfully as a form of treatment. When individuals have strong beliefs regarding health and illness, their beliefs must be respected. At times, these individuals may accept traditional health care but add their own cultural remedies to the treatment plan. It is important to remember that they have the right to determine their treatment plans and to even refuse traditional treatments.

In addition to beliefs regarding health and illness, cultural diversity may interfere with communication in other ways. Common examples relate to language differences, eye contact while communicating, ways of dealing with terminal illnesses, and the use of touch. Language differences can create major barriers. In the United States, English is a primary language used in health care. If a person has difficulty communicating in English, and a health care worker is not fluent in another language, a barrier exists. When providing care to people who have limited English-speaking abilities, speak slowly, use simple words, use gestures or pictures to clarify the meaning of words, use nonverbal communication in the form of a smile or gentle touch, and avoid the tendency to speak louder because this does not improve comprehension. Whenever possible, try to find an interpreter who speaks the language of the patient. Frequently, another health care worker, a consultant, or a family member may be able to assist in the communication process. Another example of a communication barrier related to cultural diversity is eye contact. In some cultures, direct eye-to-eye contact while communicating is not acceptable. These cultures believe that looking down shows proper respect for another individual. A health care worker who feels that eye contact is important must learn to accept and respect this cultural difference and a person's inability to engage in eye contact while communicating. The presence of a terminal illness, or an illness that will probably result in death, can lead to another communication barrier. In the United States, a traditional health care belief is that the patient should be told the truth about his or her diagnosis and informed about the expected outcome. Some cultural groups believe that a person should not be told of a fatal diagnosis or be burdened with making decisions about treatment. In these cultures, the family, the mother or father, or another designated individual is expected to make decisions about care, treatment, and information given to the patient. In such instances, it is important for health care workers to recognize and respect this and to involve these individuals in the patient's care. At times, it may be necessary for a patient to use legal means, such as power of attorney for health care, in order to designate responsibility for his or her care to another person. The use of touch can also create a communication barrier. In some cultures, it is inappropriate to touch someone on the head. Other cultures have clearly defined areas of the body that can be touched or that should be avoided. Even a simple handshake can be regarded as showing lack of respect. In some cultures, only family members provide personal care. For this reason, health care workers should always get permission from the patient before providing care and should avoid any use of touch that seems to be inappropriate for the individual.

Respect for and acceptance of cultural diversity is essential for any health care worker. When beliefs, ideas, concepts, and ways of life are different, communication barriers can result. By making every attempt to learn about cultural differences and by showing respect for an individual's right to cultural beliefs, a health care worker can provide quality health care.

RECORDING AND REPORTING

In health care, an important part of effective communication is reporting or recording all observations while providing care. In order to do this, it is important to not only listen to what the patient is saying, but to make objective observations about the patient. All senses are used to make observations. The sense of sight notes the color of skin, swelling or edema, the presence of a rash or sore, the color of urine or stool, the amount of food eaten, and other similar factors. The sense of smell alerts a health care worker to body odor or unusual odors of breath, wounds, urine, or stool. The sense of touch is used to feel the pulse, dryness or temperature of the skin, perspiration, and swelling. The sense of hearing is used while listening to respirations, abnormal body sounds, coughs, and speech. By using all senses, the health care worker can learn a great deal about a patient's condition and be able to report observations objectively.

Observations should be reported promptly and accurately to an immediate supervisor. If a health care worker is reporting a patient's statement, this is a subjective observation. It should be repeated in the exact words the patient used. If a health care worker is reporting an observation made, this is an objective observation. For example, the health care worker should not state, "I think Mr. B. has a fever." The report should state, "Mr. B. is complaining of feeling hot. His skin is red and flushed, and his temperature is 102°."

In some health care facilities, observations are recorded on a patient's health care record. Effective communication requires these written observations to be accurate, concise, and complete. The writing should be neat and legible, and spelling and grammar should be correct. Only objective observations should be noted. Subjective observations that the health care worker feels or thinks should be avoided. If a patient's statement is recorded, the statement should be written in the patient's own words and enclosed in quotation marks. All information should be signed with the name and title of the person recording the information. Errors should be crossed out neatly with a straight line, have "error" recorded by them, and show the initials of the person making the error. In this way, recorded communication will be effective communication.

Figure 7-16 What aspects of listening and nonverbal behavior can you see in this picture?

Good communication skills allow health care workers to develop good interpersonal relationships (see figure 7-16). Patients feel accepted, they feel that others have an interest and concern in them, they feel free to express their ideas and fears, they develop confidence in the health care workers, and they feel they are receiving quality health care. In addition, the health care worker will relate more effectively with coworkers and other individuals.

STUDENT *Go to the workbook and complete the assignment sheet for 7:4, Effective Communications.*

UNIT 7 SUMMARY

Human growth and development is a process that begins at birth and does not end until death. Each individual passes through certain stages of growth and development, frequently called life stages. Each stage has its own characteristics and has specific developmental tasks that an individual must master. Each stage also establishes the foundation for the next stage.

Death is often called "the final stage of growth." Dr. Elizabeth Kübler-Ross has identified five stages that dying patients and their families may experience prior to death. These stages are denial, anger, bargaining, depression, and acceptance. The health care worker must be aware of these stages in order to provide supportive care to the dying patient. In addition, the health care worker must understand the concepts represented by hospice care and the right to die.

Each life stage creates needs that must be met by the individual. Abraham Maslow, a noted psychologist, developed a hierarchy of needs that is frequently used to classify and define the needs experienced by human beings. The needs are classified into five levels, and according to Maslow, the lower needs must be met before an individual can strive to meet the higher needs. The needs, beginning at the lowest level and progressing to the highest, are physiological, or physical, needs; safety and security; love and affection; esteem; and self-actualization.

Needs are met or satisfied by direct and indirect methods. Direct methods meet and eliminate a need. Indirect methods, usually the use of defense mechanisms, reduce the need and help relieve the tension created by the unmet need.

Effective communication is an important aspect of helping individuals through stages of growth and development and in meeting needs. A health care worker must have an understanding of the communication process, factors that interfere with communication, the importance of listening, and verbal and nonverbal communication. Another important aspect of communication is the proper reporting or recording of all observations noted while providing care.

Communication barriers such as physical disabilities, psychological attitudes, and cultural diversity can interfere with the communication process. Special consideration must be given to these barriers to improve communication. Some cultural groups have beliefs and practices that may relate to health and illness. Because individuals will respond to health care according to their cultural beliefs, a health care worker must be aware of and show respect for different cultural values in order to provide optimal patient care.

Mastering these concepts will allow health care workers to develop good interpersonal relationships and provide more effective health care.

UNIT 7
SUGGESTED REFERENCES

Backer, Barbara A., Natalie Hannon, and Noreen A. Russell. *Death and Dying: Understanding and Care.* 2nd ed. Albany, NY: Delmar Publishers, 1994.

Caldwell, Esther, and Barbara Hegner. *Geriatrics: A Study of Maturity.* 5th ed. Albany, NY: Delmar Publishers, 1991.

Carr, Jacquelyn B. *Communicating and Relating.* 3rd ed. Dubuque, IA: Wm. C. Brown Publishers, 1991.

Dacey, John, and John Travers. *Human Development Across the Life Span.* Dubuque, IA: Wm. C. Brown Publishers, 1991.

Gwyn, Jack, and Robert J. Gwyn. *The Business of Oral Communication.* 2nd ed. Cincinnati, OH: Southwestern, 1989.

Kalman, Natalie, and Claire G. Waughfield. *Mental Health Concepts.* 3rd ed. Albany, NY: Delmar Publishers, 1993.

Kübler-Ross, Elizabeth. *Death: The Final Stage of Growth.* Englewood Cliffs, NJ: Prentice-Hall, 1975.

Kübler-Ross, Elizabeth. *On Death and Dying.* New York, NY: Macmillan, 1977.

Kübler-Ross, Elizabeth. *Questions and Answers to Death and Dying.* New York, NY: Macmillan, 1974.

Masters, L. Ann. *Listening Skills.* Cincinnati, OH: Southwestern, 1993.

Milliken, Mary Elizabeth. *Understanding Human Behavior.* 5th ed. Albany, NY: Delmar Publishers, 1993.

Morrison, George S. *The World of Child Development: Conception to Adolescence.* Albany, NY: Delmar Publishers, 1990.

Quill, Timothy. *Death and Dignity.* New York, NY: W.W. Norton and Co., 1993.

Rybash, John. *Adult Development and Aging.* 2nd ed. Dubuque, IA: Wm. C. Brown Publishers, 1991.

Sherman, Karen. *Communication and Image in Nursing.* Albany, NY: Delmar Publishers, 1994.

Tamparo, Carol, and Wilburta Lindh. *Therapeutic Communications for Allied Health Professions.* Albany, NY: Delmar Publishers, 1993.

UNIT 8

Geriatric Care

UNIT OBJECTIVES

After completing this unit of study, you should be able to:

- Differentiate between the myths and facts of six aspects of aging
- Identify at least two physical changes of aging in each body system
- Demonstrate at least ten methods of providing care to the elderly person who is experiencing physical changes of aging
- List five factors that cause psychosocial changes of aging
- Describe at least six methods to assist an elderly individual in adjusting to psychosocial changes
- Recognize the causes and effects of confusion and disorientation in the elderly
- Create a reality orientation program
- Justify the importance of respecting cultural and religious differences
- Explain the role of an ombudsman
- Define, pronounce, and spell all of the key terms

KEY TERMS

Alzheimer's disease
(Altz´-high-merz″)
arteriosclerosis
(r-tear-ee-o-skleh-row´-sis)
arthritis
atherosclerosis
(ath-eh-row″-skleh-row´-sis)
cataracts
cerebrovascular accident
culture
dementia
(d-men´-she-a)
disability

disease
dysphagia
(dis-fay´-she-ah)
geriatric care
gerontology
(jer-un-tahl´-oh-gee)
glaucoma
(glaw-ko´-mah)
incontinence
myths
nocturia
(nok-tur´-ee-ah)
ombudsman

osteoporosis
(os-tee´-oh-pour-oh´-sis)
reality orientation (RO)
religion
senile lentigines
(seen´-ile len-ti´-jeans)
thrombus
transient ischemic attacks
(TIAs)
(tran´-z-ent is-ke´mik)

INTRODUCTION

Just like they experienced the "baby boom," the United States and most other countries are now experiencing an "aging boom." In the 1900s, most individuals died before age 60. Today, most individuals can expect to live into their seventies, and many individuals enjoy healthy and happy lives as 80- and 90-year-olds. This age group uses health care services frequently, so it is essential for a health care worker to understand the special needs of the elderly population.

INFORMATION
8:1 Myths on Aging

Aging is a process that begins at birth and ends at death. It is a normal process and leads to normal changes in body structure and function. Even though few people want to grow old, it is a natural event in everyone's life. Gerontology is the scientific study of aging and the problems of the old. Geriatric care is care provided to elderly individuals. Through the study of the aging process and the elderly, many facts on aging have been established. However, many myths, or false beliefs, still exist regarding aging and elderly individuals. It is essential

for the health care worker to be able to distinguish fact from myth when providing geriatric care.

One of the most common myths concerning elderly individuals is that most are cared for in institutions or long-term care facilities. In fact, only approximately 5 percent of the elderly population lives in long-term care facilities. Most elderly individuals live in their own homes or apartments or with other family members (see figure 8-1).

According to another common myth, anyone over a certain set age, such as 65, is "old." In fact, old is determined less by the number of years lived and more by how an individual thinks, feels, and behaves. For example, to a 10-year-old, a 35-year-old is old. It is important to remember that many individuals are active, productive, and self-

Figure 8-1 Most elderly individuals live in their own homes or apartments.

sufficient into their eighties and even nineties. Too often, the term *old* becomes synonymous with *worthless* or *worn-out.* A better term would be *experienced* or *mature.*

It is a myth that elderly people are incompetent and incapable of making decisions or handling their own affairs. Even though some experience confusion and disorientation, the majority of elderly individuals remain mentally competent until they die. In fact, older individuals may make better decisions and judgments because they frequently base their decisions on many years of experience and knowledge. In addition, studies have proven that older people are able to concentrate, learn new skills, and evaluate new information.

It is also a myth that all elderly people live in poverty. Even though many older individuals have limited incomes, most also have comparatively low expenses. Many own their own homes, and their children are raised and out on their own. With social security, savings, retirement pensions, and other sources of income, some elderly individuals are financially secure and enjoy comfortable lifestyles. Although it is true that some elderly individuals live in poverty, this is true of some individuals in all age groups. The financial status of the elderly varies just as the financial status of young or middle-age people varies.

Another myth suggests that older people are unhappy and lonely. Studies have shown that most elderly individuals live with someone and/or associate frequently with friends or family members. Many elderly individuals are active in civic groups, charities, social activities, and volunteer programs (see figure 8-2). Others provide care for grandchildren and remain active as heads of extended families. Although it is true that some elderly individuals are lonely and unhappy, the percentage is small, and many social agencies exist to assist these individuals.

Some falsely believe that elderly individuals do not want to work—that the goal of the elderly is to retire and, prior to retirement, they lose interest in work. Although this may be true in some cases, many individuals remain employed and productive into their seventies and even eighties. Studies have shown that the older worker has good attendance, performs efficiently, readily learns new skills, and shows job satisfaction. Many retired individuals return to part-time positions or serve as consultants or volunteer workers. Along a similar line, a myth persists that retired people are bored and have

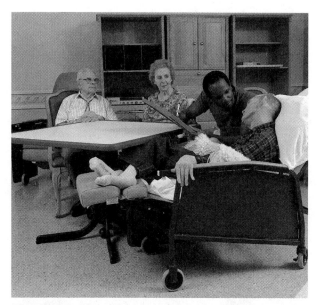

Figure 8-2 Most elderly individuals enjoy social activities.

nothing to do with their lives. Many retired people enjoy full and active lives. They engage in travel, social activities, family events, and many other activities. In fact, many retired individuals say, "I don't know how I found time to work."

Many other myths also exist. It is important for the health care worker to both recognize problems that do exist for the elderly and understand that the needs of the elderly vary according to many circumstances. Even the fact that only 5 percent of the elderly are in long-term care facilities means that over 2 million people will be in these facilities by the year 2000. Many health care workers at all levels will provide needed services for these individuals. Geriatric care is and will continue to be a major aspect of health care.

STUDENT *Go to the workbook and complete the assignment sheet for 8:1, Myths on Aging.*

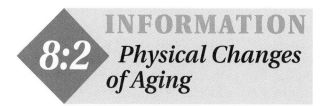

INFORMATION
8:2 *Physical Changes of Aging*

As aging occurs, certain physical changes also occur in all individuals. These changes are a normal part of the aging process. It is important to note that most of the changes are gradual and take place over a long period of time. In addition, the rate and degree of change varies among individuals. Factors such as disease can increase the speed and degree of the changes. Lifestyle, nutrition, economic status, and social environment can also have effects.

Most physical changes of aging involve a decrease in the function of body systems. Body processes slow down. There is a corresponding decrease in energy level. If an individual can recognize these changes as a normal part of aging, the individual can usually learn to adapt to and cope with the changes.

INTEGUMENTARY SYSTEM

Some of the most obvious effects of aging are seen in the integumentary system (see figure 8-3). Production of new skin cells decreases with age. The sebaceous (oil) and sudoriferous (sweat) glands become less active. Circulation to the skin decreases and causes coldness, dryness, and poor healing of injured tissue. The hair loses color, and hair loss occurs.

The decreases in body function lead to the physical changes. The skin becomes less elastic and dry. Itching is common. Dark yellow- or brown-colored spots, called **senile lentigines,** appear. Although these are frequently called "liver spots," they are not related to the liver. When the fatty tissue layer of the skin diminishes, lines and wrinkles develop. The nails become thick, tough, and brittle. An increased sensitivity to temperature develops, and the elderly individual frequently feels cold. Hypothermia, a below normal body temperature, can be a serious problem for the elderly.

Good skin, nail, and hair care are essential. Mild soaps should be used because many soaps cause dryness. Frequently, bath oils or lanolin lotions are recommended to combat dryness and itching. Daily baths can also contribute to dry, itchy skin; baths or showers once or twice a week with partial baths on other days are recommended. Brushing of the hair helps stimulate circulation and production of oil. Shampooing is usually done less frequently, but should be done as often as needed for cleanliness and comfort. Any sores or injuries to the skin should be cared for immediately. It is important to keep injured areas clean and free from

Figure 8-3 Note the physical signs of aging.

infection. When elderly people notice sores or injuries that do not heal, they should get medical help. Frequently, the elderly person requires a room temperature that is higher than normal and free from drafts. Socks, sweaters, lap blankets, and layers of clothing can all help alleviate the feeling of coldness. The use of hot water bottles or heating pads is not recommended because the decreased sensitivity to temperature can result in burns.

Proper diet, exercise, good hygiene, decreased sun exposure, and careful skin care can help slow and even decrease the normal physical changes in the integumentary system.

MUSCULOSKELETAL SYSTEM

As aging occurs, muscles lose tone, volume, and strength. **Osteoporosis,** a condition in which calcium and other minerals are lost from the bones, causes the bones to become brittle and more likely to fracture or break. **Arthritis,** an inflammation of the joints, causes the joints to become stiff, less flexible, and painful. The rib cage becomes more rigid, and the bones in the vertebral column press closer together (compress).

These changes cause the elderly individual to experience a gradual loss in height, decreased mobility, and weakness. Movement is slower, and the sense of balance is less sure. Falls occur easily and often result in fractures of the hips, arms, and/or legs. Fine finger movements, such as those required when buttoning clothes or tying shoes, are often difficult for the elderly individual.

Elderly individuals should be encouraged to exercise as much as their physical conditions permit (see figure 8-4). This helps keep muscles active and joints as flexible as possible. Even slow, daily walks help maintain muscle tone. Range-of-motion exercises can also maintain muscle strength. A diet rich in protein, calcium, and vitamins can slow the loss of minerals from the bones and maintain muscle structure. Extra attention must be paid to the environment so it is safer for the elderly person. Grab bars in the bathroom, hand rails in halls and on stairs, and other similar devices aid in ambulation. When the sense of balance is poor, an elderly person may need assistance and support during ambulation. The use of walkers and quad canes is frequently recommended. In addition, well-fitting shoes with non-slip soles and flat heels can help prevent falls. Self-stick strips and bands can replace buttons and shoestrings to make dressing easier.

Figure 8-4 Elderly individuals should be encouraged to exercise as much as their physical conditions permit.

CIRCULATORY SYSTEM

In the circulatory system, the heart muscles become less efficient at pushing blood into the arteries, and cardiac output decreases with aging. The blood vessels narrow and become less elastic. Blood flow to the brain and other vital organs may decrease. Blood pressure may increase.

Many elderly individuals do not notice any changes while at rest. They are more aware of changes when exercise, stress, excitement, illness, and other similar events call for increases in the body's need for oxygen and nutrients. During these periods, they experience weakness, dizziness, numbness in the hands and/or feet, and a rapid heart rate.

Elderly individuals who experience circulatory changes should avoid strenuous exercise or overexertion. They need periods of rest during the day. Moderate exercise, according to the individual's ability to tolerate it, does stimulate circulation and help prevent the formation of a thrombus, or blood clot. Support stockings, anti-embolism hose, and not using garters or tight bands around the legs also help prevent blood clots. If an individual is confined to bed, range-of-motion exercises help circulation. If high blood pressure is present, a diet low in salt or sodium and, in some cases, fat may be recommended. Individuals with circulatory system disease should follow the diet and exercise plans recommended by their doctors.

RESPIRATORY SYSTEM

Respiratory muscles become weaker with age. The rib cage becomes more rigid. The alveoli, or air sacs in the lungs, become thinner and less elastic, which decreases the exchange of gases between the lungs and bloodstream. The bronchioles, or air tubes in the lungs, also lose elasticity. Changes in the larynx lead to a higher-pitched and weaker voice. Chronic conditions such as emphysema, in which the alveoli lose their elasticity, or bronchitis, in which the bronchioles become inflamed, decrease the efficiency of the respiratory system even more severely.

These changes frequently cause the elderly individual to experience dyspnea, or difficult breathing. Breathing becomes more rapid, and they have difficulty coughing up secretions from the lungs.

This makes them more susceptible to respiratory infections such as colds and pneumonia.

Learning to alternate activity with periods of rest is important to avoid dyspnea. Proper body alignment and positioning can also ease breathing difficulties. The elderly individual with respiratory problems frequently sleeps in a semi-Fowler's position. Two or three pillows elevate the upper body and make breathing easier. Avoiding polluted air, such as that in smoke-filled rooms, is essential. Breathing deeply and coughing at frequent intervals helps clear the lung passages and increase lung capacity. Elderly individuals with chronic respiratory problems often use oxygen on a continuous basis. Portable oxygen units allow these individuals to still lead active lives.

Figure 8-5 Individuals who remain mentally active usually show fewer mental changes.

NERVOUS SYSTEM

Physical changes in the nervous system affect many body functions. Blood flow to the brain decreases, and there is a progressive loss of brain cells. This interferes with thinking, reacting, interpreting, and remembering. The senses of taste, smell, vision, and hearing diminish. Nerve endings are less sensitive, and there is a decreased ability to respond to pain and other stimuli.

As these physical changes occur, the elderly individual may experience memory loss. Short-term memory is usually affected. For example, an individual may not remember what he or she ate for breakfast, but does remember the entire menu from his or her retirement party. Long-term memory and intelligence do not always decrease. It may take elderly individuals longer to react, but given enough time, they can think and react appropriately. Individuals who remain mentally active and involved in current events usually show fewer mental changes (see figure 8-5).

Changes in vision cause problems in reading small print or seeing objects at a distance. There is a decrease in peripheral (side) vision and night vision. The eyes take longer to adjust from light to dark, and there is an increased sensitivity to glare. Elderly individuals are also more prone to the development of **cataracts,** where the normally transparent lens of the eye becomes cloudy or opaque. **Glaucoma,** a condition in which the intraocular pressure of the eye increases and interferes with vision, is also more common in the elderly. Proper

Figure 8-6 Good lighting and large numbers on a telephone can help improve vision.

eye care, prescription glasses/lenses, medical treatment of cataract or glaucoma, and proper lighting can all improve vision (see figure 8-6).

Hearing loss usually occurs gradually in the elderly. The individual may speak louder than usual, ask for words to be repeated, and not hear high-frequency sounds such as the ringing of a telephone. Problems may be more apparent when there is a lot of background noise. For example, an elderly person may not hear well in a crowded restaurant where music is playing and many other people are talking. A hearing aid can help some hearing problems. However, in cases of severe nerve damage, a hearing aid will not eliminate the problem. In addition, many individuals resist using hearing aids. If a person wears a hearing aid, it is important to keep the aid in good working condition by changing batteries, keeping the aid clean, and checking to make sure the individual is wearing it correctly. When a person has a hearing impairment, it is important to talk slowly and clearly. Avoid yelling or speaking excessively loudly. Facing individuals while talking to them also helps in many situations. Eliminating background noise, such as that produced by a radio or television, also increases the ability to hear.

The decrease in the sense of taste and smell frequently affects the appetite. Elderly individuals often complain that food is tasteless and add sugar, salt, or pepper (see figure 8-7). Attractive foods with a variety of textures and tastes may help stimulate the appetite. The decrease in the sense of smell may also make the elderly individual less sensitive to the smell of gas, chemicals, smoke, and other dangerous odors. A smoke detector, chemical detectors, and careful monitoring of the environment can help eliminate this danger.

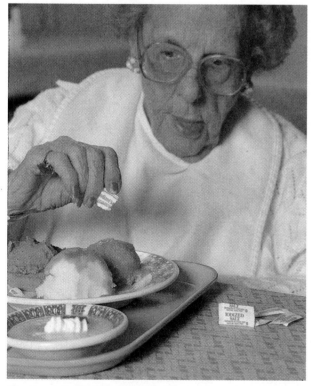

Figure 8-7 Elderly individuals may want to add salt to food due to their decreased sense of taste.

Decreased sensation to pain and other stimuli can lead to injuries. The elderly are more susceptible to burns, frostbite, cuts, fractures, muscle strain, and many other injuries. At times, elderly people are not even aware of injury or disease because they do not sense pain. It is important for elderly individuals to handle hot or cold items with extreme care, and to be aware of dangers in the environment.

Changes in the nervous system usually occur gradually over a long period of time. This allows an individual time to adapt to the changes and learn to accommodate them. However, it is sometimes necessary for someone else to assist when the changes become severe. For example, many elderly individuals continue to drive cars. Due to slower reaction times, however, these individuals may be more prone to having automobile accidents. When an elderly person shows impaired driving ability, it often becomes necessary for a family member or the law to prevent the individual from driving.

DIGESTIVE SYSTEM

Physical changes in the digestive system occur when fewer digestive juices and enzymes are produced, muscle action becomes slower and peristalsis decreases, teeth are lost, and liver function decreases.

Dysphagia, or difficult swallowing, is a frequent complaint of the elderly. Less saliva and a slower gag reflex contribute to this problem. In addition, the loss of teeth or use of poor-fitting dentures makes it more difficult to chew food properly. Another common complaint is indigestion, which results from slower digestion of foods due to decreased digestive juices. Flatulence (gas) and constipation are common due to decreased peristalsis and poor diet. The decreased sensation of taste also contributes to a poor appetite and diet.

Good oral hygiene, repair or replacement of damaged teeth, and a relaxed eating atmosphere can contribute to better chewing and digestion of food. Most elderly people find it is best to avoid dry, fried, and/or fatty foods because such foods are difficult to chew and digest. High-fiber and high-protein foods with different tastes and textures are recommended. Careful use of seasonings to improve taste also increases appetite. It is important to avoid excessive seasonings because they can cause indigestion. Increasing fluid intake makes swallowing easier, helps prevent constipation, and aids kidney function.

Urinary System

With aging, the kidneys decrease in size and become less efficient at producing urine. Poor circulation to the kidneys and a decrease in the number of nephrons results in a loss of ability to concentrate the urine, which causes a loss of electrolytes and fluids. The ability of the bladder to hold urine decreases. Sometimes the bladder does not empty completely and urine is retained in the bladder.

The elderly person may find it necessary to urinate more frequently. Nocturia, or urination at night, is common and disrupts the sleep pattern. Retention of urine in the bladder causes bladder infections. Males frequently experience enlargement of the prostate gland, which makes urination difficult and causes urinary retention. Loss of muscle tone results in incontinence, or the inability to control urination.

Many elderly individuals decrease fluid intake to cut down on the frequent need to urinate. This can cause kidney disease and infection. Elderly individuals should be encouraged to increase fluid intake to improve kidney function. To decrease incidents of nocturia, most fluids should be taken before evening. Regular trips to the bathroom, wearing easy-to-remove clothing, and using absorbent pads as needed can help the individual who has mild incontinence. Bladder training programs can also help increase bladder capacity and lead to more control over urination in incontinent persons. An indwelling catheter may be needed if all urinary control is lost.

When changes in the urinary system cause poor functioning of the kidneys, waste substances can build up in the bloodstream and cause serious illness. Therefore, it is important to keep the kidneys functioning as efficiently as possible.

Endocrine System

Changes in the endocrine system result in increased production of some hormones, such as parathormone and thyroid stimulating hormone, and decreased production of other hormones, such as thyroxin, estrogen, progesterone, and insulin. The actions of these hormones is listed in Unit 6:13 of this text.

Because hormones affect many body functions, several physical changes often occur. The immune system of the body is less effective, and elderly individuals are more prone to disease. The basal metabolic rate decreases, resulting in complaints of feeling cold, tired, and less alert. Intolerance to glucose can develop, resulting in increased blood glucose levels.

As with the other body systems, changes in the endocrine system occur slowly over a long period of time. Many elderly individuals are not as aware of changes in this system. Proper exercise, adequate rest, medical care for illness, a balanced diet, and a healthy lifestyle all help decrease the effects caused by changes in hormone activity.

Reproductive System

In the reproductive system, the decrease of estrogen and progesterone in the female causes a thinning of the vaginal walls and a decrease in vaginal secretions. Vaginal infections or inflammations become more common. In some cases, a weakness in its supporting tissues causes the uterus to sag downward, a condition known as *prolapsed uterus.* The breasts sag when fat is redistributed.

Slowly decreasing levels of testosterone in the male slow the production of sperm. Response to sexual stimulation of the penis is slower, and ejaculation may take longer. The testes become smaller and less firm. The seminal fluid becomes thinner, and smaller amounts are produced.

Sexual desire and need do not necessarily diminish with age (see figure 8-8). Many elderly individuals are sexually active. Studies have shown that sex improves muscle tone and circulation. Even pain from arthritis seems to decrease after sexual activity, probably because of increased hormone levels. When elderly individuals are in long-term care facilities, it is important for the health care worker to understand both the physical and psychological sexual needs of the resident. Long-term care facilities now allow married couples to each live in the same room. The health care worker must

Figure 8-8 Elderly individuals still experience a need for companionship and sexuality.

Figure 8-9 To respect the right to privacy, always knock before entering a resident's room.

respect the privacy of these residents and allow them to meet their sexual needs (see figure 8-9).

Aging causes many physical changes in all body systems. The rate and degree of the changes vary in different individuals, but all elderly individuals experience some degree of change. Providing means of adapting to and coping with changes allows elderly people to enjoy life even with physical limitations. It is important for all health care workers to learn to recognize changes and provide methods for dealing with them. Tolerance, patience, and empathy are essential.

STUDENT *Go to the workbook and complete the assignment sheet for 8:2, Physical Changes of Aging.*

8:3 INFORMATION
Psychosocial Changes of Aging

In addition to physical changes, elderly individuals also experience psychological and social changes. Some individuals cope with these changes effectively, but others experience extreme frustration and mental distress. It is important for the health care worker to be aware of the psychosocial changes and stresses experienced by the elderly.

WORK AND RETIREMENT

Most adults spend a large portion of their days working. Many associate their feelings of self-worth with the jobs they perform. They are proud to state that they are nurses, electricians, teachers, lawyers, or secretaries. In addition, social contact while working is a major form of interaction with others.

Retirement is often viewed as an end to the working years. Many individuals are able to enjoy retirement and find other activities to replace job roles. Some individuals find other part-time or consultant-type jobs after retirement from their primary jobs. Other individuals become active in volunteer work or take part in community or club activities. These individuals find satisfactory replacements for the feelings of self-worth once provided by their jobs.

However, some elderly individuals feel a major sense of loss upon retirement. They lose social contacts, develop feelings of uselessness, and, in some cases, experience financial difficulties. This causes them to experience stress, and they frequently become depressed. Until other sources of restoring the individual's sense of self-worth are found, these elderly individuals can have difficulty coping with life.

SOCIAL RELATIONSHIPS

Social relationships change throughout life. Among the elderly, these changes may occur more frequently. Often, children marry and move away. This brings about a loss of contact with the family. If a spouse dies, the "couple" image is replaced by one of "widow" or "widower." As a person ages, more friends and relatives die, and social contacts decrease.

Some elderly individuals are able to adjust to these changes by making new friends and establishing new social contacts (see figure 8-10). Church and community groups provide many social activities for the elderly. By taking part in these activities, individuals who made friends readily throughout their lives usually can continue to do so as they grow older.

Some elderly individuals cannot cope with the continuous loss of friends and relatives. They become withdrawn and depressed. They avoid social events and isolate themselves from others. The death of a spouse is frequently devastating to an elderly individual, especially when a couple has had a close relationship for many years. A surviving spouse may even attempt suicide. Psychological help is essential in these cases.

LIVING ENVIRONMENTS

Changes in living environments create different psychosocial changes. Most elderly individuals prefer to remain in their own homes. They feel secure surrounded by familiar environments. Many elderly individuals express fear at the thought of losing their homes.

Some elderly people leave their homes by personal choice. They find the burden of maintaining their homes too great, and move to apartments or retirement communities. The elderly individual may even move to another state with a better climate. These individuals often cope well with the change in living environment and feel the change is beneficial.

Financial problems or physical disabilities may force some people to move from their homes, sometimes to retirement communities or apartments. If they can maintain their independence, coping is usually good. In other cases, an elderly individual may be forced to move in with a son or

Figure 8-10 After the death of a spouse, the elderly individual sometimes can adjust by making new social contacts.

daughter. This move creates a change in roles, where the child becomes the caretaker of the parent. If the elderly person feels secure in this situation, coping occurs. However, if the elderly person feels unwanted or useless, conflicts and tension may develop.

Moving to a long-term care facility usually creates stress in elderly individuals. They feel a loss of independence and become frightened by their lack of control over environment. Many elderly individuals view long-term care facilities as "places to die," even when they may only require the use of the facility for a short period of time. For this reason, it is important to allow individuals to create their own "home" environments in the facility (see figure 8-11). Most long-term care facilities refer to the individuals as "residents." They allow the residents to bring favorite pieces of furniture, pictures, televisions, radios, and personal items. By being allowed choices in the arrangement of their items, residents are able to create comfortable, homelike environments. Factors such as these allow the elderly individual to adjust to the new environment and to cope with the changes it brings.

INDEPENDENCE

Most individuals want to be independent and self sufficient. Even 2-year-olds begin to assert their right to choose and strive to be independent. Just as

Figure 8-11 It is important to allow residents to create their own "home" environments in the long-term care facility.

Figure 8-12 To encourage independence, encourage elderly individuals to make as many decisions as possible.

children learn that there are limits to independence, the elderly learn that independence can be threatened with age. Physical disability, illness, decreased mental ability, and other factors can all lead to a loss of independence in the elderly.

Individuals who once took care of themselves find it necessary to ask others for assistance. After driving for a lifetime, elderly individuals might find that they can no longer drive safely. They have to depend on others to take them where they need to

go. Physical limitations prevent them from mowing lawns, cooking meals, washing, cleaning, and, in some cases, even taking care of themselves. Frustration, anger, and depression can develop.

Any care provided to elderly individuals should allow as much independence as possible. Assistance should be provided as needed for the individual's safety, but the individual should be allowed to do as much as possible. For example, a health care worker should encourage elderly persons to choose their clothing and dress themselves, even if this takes longer (see figure 8-12). Self-stick strips can replace buttons to make the task of dressing easier and to provide more independence. This helps the elderly individual adapt to the situation and maintain a sense of self-worth. At all times, elderly individuals should be allowed as much choice as possible to help them to maintain individuality.

DISEASE AND DISABILITY

Elderly people are more prone to disease and disability. **Disease** is usually defined as "any condition that interferes with the normal function of the body." Common examples in the elderly include diabetes, heart disease, emphysema, arthritis, and osteoporosis. A **disability** is defined as "a physical or mental defect or handicap that interferes with normal functions." Hearing impairments, visual defects, or the inability to walk due to a fractured hip are examples. Diseases sometimes cause permanent disabilities. For example, a cerebrovascular accident, or stroke, can result in permanent paralysis of one side of the body, or hemiplegia.

When disease or disability affects the functioning of the body, an individual may experience psychological problems. When this occurs in an elderly individual already stressed by other changes or circumstances, it can be traumatic. A fractured hip can cause an elderly individual who had been living independently in his or her own home to be admitted to a long-term care facility. Disease or disability frequently occurs suddenly and does not allow for gradual adjustment to and coping with change.

Sick people often have fears of death, chronic illness, loss of function, and pain. These are normal fears, and these individuals need time to adjust to their situations. Listen to them as they express these fears and be patient and understanding. If

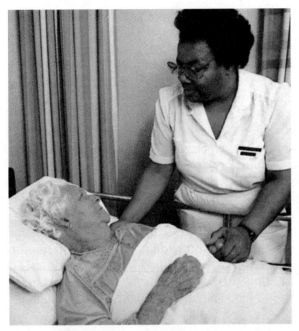

Figure 8-13 Provide supportive care and listen to sick individuals as they express their fears.

they cannot discuss their feelings, accept this and provide supportive care (see figure 8-13).

Psychosocial changes can be major sources of stress in the elderly. As changes occur, the individual must learn to accommodate the changes and function in new situations. With support, understanding, and patience, the health care worker can assist elderly individuals as they learn to adapt.

STUDENT   *Go to the workbook and complete the assignment sheet for 8:3, Psychosocial Changes of Aging.*

◆ **8:4** **INFORMATION**
Confusion and Disorientation in the Elderly

Although most elderly individuals remain mentally alert until death, some experience periods of confusion and disorientation. Signs of confusion or disorientation include talking incoherently, not knowing their own names, not recognizing others, wandering aimlessly, lacking awareness of time or place, displaying hostile and combative behavior (see figure 8-14), hallucinating, regressing in behavior, paying less attention to personal hygiene,

and being unable to respond to simple commands or follow instructions.

Confusion or disorientation is sometimes a temporary condition. Stress and/or depression due to physical or psychosocial changes is one possible cause. Use of alcohol or chemicals is another. Kidney disease, which interferes with electrolyte balance; respiratory disease, which decreases oxygen; or liver disease, which interferes with metabolism, are other causes. Elderly individuals are also more sensitive to medications, and drugs can sometimes accumulate in the body and cause confusion and disorientation. Even poor nutrition or lack of fluid intake can interfere with mental ability. Frequently, identification and treatment of any of these conditions decreases and even eliminates the confusion and disorientation. For example, changing a medication or giving it in smaller doses may restore normal function.

Disease and/or damage to the brain can sometimes result in chronic confusion or disorientation. A **cerebrovascular accident,** or stroke, which damages brain cells, is one possible cause. A blood clot can obstruct blood flow to the brain, or a vessel can rupture and cause hemorrhaging in the brain. **Arteriosclerosis,** a condition in which the walls of blood vessels become thick and lose their elasticity, is common in elderly individuals. If the vessels become narrow due to deposits of fat and minerals, such as calcium, the condition is called **atherosclerosis.** These conditions can cause **transient**

Figure 8-14 Hostile or combative behavior often signals feelings of frustration or confusion.

ischemic attacks (TIAs), or ministrokes, which result in temporary periods of diminished blood flow to the brain. Each time an attack occurs, more damage to brain cells results.

Dementia, also called *brain syndrome*, is a loss of mental ability characterized by a decrease in intellectual ability, loss of memory, impaired judgment, personality change, and disorientation. When the symptoms are caused by high fever, kidney infection, dehydration, hypoxia (lack of oxygen), drug toxicity, or other treatable conditions, the condition is called *acute*. When the symptoms are caused by permanent, irreversible damage to brain cells, the condition is called *chronic*. Cerebral vascular accidents, arteriosclerosis, and TIAs can be contributing causes to chronic dementia. One modern theory suggests that chronic dementia is caused by either a complete lack or an inadequate amount of an enzyme. Whatever the cause, chronic dementia is usually regarded as a progressive, irreversible disease.

Alzheimer's disease is a form of dementia that causes progressive changes in brain cells. It can occur in individuals as young as 40 years of age, but frequently occurs in those in their sixties. The cause is unknown, but there are many theories currently being researched. A genetic defect, a missing enzyme, toxic effects of aluminum, a virus, and the faulty metabolism of glucose have all been implicated as possible causes. Whatever the cause, Alzheimer's disease is viewed as a terminal, incurable brain disease usually lasting from 3 to 10 years. In the early stages, the individual exhibits memory loss, mood and personality changes, depression, poor judgment, confusion regarding time and place, and an inability to plan and follow through with many activities of daily living. As the disease progresses, nighttime restlessness occurs, mood swings become frequent, personal hygiene is ignored, weight fluctuates, paranoia and hallucinations increase, and full-time supervision becomes necessary. In the terminal stages, the individual experiences total disorientation regarding person, time, and place; becomes incoherent and is unable to communicate with words; loses control of bladder and bowel functions; develops seizures; loses weight despite eating a balanced diet; becomes totally dependent; and, finally, lapses into a coma and dies. Death is frequently caused by pneumonia, infections, and kidney failure. Progress through the various stages of this disease varies among individuals.

Whatever the cause of confusion or disorientation, certain courses of care should be followed. A primary concern is to provide a safe and secure environment. Dangerous objects such as drugs, poisons, scissors, knives, and cleaning solutions should be kept out of reach and in a locked area. If the individual tends to wander, doors and windows should be secure. In severe cases, special sensors may be attached to the leg or wrist of the disoriented individual (see figure 8-15). The sensors alert others if the individual starts to leave a specific area.

Following the same routine is also important. Meals, baths, dressing, walks, and bedtime should each occur at approximately the same time each day. Any change in routine can cause stress and confusion. Even though the individual should be encouraged to be as active as possible, activities should be kept simple and last for short periods of time (see figure 8-16). A calm, quiet environment is also important. Loud noises, crowded rooms, and excessive commotion can cause the individual to become agitated and more disoriented.

Reality orientation (RO) consists of activities that help promote awareness of person, time, and place. The activities should be followed by anyone caring for the confused individual, whether the care

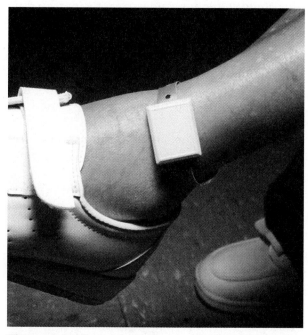

Figure 8-15 Special sensors may be attached to the leg or wrist of a wandering or disoriented individual.

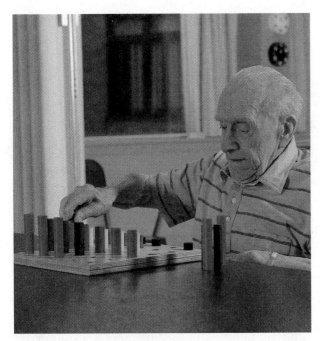

Figure 8-16 Activities for a confused or disoriented individual should be kept simple and last for short periods of time.

is in the home or in a long-term care facility. Some aspects of reality orientation are the following:

1. Address the person by the name they prefer, for example, "Mr. Smith" or "Mike."
2. Avoid terms such as "sweetie," "baby," and "honey."
3. State your name and correct the person if he or she calls you a wrong name. For example, if a patient thinks you are his or her daughter, say "I am not your daughter Lisa. I am Mrs. Simmers, your nurse for today."
4. Make constant references to day, time, and place. "It is 8:00 Tuesday morning and time for breakfast."
5. Use clocks, calendars, and information boards to point out time, day, and activities (see figure 8-17).
6. Keep the individual oriented to day-night cycles. During the day, encourage the person to wear regular clothes. Also, open the curtains and point out the sunshine. At night, close the curtains, use night lights if necessary, and promote quiet and rest.
7. Speak slowly and clearly and ask clear and simple questions.
8. Never rush or hurry the individual.
9. Repeat instructions patiently. Allow time for the individual to respond.

10. Encourage conversations about familiar things or current events.
11. Encourage the use of a television or radio, but avoid overstimulating the individual.
12. Make sure the individual uses sensory aids such as glasses and hearing aids (if needed), and that the devices are in good working order.
13. Keep familiar objects and pictures within view. Avoid moving the person's furniture or belongings.
14. Do not agree with incorrect statements. Gently provide correct information. For example, when a person states it is time to dress for work, say, "You don't have to go to work today. You retired 7 years ago."
15. Do not hesitate to use touch to communicate with the person.
16. Avoid arguments or recriminations. When you find an elderly resident in the wrong area, do not say, "You know you are not supposed to be here." Instead, say, "Let me show you how to get to your room."
17. Encourage independence and self help whenever possible.

Caring for a confused or disoriented individual can be frustrating and even frightening at times. Continual assessment of the individual's abilities and problems is needed to design a health care

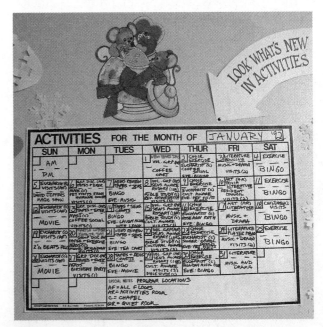

Figure 8-17 An information board can help point out day, date, and scheduled activities.

program that will allow the individual to function within the level of his or her ability. Patience, consistency, and sincere caring are essential on the part of the health care provider.

STUDENT   *Go to the workbook and complete the assignment sheet for 8:4, Confusion and Disorientation in the Elderly.*

INFORMATION
8:5 *Meeting the Needs of the Elderly*

Providing care to the elderly can be a challenging but rewarding experience. It is important to remember that the needs of the elderly do not differ greatly from the needs of any other individual. They have the same physical and psychological needs of any person at any age. However, these needs are sometimes intensified by physical or psychosocial changes that disrupt the normal life pattern. When this occurs, the elderly individual needs understanding, acceptance, and the knowledge that someone cares.

A few other factors must be considered when caring for elderly individuals. One is the importance of meeting cultural needs. Culture can be defined as "the values, beliefs, ideas, customs, and characteristics that are passed from one generation to the next." An individual's culture can affect language, food habits, dress, work, leisure activities, and health care. Culture creates differences in individuals. For example, a person may speak a different language or have specific likes or dislikes about food or dress. It is important for the health care worker to learn about a person's culture, and about the person's likes, dislikes, and beliefs. This allows the health care worker to provide care that shows a respect and acceptance of the cultural differences. (Cultural diversity is also discussed in Unit 7:4 of this text.)

Religious needs are another important aspect of care. Religion can be defined as "the spiritual beliefs and practices of an individual." Like culture, religious or spiritual beliefs can affect the lifestyle of an individual. Diet, days of worship, practices relating to birth and death, and even acceptance of medical care can be affected. It is important to accept an individual's beliefs without bias. It is

equally important that health care workers do not force their own religious beliefs on the individuals to whom they provide care. For example, if a patient asks, "Do you believe in life after death?" a health care worker may respond by saying, "How do you feel?" or "You have been thinking about the meaning of life." This allows patients to express their own feelings and thoughts. Other ways the health care worker can show respect and consideration for a person's religious beliefs include proper treatment of religious articles, such as a Bible or Koran; allowing a person to practice religion with prayer, observance of religious holidays, or participation in religious services; honoring a patient's requests for special foods; and providing privacy during clergy visits (see figure 8-18).

Freedom from abuse is another important aspect of care. Abuse of the elderly can be physical, verbal, psychological, or sexual. Handling the individual roughly; denying food, water, or medication; yelling or screaming at the person; or causing fear are all forms of abuse. Abuse is sometimes difficult to prove. Frequently, the abuser is a family member or caretaker. Elderly individuals may want to protect the abuser or may even feel that they deserve the abuse. Most states have laws requiring the reporting of any suspected abuse. It is

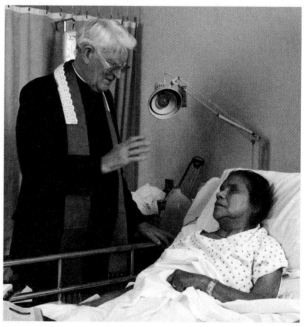

Figure 8-18 Respect religious needs and provide privacy while a resident is visiting with a member of the clergy.

important for any health care worker who sees or suspects abuse of the elderly to report it to the proper agency.

A final aspect of meeting the needs of the elderly is to respect and follow the patient's rights. Patients' rights are discussed in Unit 4:3 of this textbook. These rights assure the elderly individual of "kind and considerate care" and provide for meeting individual needs. One program that exists to ensure the rights of the elderly is the Ombudsman Program. It was developed by the federal government in its Older American Act. Each state has its own program designed to meet federal standards. Basically, an ombudsman is a specially trained individual who works with the elderly and their families, health care providers, and other concerned individuals to improve quality of care and quality of life. The ombudsman may investigate and try to resolve complaints, suggest improvements for health care, monitor and enforce state and/or federal regulations, report problems to the correct agency, and provide education for individuals involved in the care of the elderly. Although the role of the ombudsman may vary from state to state, it is important for the health care worker to cooperate and work effectively with the ombudsman in order to ensure that the needs of the elderly are met.

STUDENT *Go to the workbook and complete the assignment sheet for 8:5, Meeting the Needs of the Elderly.*

Unit 8 Summary

Geriatric care is care provided to elderly individuals. Because this age group uses health care services frequently, and many individuals are now living longer, it is important for the health care worker to understand the special needs of the elderly population.

Many myths, or false beliefs, exist regarding elderly individuals. Examples include the belief that most elderly individuals are cared for in long-term care facilities, are incompetent and incapable of making decisions, live in poverty, do not want to work, and are unhappy and lonely. Although these beliefs may be true for some elderly individuals, they are not true for the majority.

Physical changes occur in all individuals as a normal part of the aging process. It is important to remember that most of the changes are gradual and occur over a long period of time. The physical changes may impose some limitations on the activities of the individual. If the health care worker is aware of these changes and is able to provide individuals with ways to adapt to and cope with the changes, many elderly individuals can enjoy life even with physical limitations.

Psychosocial changes also create special needs in the elderly. Retirement, death of a spouse and of friends, changes in social relationships, new living environments, loss of independence, and disease and disability can all cause stress and crisis for an individual. With support, understanding, and patience, health care workers can assist elderly individuals as they learn to accommodate the changes and to function in new situations.

Although most elderly individuals remain mentally alert until death, some have periods of confusion and disorientation. This is sometimes a temporary condition that can be corrected. Other times, disease and/or damage to the brain results in chronic confusion or disorientation. Special techniques should be used in dealing with these individuals. Providing a safe and secure environment, following a set routine, promoting reality orientation, and giving supportive care can allow individuals to function to the best of their abilities.

Meeting the cultural and religious needs of the elderly is also essential. In addition, it is important for health care workers to respect and follow the "rights" of elderly individuals and to protect the elderly from abuse.

Unit 8
Suggested References

Badasch, Shirley, and Doreen Chesebro. *Essentials for the Nursing Assistant in Long-Term Care.* 2nd ed. Albany, NY: Delmar Publishers, 1994.

Carr, Jacquelyn B. *Communicating and Relating.* 3rd ed. Dubuque, IA: Wm. C. Brown Publishers, 1991.

Dacey, John, and John Travers. *Human Development Across the Life Span.* Dubuque, IA: Wm. C. Brown Publishers, 1991.

Fasano, Marie A. *Creative Care for the Person with Alzheimer's.* Old Tappan, NJ: Brady Company, 1986.

Hampton, John K. *The Biology of Human Aging.* Dubuque, IA: Wm. C. Brown Publishers, 1991.

Hegner, Barbara R., and Esther Caldwell. *Assisting in Long-Term Care.* 2nd ed. Albany, NY: Delmar Publishers, 1994.

Hegner, Barbara, and Esther Caldwell. *Geriatrics: A Study of Maturity.* 5th ed. Albany, NY: Delmar Publishers, 1991.

Hogstel, Mildred. *Nursing Care of the Older Adult.* 3rd ed. Albany, NY: Delmar Publishers, 1994.

Kalman, Natalie, and Claire G. Waughfield. *Mental Health Concepts.* 3rd ed. Albany, NY: Delmar Publishers, 1993.

Milliken, Mary Elizabeth. *Understanding Human Behavior: A Guide for Health Care Providers.* 5th ed. Albany, NY: Delmar Publishers, 1993.

Ringsven, Mary K., and Donna Bond. *Gerontology and Leadership Skills for Nurses.* Albany, NY: Delmar Publishers, 1991.

Rybash, John. *Adult Development and Aging.* 2nd ed. Dubuque, IA: Wm. C. Brown Publishers, 1991.

Walston, Betty, and Keith Walston. *The Nurse Aide in Long Term Care.* Albany, NY: Delmar Publishers, 1995.

Zins, Sandra. *Aging in America: An Introduction to Gerontology.* Albany, NY: Delmar Publishers, 1987.

UNIT 9

Nutrition and Diets

UNIT OBJECTIVES

After completing this unit of study, you should be able to:

♦ Define the term *nutrition* and list the effects of good nutrition
♦ Name the six groups of essential nutrients and their functions and sources
♦ Create a sample daily menu using the five major food groups
♦ Differentiate between the processes of digestion, absorption, and metabolism
♦ Name, describe, and explain the purposes of at least eight therapeutic diets
♦ Define, pronounce, and spell all of the key terms

KEY TERMS

absorption

anorexia
   (an-oh-rex´-ee˝-ah)

atherosclerosis
   (ath-eh-row˝-skleh-row´-sis)

basal metabolic rate (BMR)
   (base´-al met˝-ah-ball´-ik)

bland diet

calorie

calorie-controlled diets

carbohydrates

cellulose

cholesterol
   (co˝-less´-ter-all)

diabetic diet

digestion

essential nutrients

fat-restricted diets

fats

hypertension
   (high˝-purr-ten´-shun)

kilocalorie (kcal)
   (kill´-oh-kall˝-oh-ree)

liquid diets

low-cholesterol diet

low-residue diet

malnutrition

metabolism
   (meh-tab´-oh-liz˝-em)

minerals

nutrition

nutritional status

osteoporosis
   (os-tee˝-oh-pour-oh´-sis)

peristalsis
   (per-eh-stall˝-sis)

protein diets

proteins

regular diet

sodium-restricted diets

soft diet

therapeutic diets
   (ther˝-ah-pew´-tick)

vitamins

wellness

INFORMATION 9:1 *Fundamentals of Nutrition*

People enjoy food and like to discuss it. Most people know that there is an important relationship between food and good health. However, many people do not know which nutrients are needed or why they are necessary. They are not able to select proper foods in their daily diets in order to promote optimum health. Therefore, it is important for every health care worker to have a solid understanding of basic nutrition. With this understanding, the health care worker can both practice and promote good nutrition.

Nutrition includes all body processes relating to food. These include digestion, metabolism, circulation, and elimination. These processes allow the body to use food for energy, maintenance of health, and growth. Nutritional status refers to the state or condition of one's nutrition. The goal is, of course, to be in a state of good nutrition and to maintain wellness, a state of good health with optimal body function. To do this, one must choose foods that are needed by the body, and not just foods that taste good.

Nutrition plays a large role in determining height, weight, strength, skeletal and muscular development, physical agility, resistance to disease, appetite, posture, complexion, mental ability, and emotional and psychological health. The immediate effects of good nutrition include a healthy appearance, a good attitude, proper sleep and bowel habits, a high energy level, enthusiasm, and freedom from anxiety. In addition, the effects of good nutrition accumulate throughout life and may prevent or delay diseases or conditions such as the following:

◆ **Hypertension**—high blood pressure; an excess of salt in the diet seems to be one cause; can lead to diseases of the heart, blood vessels, and kidneys.

◆ **Atherosclerosis**—condition in which arteries are narrowed by the accumulation of fatty substances on their inner surfaces; thought to be caused by a diet high in saturated fats and cholesterol; can lead to heart attack or stroke.

◆ **Osteoporosis**—condition in which bones become porous (full of tiny openings) and break easily; one cause is long-term deficiencies of calcium, magnesium, and vitamin D.

◆ **Malnutrition**—the state of poor nutrition; may be caused by poor diet or illness. Symptoms include fatigue, depression, poor posture, being overweight or underweight, poor complexion, lifeless hair, and irritability. It can cause deficiency diseases, poor muscular and skeletal development, reduced mental abilities, and even death. Malnutrition is most likely to affect individuals living in extreme poverty, patients undergoing drug therapy such as treatment for cancer, infants (see figure 9-1), young children, adolescents, and the elderly.

INFORMATION
9:2 *Essential Nutrients*

Essential nutrients are composed of chemical elements found in food. They are used by the body to perform many different body functions. As the body uses the elements, they are replaced by elements in the food one eats. The essential nutrients are divided into six groups. The six groups and the specific functions of each group are shown in table 9-1.

CARBOHYDRATES

Carbohydrates are the major source of human energy. They are commonly called "starches" or "sugars." Carbohydrates are a cheaper source of energy than are proteins and fats. They are easily digested, grow well in most climates, and keep well without refrigeration. They are made of carbon, hydrogen, and oxygen.

The main sources of carbohydrates are breads, cereals, noodles or pastas, crackers, potatoes, corn, peas, fruits, sugar, and syrups.

Cellulose is the fibrous, indigestible form of carbohydrate. It is important because it provides bulk in the digestive tract and causes regular bowel movements. The best sources of cellulose are bran, whole-grain cereals, and fibrous fruits and vegetables.

FATS

Fats (lipids) are also made of carbon, hydrogen, and oxygen, but they contain more oxygen than do carbohydrates. They provide the most concentrated form of energy but are a more expensive source of energy than are carbohydrates. Fats also

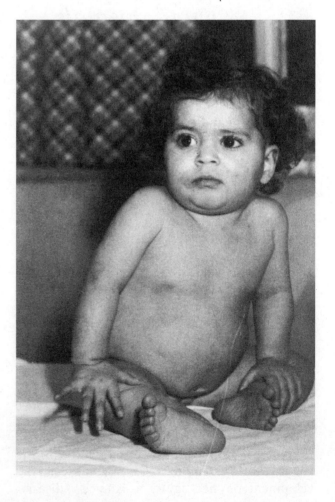

Figure 9-1 (Above) A 4-month-old baby suffering from severe malnutrition. **(Right)** The same child at the age of 10 months after having been properly fed. (*Courtesy of the Food and Agriculture Organization of the United Nations*)

TABLE 9-1 **The Six Essential Nutrient Groups**

NUTRIENT GROUPS	FUNCTIONS
Carbohydrates	Provide heat and energy; supply fiber for good digestion and elimination
Fats	Provide fatty acids needed for growth and development; provide heat and energy; carry fat-soluble vitamins (A, D, E, and K)
Proteins	Build and repair body tissue; provide heat and energy; help produce antibodies
Vitamins	Regulate body functions; build and repair body tissue
Minerals	Regulate body functions; build and repair body tissue
Water	Carries nutrients and wastes to and from body cells; regulates body functions

maintain body temperature by providing insulation; cushion organs and bones; aid in the absorption of fat-soluble vitamins; and provide flavor to meals. The main sources of fats include butter, margarine, oils, cream, fatty meats, cheeses, and egg yolk.

Fats are also classified as saturated or polyunsaturated. Saturated fats are usually solid at room temperature. Examples include the fats in meats, eggs, whole milk, cream, butter, and cheeses. Polyunsaturated fats are usually soft or oily at room temperature. Examples include vegetable oils, margarines and other products made from vegetable oils, fish, and peanuts.

Cholesterol is a fatty substance found in body cells and animal fats. Common sources are egg yolk, fatty meats, shellfish, butter, cream, cheeses, whole milk, and organ meats (liver, kidney, and brains). In addition, cholesterol is synthesized (manufactured) by the liver. It is essential to life, but an excess is believed to contribute to atherosclerosis. Consequently, it is advisable to limit the intake of foods containing fats from animal sources.

PROTEINS

Proteins are the basic components of all body cells. They are essential for building and repairing tissue, regulating body functions, and providing energy and heat. They are made of carbon, hydrogen, oxygen, and nitrogen, and some also contain sulfur, phosphorus, iron, and iodine.

Proteins are made up of twenty-two "building blocks" called *amino acids*. Nine of these amino acids are essential to life. The proteins that contain these nine are called *complete proteins*. The best sources of complete proteins are animal foods such as meats, fish, milk, cheeses, and eggs. Proteins that contain any of the remaining thirteen amino acids and some of the nine essential amino acids are called *incomplete proteins*. Sources of incomplete proteins are usually vegetable foods such as cereals, soybeans, dry beans, peas, and peanuts.

VITAMINS

Vitamins are organic compounds that are essential to life. They are important for metabolism, tissue building, and body processes regulation. They allow the body to use the energy provided by carbohydrates, fats, and proteins. Only small amounts of vitamins are required, and a well-balanced diet usually provides the required vitamins. An excess amount of vitamins or a deficiency of vitamins can cause poor health.

Vitamins are usually classified as water soluble or fat soluble. Water-soluble vitamins dissolve in water, are not normally stored in the body, and are easily destroyed by cooking, air, and light. Fat-soluble vitamins dissolve in fat, can be stored in the body, and are not easily destroyed by cooking, air, and light. Some of the vitamins along with their sources and functions are listed in table 9-2.

MINERALS

Minerals are inorganic (nonliving) elements found in all body tissues. They regulate body fluids, assist in various body functions, contribute to growth, and aid in building tissues. Table 9-3 lists some of the minerals essential to life, their sources, and their main functions.

TABLE 9-2 **Vitamins**

VITAMINS	BEST SOURCES	FUNCTIONS
Fat-Soluble Vitamins		
Vitamin A	Liver Butter, margarine Whole milk, cream, cheese Egg yolk Leafy green and yellow vegetables	Growth Health of eyes Structure and functioning of the cells of the skin and mucous membranes
Vitamin D	Sunshine Fatty fish Egg yolk Liver Butter, cream Fortified milk	Growth Regulates calcium and phosphorous metabolism Builds and maintains bones and teeth
Vitamin E	Vegetable oils Butter, margarine Peanuts Egg yolk Dark-green leafy vegetables	Necessary for protection of cell structure, especially red blood cells Inhibits breakdown of some unsaturated fatty acids
Vitamin K	Spinach, kale, cabbage Liver Soybean oil Cereals	Normal clotting of blood
Water-Soluble Vitamins		
Thiamine (B_1)	Lean pork Enriched bread and cereals Liver, heart, kidney Potatoes, legumes	Carbohydrate metabolism Promotes normal appetite and digestion Normal function of nervous system
Riboflavin (B_2)	Milk, cheese, yogurt, eggs Enriched breads and cereals Green leafy vegetables Liver, kidney, heart	Carbohydrate, fat, and protein metabolism Health of mouth tissue Healthy eyes
Niacin (B_3)	Meats (especially organ meats) Poultry and fish Enriched breads and cereals Peanuts	Carbohydrate, fat, and protein metabolism Healthy skin, nerves, and digestive tract
Vitamin B_{12}	Liver, kidney, muscle meats Milk, cheese Eggs	Metabolism Healthy red blood cells Maintains nerve tissue
Vitamin C (Ascorbic Acid)	Citrus fruits, pineapple Melons and berries Tomatoes Cabbage, broccoli Green peppers	Healthy gums Aids in wound healing Aids in absorption of iron
Folic Acid (Folacin)	Green leafy vegetables Citrus fruits Organ meats, liver Whole-grain cereals Yeast	Protein metabolism Maturation of red blood cells Formation of hemoglobin

TABLE 9-3 **Minerals**

MINERALS	BEST SOURCES	FUNCTIONS
Calcium	Milk Cheese Some dark-green leafy vegetables	Develops/maintains bones and teeth Clotting of the blood Normal heart and muscle action Nerve irritability
Phosphorus	Milk and cheese Meat, poultry, fish Nuts, legumes Whole-grain cereals	Develops/maintains bones and teeth Maintains blood acid-base balance Metabolism of carbohydrates, fats, and proteins Constituent of body cells
Magnesium	Meat, seafood Nuts Milk Cereal grains Fresh green vegetables	Constituent of bones, muscles, and red blood cells Healthy muscles and nerves Metabolism
Sodium	Salt Meat and fish Poultry and eggs Milk, cheese	Fluid balance, acid-base balance Regulates muscles and nerves Glucose (sugar) absorption
Potassium	Meat Milk Vegetables Oranges, bananas, prunes Cereals	Fluid balance Regular heart rhythm Cell metabolism Proper nerve function
Chlorine (Chloride)	Salt Meat Milk, eggs	Fluid balance Acid-base balance Formation of hydrochloric acid
Iron	Liver, muscle meats Dried fruits Egg yolk Enriched breads and cereals Dark-green leafy vegetables	Formation of hemoglobin on red blood cells Part of cell enzymes Aids in production of energy
Iodine	Saltwater fish Iodized salt	Formation of hormones in thyroid gland
Copper	Liver, organ meats Nuts, legumes Whole-grain cereals	Utilization of iron Component of enzymes
Fluorine (Fluoride)	Fluoridated water Fish, meat	Healthy teeth and bones

WATER

Water is found in all body tissues. It is essential for the digestion (breakdown) of food, makes up most of the blood plasma, helps body tissues absorb nutrients, and helps move waste material through the body. Although water is found in almost all foods, the average person should still drink six to eight glasses of water each day to provide the body with the water it needs.

9:3 INFORMATION
Utilization of Nutrients

Before the body is able to use nutrients, it must break down the foods that are eaten to obtain the nutrients and then absorb them into the circulatory system. These processes are called *digestion* and *absorption* (see figure 9-2). The actual use of the nutrients by the body is called *metabolism*.

DIGESTION

Digestion is the process by which the body breaks down food into smaller parts, changes the food chemically, and moves the food through the digestive system. There are two types of digestive action: mechanical and chemical. During mechanical digestion, food is broken down by the teeth and moved through the digestive tract by a process called **peristalsis,** a rhythmic, wavelike motion of the muscles. During chemical digestion, food is mixed with digestive juices secreted by the mouth, stomach, small intestine, and pancreas. The digestive juices contain enzymes, which break down the food chemically so the nutrients can be absorbed into the blood.

ABSORPTION

After the food is digested, absorption occurs. **Absorption** is the process in which blood capillaries pick up the digested nutrients. The nutrients are then carried by the circulatory system to every cell

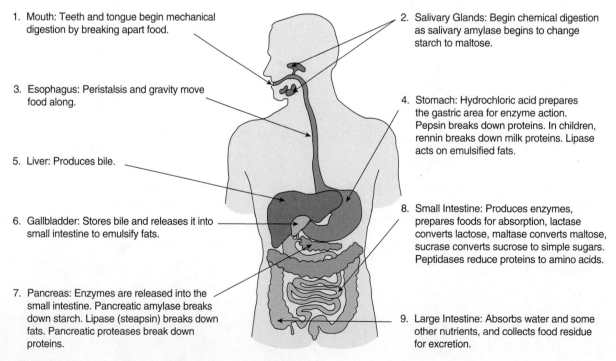

1. Mouth: Teeth and tongue begin mechanical digestion by breaking apart food.

2. Salivary Glands: Begin chemical digestion as salivary amylase begins to change starch to maltose.

3. Esophagus: Peristalsis and gravity move food along.

4. Stomach: Hydrochloric acid prepares the gastric area for enzyme action. Pepsin breaks down proteins. In children, rennin breaks down milk proteins. Lipase acts on emulsified fats.

5. Liver: Produces bile.

6. Gallbladder: Stores bile and releases it into small intestine to emulsify fats.

7. Pancreas: Enzymes are released into the small intestine. Pancreatic amylase breaks down starch. Lipase (steapsin) breaks down fats. Pancreatic proteases break down proteins.

8. Small Intestine: Produces enzymes, prepares foods for absorption, lactase converts lactose, maltase converts maltose, sucrase converts sucrose to simple sugars. Peptidases reduce proteins to amino acids.

9. Large Intestine: Absorbs water and some other nutrients, and collects food residue for excretion.

Figure 9-2 The processes of digestion and absorption.

in the body. Most absorption occurs in the small intestine, but water, salts, and some vitamins are absorbed in the large intestine.

METABOLISM

After nutrients have been absorbed and carried to the body cells, metabolism occurs. This is the process in which nutrients are used by the cells for building tissue, providing energy, or regulating various body functions. During this process, nutrients are combined with oxygen, and energy and heat are released. Energy is required for voluntary work, such as swimming or housecleaning, and for involuntary work, such as breathing and digestion. The rate at which the body uses energy just for maintaining its own tissue, without doing any voluntary work, is called the basal metabolic rate, or BMR. The body needs energy continuously, so it stores nutrients for future use. These stored nutrients are used to provide energy when food intake is not adequate for energy needs.

MEASURING FOOD ENERGY

Foods vary in the amount of energy they contain. For example, a candy bar provides more energy than does an apple. When the body metabolizes nutrients to produce energy, heat is also released. The amount of heat produced during metabolism is the way the energy content of food is measured. This heat is measured by a unit called a kilocalorie (kcal), or just calorie. The number of kilocalories, or calories, in a certain food is known as that food's *caloric value.*

An individual's caloric requirement is the number of kilocalories, or calories, needed by the body during a 24-hour period. Caloric requirements vary from person to person, depending on activity, age, size, sex, physical condition, and climate. The amount of physical activity or exercise is usually the main factor determining caloric requirement, because energy used must be replaced. An individual who wants to gain weight can decrease activity and increase caloric intake. An individual who wants to lose weight can increase activity and decrease caloric intake.

1/2 A general guideline for weight loss or gain is that 1 pound of body fat equals approximately 3,500 calories. To lose 1 pound, a decrease of 3,500 calories is required, either by consuming 3,500 fewer calories or by using 3,500 calories through increased exercise. To gain 1 pound, an increase of 3,500 calories is required. A general guideline to maintain weight is that a person consume 15 calories per pound per day. For example, if a person weighs 120 pounds, maintaining this weight would require a daily intake of 15 x 120, or 1,800, calories daily. By decreasing caloric intake by 500 calories per day, a person would lose 1 pound per week (500 calories per day times 7 days equals 3,500 calories, or 1 pound of fat). By increasing caloric intake by 500 calories per day, a person would gain 1 pound per week. It is important to note that increasing or decreasing exercise along with controlling calorie intake is essential. Also, a slow, steady gain or loss of 1 to 2 pounds per week is an efficient and safe form of weight control.

INFORMATION 9:4 *Maintenance of Good Nutrition*

Good health is everyone's goal, and good nutrition is the best way of achieving and maintaining it. Normally, this is accomplished by eating a balanced diet in which all of the required nutrients are included in correct amounts. The simplest guide for planning healthy meals is the *U.S. Department of Agriculture (USDA) Food Guide,* which classifies foods into five major food groups. Foods are arranged in groups containing similar nutrients. This is known as the Food Guide Pyramid (see figure 9-3). Portion sizes vary according to the caloric requirements of individuals.

The five major food groups, number of daily recommended servings, and nutrient contents of the foods are shown in table 9-4. A sample menu using the five major food groups is shown in table 9-5.

Although the major food groups are a key to healthy meal plans, variety, taste, color, aroma, texture, and general food likes and dislikes must also be considered. If food is not appealing, people will usually not eat it even though it is healthy.

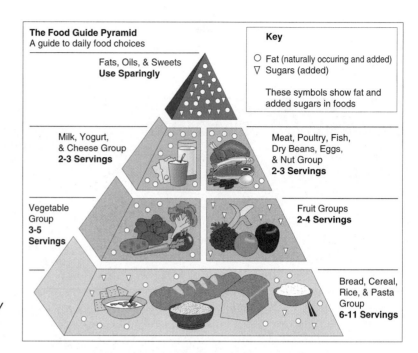

Figure 9-3 The Food Guide Pyramid shows the five major food groups and recommended daily servings. (*Courtesy of the U.S. Department of Agriculture*).

TABLE 9-4 **The Five Major Food Groups**

FOOD GROUP	NUMBER OF SERVINGS	NUTRIENT CONTENT
Milk, Milk Products, Yogurt & Cheese	2–3	Protein; calcium; carbohydrate; fat; phosphorus; vitamins A, D, B_{12}, and riboflavin
Vegetables	3–5	Carbohydrates; vitamins A, E, K, B, and C; iron; calcium; potassium
Fruits	2–4	Carbohydrates, vitamin C, folic acid, potassium
Bread, Cereals, Rice, & Pasta	6–11	Carbohydrates, B vitamins, iron, phosphorus, magnesium
Meats, Fish, Poultry, Dry Beans, Eggs, & Nuts	2–3	Proteins; fats; vitamins A, B, D; iron; sulfur; copper; iodine; sodium; magnesium; zinc

TABLE 9-5 **Sample Menu Using The Five Major Food Groups**

BREAKFAST	LUNCH	DINNER
Orange juice	Tuna sandwich	Roast chicken
Cereal	with	Rice
Toast	Lettuce and tomato	Broccoli
Margarine	Carrot and celery sticks	Green salad
Milk	Cookies	Oil dressing
	Milk	Rolls and margarine
	Fresh fruit	Milk
		Fruit sherbert

Suggested snacks: fresh fruit, pizza, milkshake

Sound and sensible nutritional principles can be found in the booklet published by the USDA and entitled *Nutrition and Your Health: Dietary Guidelines for Americans*. This booklet lists the following seven guidelines to help establish good eating habits based on moderation and variety:

1. Eat a variety of foods. Choose different foods from each of the five major food groups each day. Adjust the number and size of portions based on body weight and nutritional needs. This helps provide the wide variety of nutrients required for good health.
2. Maintain healthy weight. Determine your proper body weight and try to maintain this weight by proper eating habits and exercise.
3. Choose a diet-low in fat, saturated fat, and cholesterol. Eat lean meat, poultry without skin, fish, and low-fat dairy products. Use fats and oils sparingly and limit fried foods.
4. Choose a diet with plenty of vegetables, fruits, and grain products.
5. Use sugars only in moderation. Limit cookies, candy, cakes, and soft drinks. Brush and floss your teeth after eating sweet foods.
6. Use salt and sodium only in moderation. Flavor foods with herbs and spices. Reduce the amount of salty foods.
7. If alcohol is consumed, it should be in moderation. Alcohol should be avoided by pregnant women, individuals using medications, children and adolescents, and individuals who are driving or engaging in an activity that requires attention or skill.

Following the preceding guidelines will result in a diet that will maintain and may even improve health.

Food habits also affect nutrition. At times, habits are based on cultural or religious beliefs. Different cultures and races have certain food preferences. Some religions require certain dietary restrictions that must be observed (see figure 9-4). Unusual habits are not necessarily bad. They should be evaluated using the five major food groups as a guide. When habits do require changing in order to improve nutrition, the person making suggestions must use tact, patience, and imagination. Many food habits are formed during youth, and changing them is a difficult and slow process.

Faith ➡	Christian Science	Roman Catholic	Muslim Moslem	Seventh Day Adventist	Some Baptists	Greek Orthodox (on fast days)
Restricted Food						
Coffee	●			●	●	
Tea	●			●	●	
Alcohol	●		●	●	●	
Pork/pork products			●	●		
Caffeine-containing foods				●		
Dairy products						●
All meats		1 hour before Communion; Ash Wed., Good Friday		Some groups		●

In addition, the Jewish Orthodox faith;
- ■ forbids the serving of milk and milk products with meat.
- ■ forbids cooking of food on the Sabbath.
- ■ forbids eating of leavened bread during Passover.
- ■ observes specific fast days.

Figure 9-4 Some religions require certain dietary restrictions that must be respected. This chart represents only a small sampling of some of these restrictions. As a health care worker, you should check with the dietary supervisor to ensure whether or not an individual patient observes any religious dietary restrictions.

9:5 INFORMATION *Therapeutic Diets*

Therapeutic diets are modifications of the normal diet and are used to improve specific health conditions. They are normally prescribed by a doctor and planned by a dietitian. These diets may change the nutrients, caloric content, and/or texture of the normal diet. They may seem strange and even unpleasant to patients. In addition, a patient's appetite may be affected by **anorexia** (loss of appetite), weakness, illness, loneliness, self pity, and other factors. Therefore, it is essential that the health care worker use patience and tact to convince the patient to eat the foods on the diet. An understanding of the purposes of the various diets will also help the health care worker provide simple explanations to patients.

REGULAR DIET

A **regular diet** is a balanced diet usually used for the ambulatory patient. At times, it has a slightly reduced calorie content. Foods such as rich desserts, cream sauces, salad dressings, and fried foods may be decreased or omitted.

LIQUID DIETS

Liquid diets include both clear liquids and full liquids. Both are nutritionally inadequate and should be used only for short periods of time. All foods served must be liquid at body temperature. Foods included on the clear-liquid diet are mainly carbohydrates and water, including apple or grape juice, fat-free broths, plain gelatin, fruit ice, ginger ale, and tea or black coffee with sugar. The full-liquid diet includes the liquids allowed on the clear-liquid diet plus strained soups and cereals, fruit and vegetable juices, yogurt, hot cocoa, custard, ice cream, pudding, sherbet, and eggnog. These diets may be used after surgery or a heart attack, for patients with acute infections or digestive problems, and before some X rays of the digestive tract.

SOFT DIET

A **soft diet** is similar to the regular diet, but foods must require little chewing and be easy to digest (see figure 9-5). Foods to avoid include meat and shellfish with tough connective tissue, coarse cereals, spicy foods, rich desserts, fried foods, raw fruits and vegetables, nuts, and coconut. This diet may be used following surgery, or for patients with infections, digestive disorders, or chewing problems.

DIABETIC DIET

A **diabetic diet** is used for patients with diabetes mellitus. In this condition, the body does not produce enough of the hormone insulin to metabolize carbohydrates. Patients frequently take insulin by injection. The diet contains exchange lists that group foods according to type, nutrients, and caloric content. Patients are allowed a certain number of items from each exchange list according to their individual needs. Sugar-heavy foods such as candy, soft drinks, desserts, cookies, syrup, honey, condensed milk, chewing gum, and jams and jellies are usually avoided.

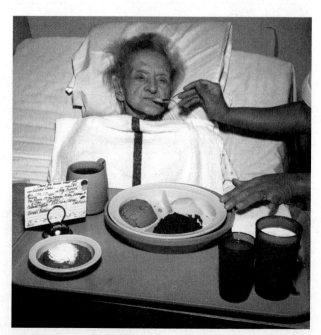

Figure 9-5 Soft diets include foods that require little chewing and are easy to digest.

CALORIE-CONTROLLED DIETS

Calorie-controlled diets include both low-calorie and high-calorie diets. Low-calorie diets are frequently used for patients who are overweight. High-calorie foods are either avoided or very limited. Examples of such foods include butter, cream, whole milk, cream soups or gravies, sweet soft drinks, alcoholic beverages, salad dressings, fatty meats, candy, and rich desserts. High-calorie diets are used for patients who are underweight or have anorexia nervosa, hyperthyroidism (overactivity of thyroid gland), or cancer. Extra proteins and carbohydrates are included. High-bulk foods such as green salads, watermelon, and fibrous fruits are avoided because they fill up the patient too soon. High-fat foods such as fried foods, rich pastries, and cheese cake are avoided because they digest slowly and spoil the appetite.

LOW-CHOLESTEROL DIET

A **low-cholesterol diet** restricts foods containing cholesterol. It is used for patients with atherosclerosis and heart disease. Foods high in saturated fat, such as beef, liver, pork, lamb, egg yolk, cream cheese, natural cheeses, shellfish (crab, shrimp, lobster), and whole milk, are limited, as are coconut and palm oil products.

FAT-RESTRICTED DIETS

Fat-restricted diets are also called *low-fat diets*. Examples of foods to avoid include cream, whole milk, cheeses, fats, fatty meats, rich desserts, chocolate, nuts, coconut, fried foods, and salad dressings. Fat-restricted diets may be used for obese patients or patients with gallbladder and liver disease or atherosclerosis.

SODIUM-RESTRICTED DIETS

Sodium-restricted diets are also called *low-sodium* or *low-salt diets*. Frequently, patients use low-sodium-diet lists similar to the carbohydrate-exchange lists used by diabetic patients. Patients should avoid or limit adding salt to food; smoked meats or fish; processed foods; pickles; olives; sauerkraut; and some processed cheeses. This diet reduces salt intake for patients with cardiovascular diseases (such as hypertension or congestive heart failure), kidney disease, and edema (retention of fluids).

PROTEIN DIETS

Protein diets include both low-protein and high-protein diets. Protein-rich foods include meats, fish, milk, cheeses, and eggs. These foods would be limited or decreased in low-protein diets and increased in high-protein diets. Low-protein diets are ordered for patients with certain kidney or renal diseases and certain allergic conditions. High-protein diets may be ordered for children and adolescents, if growth is delayed; for pregnant or lactating (milk-producing) women; before and/or after surgery; and for patients suffering from burns, fevers, or infections.

BLAND DIET

A **bland diet** consists of easily digested foods that do not irritate the digestive tract. Foods to be avoided include coarse foods, fried foods, highly seasoned foods, pastries, candies, raw fruits and vegetables, alcoholic and carbonated beverages, smoked and salted meats or fish, nuts, olives, avocados, coconut, whole-grain breads and cereals, and, usually, coffee and tea. It is used for patients with ulcers and other diseases of the digestive system.

LOW-RESIDUE DIET

A **low-residue diet** eliminates or limits foods that are high in bulk and fiber. Examples of such foods include raw fruits and vegetables, whole-grain breads and cereals, nuts, seeds, beans, peas, coconut, and fried foods. It is used for patients with digestive and rectal diseases, such as colitis or diarrhea.

OTHER DIETS

Other therapeutic diets that restrict or increase certain nutrients may also be ordered. The health care worker should always check the prescribed diet and ask questions if foods seem incorrect. Every effort should be made to include foods the patient likes if they are allowed on a particular diet. If a patient will not eat the foods on a prescribed therapeutic diet, the diet will not contribute to good nutrition.

STUDENT *Go to the workbook and complete the assignment sheet for Unit 9, Nutrition and Diets.*

UNIT **9** SUMMARY

An understanding of basic nutrition is essential for health care workers. Good nutrition helps maintain wellness, a state of good health with optimal body function.

Essential nutrients are used by the body to perform many different functions. There are six groups of essential nutrients: carbohydrates, fats, proteins, vitamins, minerals, and water. Daily food intake should provide an individual with proper amounts of the essential nutrients.

Before the body can obtain the essential nutrients from food, the body must digest the food. After digestion, the nutrients are absorbed and carried by the circulatory system to every cell in the body. Metabolism then occurs, and the nutrients are used by cells for body functions.

The simplest guide for planning healthy meals that provide the required essential nutrients is to eat a variety of foods from the five major food groups. Portion sizes should vary according to the individual's caloric requirements. Maintaining healthy weight, choosing foods low in fat, using sugar and salt in moderation, and limiting alcoholic beverages are also important aspects of proper nutrition.

Therapeutic diets are modifications of the normal diet. They are used to improve specific health conditions. Examples of therapeutic diets include liquid, diabetic, calorie-controlled, low-cholesterol, fat- or sodium-restricted, high- or low-protein, and bland diets. An understanding of these diets will allow the health care worker to encourage patients to follow prescribed diets.

UNIT 9
SUGGESTED REFERENCES

Ehrlich, Ann. *Nutrition and Dental Health.* 2nd ed. Albany, NY: Delmar Publishers, 1994.

Guthrie, Helen A. *Principles of Human Nutrition.* St. Louis, MO: C. V. Mosby, 1994.

Lankford, T. Randall. *Foundations of Normal and Therapeutic Nutrition.* 2nd ed. Albany, NY: Delmar Publishers, 1994.

Nieman, David C. *Nutrition.* Dubuque, IA: Wm. C. Brown Publishers, 1990.

Townsend, Carolynn E. *Nutrition and Diet Therapy.* 6th ed. Albany, NY: Delmar Publishers, 1994.

U.S. Department of Agriculture. *Nutrition and Your Health: Dietary Guidelines for Americans.* 3rd ed. Washington, D.C.: U. S. Government Printing Office, 1990.

Williams, Sue. *Essentials of Nutrition and Diet Therapy.* 6th ed. St. Louis, MO: Mosby, 1994.

UNIT 10

Computers in Health Care

UNIT OBJECTIVES

After completing this unit of study, you should be able to:

◆ Identify the three major components of a computer system
◆ Compare and contrast computer capabilities and limitations
◆ Describe computer applications currently being used in today's health care computer systems
◆ Define, pronounce, and spell all of the key terms

KEY TERMS

central processing unit (CPU)

computer literacy
(come-pew´-tur lit´-er-ass-see)

computer-assisted instruction (CAI)

computerized tomography (CT)
(com-pew´-tur-eyesd toe-mawg´-rah-fee)

echocardiograph

hardware

input

interactive video (computer-assisted video)

magnetic resonance imaging (MRI)
(mag-net´-ik rez´-oh-nance im´-adj-ing)

mainframe computer

microcomputer

output

personal computer

positron emission tomography (PET)
(pos-ee´-tron ee-miss´-shun toe-mawg´-rah-fee)

random access memory (RAM)

read only memory (ROM)

software

stress test

ultrasonography
(ul-trah-sawn-ahg´-rah-fee)

INFORMATION
10:1 *Introduction*

Computer technology has been called the greatest advance in information processing since Gutenberg invented the printing press. The rapid advances in health care and the explosion of information needed for health care workers to provide quality patient care have made the use of the computer a necessity. Today, it is as common to see a computer terminal in the admissions office of your local hospital or clinic as it is to see a bar code reader being used to add up a grocery bill in your neighborhood supermarket. In fact, many hospitals use this same bar coding method to control inventories and patient costs for hospital supplies.

The computer has become essential in almost every aspect of health care. Computers are used in four general areas:

1. as hospital information systems (HIS) or medical information systems (MIS) for managing budgets, equipment inventories, patient information, laboratory reports, operating room and personnel scheduling, and general records;
2. in diagnostic testing such as analyzing blood and scanning or viewing body parts by computerized tomography (CT scan), magnetic resonance imaging (MRI), positron emission tomography (PET), and ultrasonography;
3. as educational tools in the forms of computer-assisted instruction (CAI) and computer-

assisted video instruction (interactive video) for professional nurses, physicians, and other allied health personnel;
4. and in basic and applied research, including statistical analysis of data.

It is estimated that the health care industry will spend approximately one billion dollars on computer technology within the next few years. Whether you want to be a physician, registered nurse, lab technician, nurse's aide, radiology technician, dietitian, pharmacist, occupational therapist, physical therapist, or any other type of allied health professional, a working knowledge of the computer is essential. This working knowledge is sometimes called *computer literacy*. Computer literacy means a basic understanding of how the computer works and a basic understanding of the applications used in your field or profession. Computer literacy also means feeling comfortable using a computer for your job needs. Practice and experience in using a computer are essential in order to develop computer literacy.

HISTORY OF THE COMPUTER

The first computers were installed in hospitals in the late 1950s and early 1960s. Some of these hospitals had some form of assistance from the International Business Machines (IBM) Corporation.

Today's computers have come a long way from the Electronic Numerical Integrator and Computer

(ENIAC) built in 1946 by J. P. Eckert and J. W. Mauchly at the University of Pennsylvania (see figure 10-1A). This huge computer had to be housed in a room that measured 20 by 40 feet. The ENIAC contained approximately 18,000 vacuum tubes. With the invention of the silicon chip in the 1970s, hundreds of thousands of electronic components were able to fit on a single chip smaller in size than a fingernail. These microchips paved the way for the introduction of the microcomputer.

Computer chips are found in many commonly used items such as watches, cameras, telephones, thermometers, blood pressure gauges, cars, satellite navigation equipment, stoves, burglar alarm systems, and personal desktop computers.

Computers vary in size. Computer size can range from that of a microcomputer such as a hand-held calculator, which can be held in one hand, to that of a personal computer, which can sit on a desktop (figure 10-1B), to that of a very large mainframe computer, which can control the launching of a rocket to outer space.

INFORMATION
10:2 *What is a Computer System?*

A computer system is an electronic device that can be thought of as a complete information-processing center. It can calculate, store, sort, update, manipulate, sequence, organize, and process data. It also controls logic operations and can rapidly communicate in graphics, numbers, words, and sound.

COMPONENTS OF A COMPUTER SYSTEM

All computer systems contain essentially the same parts. These parts are the hardware and software. The hardware consists of the machine components, including the keyboard, central processing unit (CPU), disk drive, and monitor with display screen. The software consists of the programs, or instructions, that run the hardware and allow the computer to perform specific tasks.

There are three major components to a computer system: input, the central processing unit, and output (see figure 10-2). Input is the information that is entered into the computer by means of an input device. The central processing unit (CPU) processes the input and performs the operations of the computer by following the instructions in the software. The output is the processed information, or final product. It can be displayed on a screen, printed as hard copy, stored on magnetic tape or disks, or transmitted to another user or users.

Figure 10-1 **(A)** The ENIAC was 10 feet tall, 3 feet deep, and 100 feet long. *(Courtesy of Unisys Corporation).* **(B)** Today's microcomputers fit easily on a desktop. *(Photo by Michael Dzaman)*

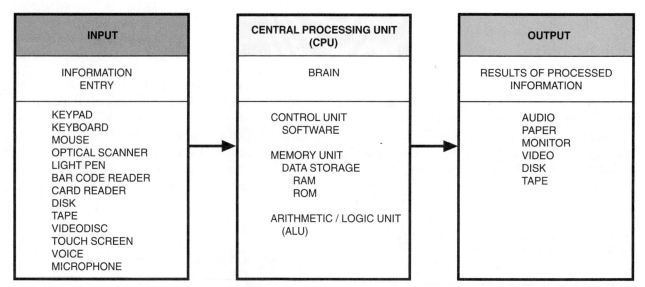

Figure 10-2 Components of a computer system.

Input Devices

In order for the computer to work, instructions and data, or input, must be entered into it using some form of input device. One of the most popular input devices is the computer keyboard. This device is similar to the familiar typewriter keyboard. Other input devices include:

◆ *Magnetic tape*—usually used to enter data on large, mainframe computers.
◆ *Touch screen monitor*—a monitor with touch-sensitive areas built into the screen. Examples are the touch screens found in many fast food outlets and on many microwave ovens.
◆ *Optical scanner*—a machine that can scan a document and read the printed text. An example is the bar code readers found in many supermarkets and used to record and total grocery items.
◆ *Mouse*—a small device that sits on a desktop, controls the cursor, and performs other functions such as creating graphics.
◆ *Light pen*—a device that looks like a pen and is used to perform functions such as selecting menus and drawing graphics on a cathode ray tube, or CRT, which is similar to a television screen.

Central Processing Unit

The central processing unit, or CPU, processes all information or data entering the computer. It acts as the "brains" of the computer. The CPU is divided into three main units: the internal memory unit, the arithmetic and logic unit, and the control unit (see figure 10-3).

1. *Internal Memory Unit.* This unit is controlled by two types of memory. A permanent program already built and stored in the computer system by the manufacturer of the computer is called **read only memory (ROM)**. A program that is *NOT* permanent because data can be stored, changed, and/or retrieved is called **random access memory (RAM),** or read/write memory.
2. *Arithmetic and Logic Unit (ALU).* This performs all of the calculations, such as addition, subtraction, multiplication, and division. It also provides for a logical, step-by-step handling of data or information as the data or information enters or leaves the computer.
3. *Control Unit.* This unit communicates with the input and output units of the computer system. It initiates, interprets, directs, and controls the processing of information.

Output Devices

Output is the finished work of the computer. Output occurs after the data has been processed by the CPU. The most common output devices are the printer, or plotter (see figure 10-4), which is similar to a typewriter, and the video display monitor, such as the *cathode-ray tube* (CRT).

Output can take the form of a hard copy (paper printout) from a printer or plotter. Output can also appear on a computer monitor display

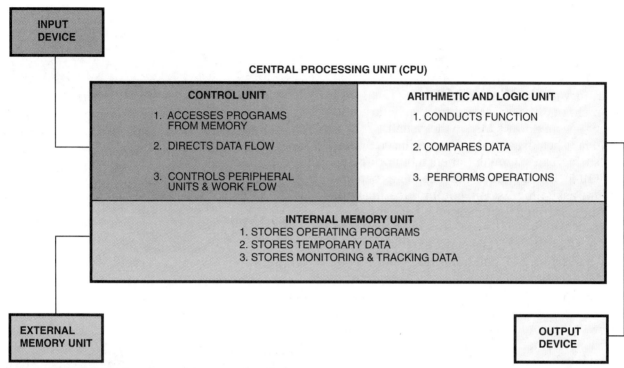

Figure 10-3 The central processing unit (CPU) is the "brains" of the computer.

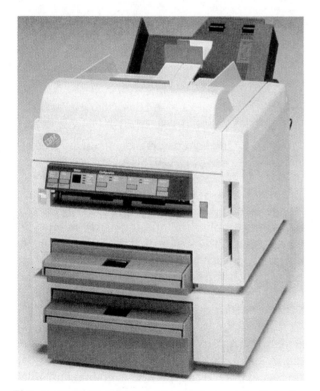

Figure 10-4 The printer is a common output device that produces a paper printout called *hard copy.* *(Courtesy of International Business Machines Corporation)*

screen. Data can be stored or transferred to magnetic tapes, to disks, or to punched cards. Data can also be displayed on a video monitor or heard as music or sound through an audio speaker.

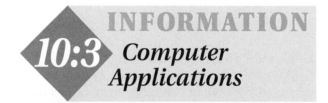

INFORMATION
10:3 Computer Applications

INFORMATION SYSTEMS

Computers were first introduced into hospitals to simplify accounting procedures such as payrolls and inventories. The introduction of computers saved both money and time. This Medical Information System (MIS)—or Hospital Information System (HIS), as it is sometimes called when used in a hospital environment—used expensive, large, mainframe computers. The software, or computer programs needed to run the hardware, was also very expensive to produce and took time to develop. Because of the expense, other departments in the hospital—such as the pharmacy (medications), hematology (blood and blood-forming tissues), clinical chemistry (chemical laboratory methods to aid in the diagnosis and treatment of disease), microbiology, dietary, and nursing—were slowly added to the system.

Today's health care providers use the computer for charting, care planning, patient monitoring (see figure 10-5), interdepartmental scheduling, personnel time assignments, and communicating with other hospital or institutional computer banks.

The Clinical Center Medical Information System established at the National Institutes of Health (NIH), a 541-bed hospital in Bethesda, Maryland, has all of its patient services computerized. Patient clinical findings (such as results of laboratory tests) and observations based on these findings are recorded directly into computer terminals. This method replaces all paper and pencil documentation.

There are approximately 6,000 computer screens at the NIH. Each nursing station is equipped with computer terminals and printers. Lightpens are used to make menu selections from televisionlike monitors (see figure 10-6), and keyboards are used to input any changes or new information. Physicians and nurses use keyboards to enter data such as vital signs, medications, nursing care plans, doctors' orders for patient care, dietary restrictions, and other procedures.

Other health care workers can then retrieve needed information from the computer. Confidentiality of patient information is strictly enforced by means of access codes. Computer users must enter special access codes to retrieve information. Only authorized workers are told the access codes.

A typical hospital information system might work as follows. When a patient enters the hospital, the admission is recorded by an admissions clerk. The patient's name, age, and all other vital information is entered, processed, and stored in the computer's memory. An electronic record is established so that the information about the patient can be retrieved whenever it is needed. For example, while sitting at a computer terminal with a typewriterlike keyboard, the physician can enter all of the findings found on the initial admitting physical examination; order all of the patient's medications from the pharmacy; order laboratory tests, including blood and urine studies; order an electrocardiogram, X-rays, dietary restrictions, and specific nurs-

Figure 10-5 Computers are used to monitor the heart and for defibrillation of abnormal heart patterns. *(Courtesy of Siemens Burdick, Inc.)*

Figure 10-6 The light pen is a common input device. *(Courtesy of USDA/ARS #K-2656-2)*

ing care. A pharmacist in the pharmacy department both checks the computer regularly for new orders and supplies the nursing departments with ordered medications. The pharmacist also uses the computer to warn physicians of drug interactions and to monitor pharmacy inventory (see figure 10-7). Laboratory technicians check the computers for their new or revised orders. When any test or procedure is completed, the laboratory technician records the results in the patient's computerized record. All this current information is then immediately accessible to the medical, nursing, and allied health teams. These teams no longer have to wait for the results of tests to be typed on a typewriter and hand delivered to the patient care area. Nurses no longer have to manually transcribe physicians'

Figure 10-7 Pharmacists can use the computer to monitor medications and maintain inventories. *(Courtesy of USDA/ARS #K-3512-3)*

orders or nurses' notes. Because patient care plans are computerized, they can be easily updated. This use of the computer decreases the time nurses spend on paperwork and away from patient care.

Hand-held portable computers are currently being tested in several hospitals (see figure 10-8). The terminal device is slightly larger than a clipboard. It contains a miniature keyboard and is linked remotely to the nurse's station. With this small terminal, the health care worker is able to record data at a patient's bedside. Patient information such as temperature, heart rate, and respirations is recorded and immediately available to other health care providers. Updated data is also received from other parts of the hospital. It is estimated that this type of device will decrease the time nurses spend on written documentation.

DIAGNOSTICS

A major problem in medicine is determining exactly what is wrong with the patient. The first step in the process is taking a medical history and doing a physical examination. Based on these findings, several tests may be ordered to diagnose or rule out disease.

Several computer-related diagnostic tests have had a real impact on patient care. These diagnostic aids or specialized technological tools are quite varied. They may be invasive, such as a blood test where a syringe is inserted into a vein and blood is removed, or noninvasive, such as an X-ray procedure where no opening into the body is required.

Some computerized instruments automate the step-by-step manual procedure of analyzing blood, urine, serum, and other body-fluid samples. Most laboratories rely heavily on computers for both blood and urine analysis. Smaller units are now used in many medical offices and other health care facilities. The computerized instruments can analyze a drop of serum, blood, urine, or body fluid placed on a slide at rates of over 500 specimens an hour. Such systems have proven to be reliable for clinical chemistry evaluations.

An electrocardiogram (ECG) computerized interpretation system produces visual pictures on a computer monitor and a printout of the electrical activity of a patient's heart. The ECG gives important information concerning the spread of electrical impulses to the heart chamber. It is very important in diagnosing heart disease. An ECG run while the patient is exercising is known as a stress test (see figure 10-9). This allows the physician to

Figure 10-8 A hand-held portable computer can be used to record information at the patient's bedside. *(Courtesy of NCR Corporation, Dayton, Ohio)*

evaluate the function of the patient's heart during activity. An echocardiograph utilizes a computer to direct ultrahigh-frequency sound waves through the chest wall and into the heart (see figure 10-10). The computer then converts the reflection of the waves into an image of the heart. This test can be used to evaluate cardiac function, reveal valve irregularities, show defects in the heart walls, and visualize the presence of fluid between the layers of the pericardium (membrane that surrounds the outside of the heart).

One of the most powerful advances in medical imaging is the computerized tomography (CT) scanner, introduced in 1972. The CT scanner was the first computer-based body and brain scanner. This noninvasive, computerized X ray permits physicians to see clear, cross-sectional views of both bone and body tissues (see figure 10-11). The CT scanner shoots a pencil-thin beam of X rays through any part of the body and from many different angles. The device's computer then creates a cross-sectional image of the body part on a screen. A CT scan provides a clear image of the soft tissues inside the body and exposes the patient to less radiation than does a conventional X ray. In addition, a regular X ray shows little depth, and the soft tissue does not appear clearly.

Another new advance in medical imaging is magnetic resonance imaging (MRI). This comput-

Figure 10-10 An echocardiograph utilizes a computer to evaluate cardiac function, reveal heart valve irregularity, and show defects or diseases of the heart. *(Photo by Marcia Butterfield, courtesy of W. A. Foote Memorial Hospital, Jackson, MI)*

Figure 10-11 This CT scan, a cross section of an abdomen, shows the presence of metastatic liver disease. *(Courtesy of Harbor-UCLA Diagnostic Imaging Center)*

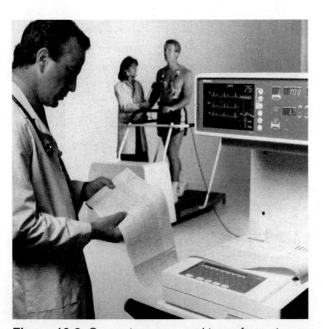

Figure 10-9 Computers are used to perform stress tests to evaluate the function of a patient's heart during exercise. *(Courtesy of Siemens Burdick,*

erized, body-scanning method uses nuclear magnetic resonance instead of X-ray radiation. Magnetic resonance imaging is the alteration of the magnetic position of hydrogen atoms to produce an image. The patient is placed in a large circular magnet, which uses the magnetic field to measure activity of hydrogen atoms within the body (see figure 10-12). A computer translates that activity into cross-sectional images of the body (see figure 10-13). For example, a lung tumor can be more easily detected by scanning with MRI than by scanning with X rays. Magnetic resonance imaging allows physicians to see blood moving through veins and arteries, to see a swollen joint shrink in response to

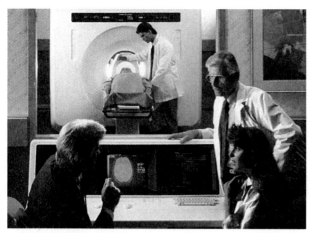

Figure 10-12 For magnetic resonance imaging (MRI), the patient is placed in the center of a large magnet that measures the activity of hydrogen ions inside the body and creates an image of the body. *(Courtesy of GE Medical Systems)*

Figure 10-13 This MRI scan shows a sagittal image of a brain. *(Courtesy of Harbor-UCLA Diagnostic Imaging Center)*

Figure 10-14 Ultrasonography is used during pregnancy to determine the size, position, sex, and even abnormalities of the fetus. *(Photo by Michael Dzaman)*

medication, and to see the reaction of cancerous tumors to treatment.

Positron emission tomography (PET) is another scanning procedure. A slightly radioactive substance is injected into the patient and detected by the PET scanner. The device's computer then composes a three-dimensional image from the radiation detected. The image allows the doctor to see an organ or bone from all sides. In this way, a PET image is similar to a model that can be picked up and examined.

Ultrasonography, figure 10-14, is another non-invasive scanning method. It uses high-frequency sound waves that bounce back as an echo when they hit different tissues and organs inside the body. A computer then uses the sound wave signals to create a picture of the body part, which can be viewed on a computer screen or processed on a photographic film that resembles an X ray. Ultrasonography can be used to detect tumors, locate aneurysms and blood vessel abnormalities, and examine the shape and size of internal organs. During pregnancy, when radiation can harm the fetus, ultrasonography is used to detect multiple pregnancies, and to determine the size, position, sex, and even abnormalities of the fetus (see figure 10-15).

EDUCATION

Computers have become commonplace as educational tools. They can be found in elementary, mid-

dle, junior high, and high schools. Research has shown that computer-based learning decreases time on the task and increases achievement and retention of knowledge. Therefore, it comes as no surprise to find computer-based learning in most schools of medicine, nursing, and allied health.

Computer-assisted instruction (CAI) is educational computer programming designed for individualized use. It is user paced, user friendly, and proceeds in an orderly, organized fashion from topic to topic. It may use animated graphics, color,

Figure 10-15 This ultrasound shows the fetus inside the uterus. *(Courtesy of Sandy Clark)*

and sound. It may be a drill-and-practice program for learning to calculate medication doses. It can also take the form of a tutorial for learning concepts about the heart. In addition, it can be a simulation that allows the learner to do a clinical procedure, such as taking a patient's blood pressure, while sitting in front of the computer. Computer programs have even been developed to allow a user to perform a simulated operation on a patient.

Patient-education software is available for the patient with osteoarthritis (inflammation of the joints), obesity (overweight), and many other diseases. Software is even available to teach people how to manage stress.

Another advance in computer learning technology is interactive video, or computer-assisted video. Interactive video is the integration of computer and video technology. It combines the advantages of video (color, sound, and motion) with the advantages of computer-assisted instruction to provide a dynamic new learning medium. Research has shown that this technology greatly enhances learning and retention. Programs available include those that teach medical terminology to health care workers, clinical skills to nurses, physical examination techniques to physicians, and anatomy and physiology. Programs are stored on compact disks, CD-ROM, that are inserted into a videodisc player.

A network of computer users can be found on the Internet. By using a modem attached to a computer, the telephone lines and specialized software, one computer operator can readily contact other operators. Many types of services and sources of information are offered on the Internet. These in-

clude CompuServe Inc., Prodigy, America Online, and the Microsoft Network. Through the Internet, health care professionals in one area can readily contact others for medical updates, information on new procedures, aid in making diagnoses and other information. A major use of the Internet relates to organ transplants. When an individual needs a transplant, vital information regarding the individual is recorded on the transplant network. The computer monitors all organs as they become available, and can immediately notify the online facility when an organ is suitable for that patient. This allows the most expedient use of donor organs and ensures that organs are given to the most compatible recipient. It is another example of modern technology providing a service that saves lives.

RESEARCH

Mainframe computers are often used to help health care professionals analyze statistics and obtain information from the National Library of Medicine database, which is the largest research library in the scientific community. It serves as a national resource for all United States health science libraries. It is located at the National Institutes of Health in Bethesda, Maryland, where it occupies two buildings, one of which is ten stories high.

The library's computer-based MEDical Literature Analysis and Retrieval System (MEDLARS) is a bibliographic biomedical information database. It can be easily accessed by computer through the Regional Medical Library Network. The MEDLARS includes twenty other databases, including Index Medicus, a monthly subject/author guide to over 3,000 journal articles, and Medline, which currently contains over 5 million references as well as information about audiovisual materials.

Statistical Package for the Social Sciences (SPSS) is a program used in many universities to prepare and analyze research data. Other programs score and analyze student test scores. Some programs can draw graphs and charts, and others help the user learn how to use the program in a step-by-step fashion.

Research using computer technology is being conducted in the areas of diabetes, arthritis, patient management systems, and speech recognition patterns. Interactive videodiscs are used to teach anatomy to medical students, and to teach health care personnel and patients about AIDS.

In addition, clinical researchers are now using microcomputers in several areas. For example, in people who have had severe spinal cord injuries, microcomputers are used to initiate the electrical impulses that stimulate skeletal muscles. This exciting application of computing was used to develop a computer-controlled walking system. This system enables paraplegics and quadriplegics to stand, sit, and walk. Electrodes are applied above the hamstring, quadriceps, and gluteus maximus muscles. These electrodes allow control of flexion and extension of the knees and hips. Sensors applied to the knee provide information to coordinate movement of the knee when the patient is standing or walking. Electrical impulses (controlled by the microcomputer) are delivered through these electrodes to stimulate the muscles through a preprogrammed exercise workout. The computer is programmed to automatically stop the exercise program when the sensors detect that the muscles have become fatigued.

Today, computers are used as cost-effective and efficient tools to enhance quality patient care. They are used to analyze blood; regulate electrical impulses to muscles; take pictures of the body; collect patient data; analyze electrocardiograms; schedule hospital personnel; keep hospital and clinic records, inventories, and budgets; and provide information on wellness to the general public. Computer technology has truly invaded the health care field.

STUDENT Go to the workbook and complete the assignment sheet for Unit 10, Computers in Health Care.

UNIT *10* SUMMARY

The use of computers in health care has almost become a necessity. Every health care worker should have basic computer literacy, meaning an understanding of how the computer works and an understanding of the applications used in their particular health careers.

A computer system is a complete information-processing center. All computer systems contain essentially the same parts: hardware and software. The hardware consists of the machine components. The software consists of the programs, or instructions, that run the hardware and allow the computer to perform specific tasks. Each computer system also requires input, or the information entered into the computer, and a central processing unit (CPU), which performs the operations of the computer by following the directions in the software. This results in output (the processed information, or final product), which can be displayed on a screen, printed, stored, or transmitted to another user.

Computers are used in many aspects of health care. They serve as information centers to provide patient information, schedule personnel, and maintain records and inventory. Computers are also used as diagnostic tools in performing blood tests or viewing body parts, among other procedures. They are major educational tools, and many computer-assisted instructional programs exist to teach both health care workers and patients. Another major use is in research. The use of computers in health care has proven they are efficient tools that enhance the quality of patient care.

UNIT 10 SUGGESTED REFERENCES

Anderson, Sandra. *Computer Literacy for Health Care Professionals.* Albany, NY: Delmar Publishers, 1992.

Carlton, Richard R., and Arlene McKenna-Adler. *Principles of Radiographic Imaging.* Albany, NY: Delmar Publishers, 1992.

Clark, James F., Warren W. Allen, and Dale H. Klooster. *Computers and Information Processing.* 2nd ed. Cincinnati, OH: Southwestern, 1990.

Duffy, Tim, and Tracy Berchelmann. *Computing Concepts.* 2nd ed. Albany, NY: Delmar Publishers, 1995.

Petrofsky, J. S., and C. A. Philips. A computer-controlled walking system: The combination of an orthosis with functional electrical stimulation. *Journal of Clinical Engineering, 11*(2):121–33, 1986.

Sanders, Donald H. *Computers Today.* 3rd ed. New York, NY: McGraw-Hill, 1988.

Shelly, Gary B., Thomas Cashman, and Gloria Waggoner. *Using Computers: A Gateway to Information.* Albany, NY: Delmar Publishers, 1995.

UNIT 11

Promotion of Safety

OBRA

UNIT OBJECTIVES

After completing this unit of study, you should be able to:

◆ Define the term *body mechanics* as it is used
◆ Use correct body mechanics while doing procedures in the laboratory or clinical area
◆ Follow safety regulations stated in the information sections while performing in the laboratory area
◆ Observe all regulations for patient safety while performing procedures on a student partner in the laboratory or clinical area or on a patient in any area
◆ List the four main classes of fire extinguishers
◆ Relate each class of fire extinguisher to the specific fire(s) for which it is used
◆ Simulate the operation of a fire extinguisher by following the directions on the extinguisher and specific measures for observing fire safety
◆ Locate and describe the operation of the nearest fire alarm
◆ Describe in detail the evacuation plan for the laboratory area according to established school policy
◆ Define, pronounce, and spell all of the key terms

KEY TERMS

base of support
body mechanics

fire extinguishers

safety standards

INFORMATION

11:1 *Using Body Mechanics*

In order to prevent injury to yourself while working in the health field, it is important that you observe good body mechanics.

Body mechanics refers to the way in which the body moves and maintains balance while making the most efficient use of all its parts. Basic rules for body mechanics are provided as guidelines to prevent strain and help maintain muscle strength.

Four main reasons for using good body mechanics include:
a. Muscles work best when used correctly.
b. Correct use of muscles makes lifting, pulling, and pushing easier.
c. Correct application of body mechanics prevents unnecessary fatigue and strain, and saves energy.
d. Correct application of body mechanics prevents injury to self.

Eight basic rules of good body mechanics include:
a. Maintain a broad **base of support** by keeping the feet 6 to 8 inches apart, placing one foot slightly forward, balancing weight on both feet, and pointing the toes in the direction of movement (see figure 11-1).
b. Bend from the hips and knees to get close to an object, and keep your back straight (see figure 11-2). Do not bend at the waist.
c. Use the strongest muscles to do the job. The larger and stronger muscles are located in the shoulders, upper arms, hips, and thighs.
d. Use the weight of your body to help push or pull an object. Whenever possible, push, slide, or pull rather than lift.
e. Carry heavy objects close to the body. Also,

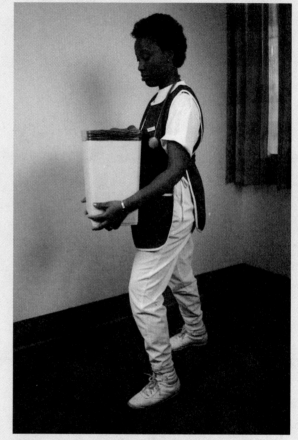

Figure 11-1 Maintain a broad base of support by keeping the feet 6 to 8 inches apart.

stand close to the object or person being moved.
f. Avoid twisting your body as you work. Turn with your feet and entire body when you change direction of movement.
g. Avoid bending for long periods of time.
h. If a patient or object is too heavy for you to lift alone, always get help.

Many health care facilities now require health care workers to wear back supports while lifting or moving patients (see figure 11-3). The supports are used to prevent back

Figure 11-2 Bend from the hips and knees to get close to an object.

Figure 11-3 Many health care facilities now require workers to wear back supports while lifting or moving patients. *(Courtesy of J. T. Posey Company).*

injuries. The support should be the correct size in order to provide the maximum benefit. When the worker is performing strenuous tasks, the support should fit snugly. At other times, it can be loosened; but it should be worn at all times, so it is in place when needed.

STUDENT: *Go to the workbook and complete the assignment sheet for 11:1, Using Body Mechanics. Then return and continue with the procedure.*

PROCEDURE

Using Body Mechanics *11:1*

EQUIPMENT AND SUPPLIES

Heavy book, bedside stand, bed with wheel locks

PROCEDURE

1. Assemble equipment.
2. Compare using a narrow base of support to using a broad base of support. Stand on your toes, with your feet close together. Next, stand on your toes with your feet further apart. Then, stand with your feet flat on the floor but close together. Finally, stand with your feet flat on the floor but approximately 6 to 8 inches apart and with one foot slightly forward. Balance your weight on both feet. You should feel the best support in the final position because of the broad base.
3. Place the book on the floor. Bend from the hips and knees (not the waist) and keep your back straight to pick up the book. Return to the standing position.
4. Place the book between your thumb and fingers, but not touching the palm of your hand, and hold your hand straight out in front of your body. Slowly move your hand toward your body, stopping several times to feel the weight of the book in different positions. Finally, hold the book with your entire hand and bring your hand close to your body. The final position should be the most comfortable.

NOTE: This illustrates the need to carry heavy objects close to your body and to use the strongest muscles to do the job.

5. Stand at either end of the bed. Release the wheel locks on the bed. Position your feet to provide a broad base of support. Get close to the bed. Use the weight of your body to push the bed forward.

6. Place the book on the bed. Pick up the book and place it on the bedside stand. Avoid twisting your body. Turn with your feet to place the book on the stand.
   NOTE: Remember that holding the book close to your body allows you to use the strongest muscles. ·

7. Practice the rules of body mechanics by setting up situations similar to those listed in the pre-vious steps. Continue until the movements feel natural to you.

8. Replace all equipment used.

PRACTICE   *Use the evaluation sheet for 11:1, Using Body Mechanics to practice this procedure. When you feel you have mastered this skill, sign the sheet and give it to your instructor for further action.*

 FINAL CHECKPOINT   Using the criteria listed on the evaluation sheet, your instructor will grade you on your performance.

INFORMATION
11:2 *Preventing Accidents and Injuries*

Safety standards have been established for your protection while you are working in the laboratory or clinical area. It is essential that you know and follow these standards.

The prevention of accidents and injury centers around people and the immediate environment. The health worker must be conscious of personal and patient/resident safety and must exercise care in handling equipment and solutions that may be used.

EQUIPMENT AND SOLUTIONS

◆ Do *not* operate or use any equipment until you have been instructed on how to use it.

◆ Read and follow the operating instructions for all major pieces of equipment. If you do not understand the instructions, ask for assistance.

◆ Do *not* operate any equipment if your instructor is not in the room.

◆ Report any damaged or malfunctioning equipment immediately. Make no attempt to use it.

◆ Do not use frayed or damaged electrical cords. Do not use a plug if the third prong for grounding has been broken off.

◆ When handling any equipment, observe all safety precautions that have been taught.

◆ Never use solutions from bottles that are not labeled.

◆ Read the labels of solution bottles at least three times during use to be sure you have the correct solution (see figure 11-4).

◆ Do *not* mix any solutions together unless instructed to do so by your instructor/immediate supervisor.

◆ Some solutions can be injurious or poisonous. Avoid contact with your eyes and skin. Use only as directed.

◆ If you break any equipment or spill any solutions, immediately report the incident to your instructor/immediate supervisor. You will be told how to dispose of the equipment or how to remove the spilled solution (see figure 11-5).

PATIENT/RESIDENT SAFETY

◆ Do *not* perform any procedure on patients unless you have been instructed to do so. Make sure you have the proper authorization. Follow instructions carefully. Ask questions if you do not understand. Use correct or approved methods while performing any procedure. Avoid shortcuts or incorrect techniques.

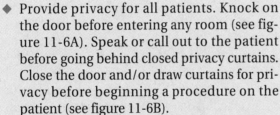

Figure 11-4 Read the label on a solution bottle at least three times to be sure you have the correct solution. *(Photo by Michael Dzaman)*

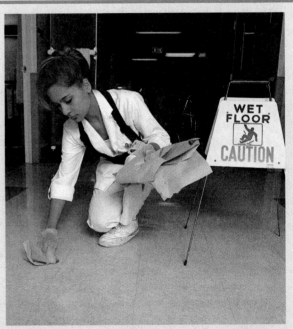

Figure 11-5 Follow proper procedure to clean up spilled solutions.

◆ Provide privacy for all patients. Knock on the door before entering any room (see figure 11-6A). Speak or call out to the patient before going behind closed privacy curtains. Close the door and/or draw curtains for privacy before beginning a procedure on the patient (see figure 11-6B).

◆ Always identify your patient. Be absolutely positive that you have the correct patient. Check the identification wristband, if present. Repeat the patient's name at least twice. Check the name on the patient's bed and on the patient's record.

◆ Always explain the procedure so the patient knows what you are going to do (see figure 11-6C). Answer any questions and make sure you have the patient's consent before performing any procedure. Never perform a procedure if a patient refuses to allow you to do it.

◆ Observe the patient closely during any procedure. If you notice any change, immediately report this. Be alert to the patient's condition at all times.

◆ Frequently check the patient area, waiting room, office rooms, bed areas, or home environment for safety hazards. Report all unsafe situations immediately to the proper person or correct the safety hazard.

◆ Before leaving a patient/resident in a bed, observe all safety checkpoints. Make sure the patient is positioned in a comfortable position. Check the bed to be sure that the side rails are elevated, if indicated; the bed is at the lowest level to the floor; and the wheels on the bed are locked to prevent movement of the bed. Place the call signal (a bell can be used in a home situation) (see figure 11-7A), and other supplies within easy reach of the patient/resident (see figure 11-7B). Open the privacy curtains if they were closed. Leave the area neat and clean and make sure no safety hazards are present.

PERSONAL SAFETY

◆ Use correct body mechanics while performing any procedure.

◆ Wear the required uniform.

◆ Walk—do *not* run—in the laboratory area or clinical area, in hallways, and especially on stairs. Keep to the right and watch carefully at intersections to avoid collisions. Use handrails on stairways.

◆ Report any injury or accident, no matter how minor, to your instructor/immediate supervisor promptly.

Figure 11-6A Always knock on the door or speak before entering a patient's room.

Figure 11-6B Close the door and draw curtains for privacy before beginning a procedure.

Figure 11-6C Explain the procedure and answer any questions to make sure you have the patient's consent.

◆ If you see an unsafe situation or a violation of a safety practice, report it to your instructor/immediate supervisor.

◆ Keep all areas clean and neat with all equipment and supplies in their proper locations at all times.

◆ Wash your hands frequently. Hands should always be washed before and after any procedure, and anytime they become contaminated during a procedure (see figure 11-8). Keep your hands away from your face, eyes, and mouth.

◆ Dry your hands thoroughly before handling any electrical equipment.

◆ Wear safety glasses when instructed to do so and in situations that might result in possible eye injury.

◆ While working with your partner in patient simulations, observe all safety precautions taught in caring for a patient. Avoid horseplay and practical jokes; they cause accidents.

◆ If any solutions come in contact with your skin or eyes, immediately flush the area with

Figure 11-7A Lower the bed and place the call signal within easy reach of the patient.

Figure 11-7B Make sure other supplies and equipment are conveniently placed within the patient's reach.

Figure 11-8 Wash your hands before and after any procedure, and anytime they become contaminated during a procedure.

water. Inform your instructor/immediate supervisor.

◆ If a particle gets in your eye, inform your instructor/immediate supervisor. Do *not* try to remove the particle or rub your eye.

STUDENT   *Go to the workbook and complete the assignment sheet for 11:2, Preventing Accidents and Injuries. Then return and continue with the procedure.*

PROCEDURE

Preventing Accidents and Injuries   11:2

EQUIPMENT AND SUPPLIES

Information section on Preventing Accidents and Injuries, several bottles of solutions, laboratory area with equipment

PROCEDURE

1. Assemble equipment.
2. Review the safety standards in the information section for Preventing Accidents and Injuries. Note standards that are not clear and ask your instructor for an explanation.
3. Examine several bottles of solutions. Read the labels carefully. Read the safety or danger warnings on the bottles.
4. Practice reading the label three times to be sure you have the correct solution. Read the label before taking the bottle off the shelf, before pouring from the bottle, and after you have poured from the bottle.
5. Look at major pieces of equipment in the laboratory. Read the operating instructions for the equipment. Do *not* operate the equipment until you are taught.
6. Role play the following situations by using another student as a patient.

   ◆ Show ways to provide privacy for the patient.
   ◆ Identify the patient.
   ◆ Explain a procedure to the patient.
   ◆ Check various patient areas in the laboratory. Note any safety hazards that may be

present. Discuss how you can correct the problems. Report your findings to your instructor.

   ◆ Observe the patient during a procedure. List points you should observe to note a change in the patient's condition.

7. Discuss the following situations with another student and decide how you would handle them:

   ◆ You see an unsafe situation or a violation of a safety practice.
   ◆ You see a wet area on the laboratory counter.
   ◆ You get a small cut on your hand while using a glass slide.
   ◆ A solution splashes on your arm.
   ◆ A particle gets in your eye.
   ◆ A piece of equipment is not working correctly.
   ◆ A bottle of solution does not have a label.
   ◆ You break a glass thermometer.

8. Observe and practice all of the safety regulations as you work in the laboratory.
9. Study the regulations in preparation for the safety examination. You must pass the safety examination.
10. Replace all equipment used.

PRACTICE   *Use the evaluation sheet for 11:2, Preventing Accidents and Injuries to practice this procedure. When you feel you have mastered this skill, sign the sheet and give it to your instructor for further action.*

✔ **FINAL CHECKPOINT**   Using the criteria listed on the evaluation sheet, your instructor will grade you on your performance.

INFORMATION
11:3 Observing Fire Safety

This information section provides you with basic facts about fires, how they start, and how to prevent them. This information is important for fire safety in the laboratory and work environment.

Fires need three things in order to start: oxygen or air, fuel (any material that will burn), and heat (sparks, matches, flames) (see figure 11-9).

The major cause of fires is carelessness with smoking and with matches. Other causes include misuse of electricity, defects in heating systems, spontaneous ignition, improper rubbish disposal, and arson.

Fire extinguishers are classified according to the kind of fire they extinguish. There are many different fire extinguishers. The main ones are:

◆ *Class A:* This extinguisher contains pressurized water. It is used on fires involving combustibles such as paper, cloth, and wood.
◆ *Class B:* This extinguisher contains carbon dioxide (CO_2). It is used on gasoline, oil, paint, liquid, and cooking fat fires. These types of fire spread if water is used to put them out. Carbon dioxide provides a smothering action. A Class B extinguisher does leave a powdery, snowlike residue that irritates the skin and eyes. The residue is also dangerous if inhaled.
◆ *Class C:* This extinguisher is a dry-chemical type. It contains potassium bicarbonate or potassium chloride. The chemical is a nonconducting agent, so it is used on electrical fires. It can also be used on burning liquids for a smothering action.
◆ *Class ABC,* or *Combination:* This extinguisher contains a graphite-type chemical. It is a multipurpose extinguisher and can be used on all fires. This type also leaves a residue irritating to skin and eyes.

In case of fire, the main rule is to remain calm. If your personal safety is endangered, evacuate the area according to the stated method and sound the alarm. If the fire is small, con-

Figure 11-9 The fire triangle shows the three things needed to start a fire.

fined to one area, and your safety is not endangered, determine what type of fire it is and use the proper extinguisher.

While working in a health care facility, know and follow the fire emergency plan established by the facility (see figure 11-10). The plan usually states that all patients and personnel in immediate danger should be moved from the area. The alarm should be activated as

Figure 11-10 All personnel should be familiar with the fire emergency plan established by the facility in which they work.

quickly as possible. All doors and windows should be closed, if possible, to prevent drafts, which cause fire to spread more rapidly. Electrical equipment and oxygen should be shut off. Elevators should never be used during a fire. By following the fire emergency plan, knowing the location of fire extinguishers and exit doors, and remaining calm, the health care worker can help prevent loss of life or serious injury during a fire.

Preventing fires is everyone's job. Constantly be alert to causes of fires, and correct all situations that can lead to fires. Some main rules for preventing fires are:

a. Obey all "No Smoking" signs. Many health care facilities are now "smoke-free" environments and do not permit smoking anywhere on the premises.

b. Extinguish matches, cigarettes, and any other flammable items completely. Do not empty ashtrays into trash cans or plastic bags that can burn. Always empty ashtrays into separate metal cans or containers partially filled with sand or water.

c. Dispose of all waste materials in proper containers.

d. Before using electrical equipment, check for damaged cords or improper grounding. Avoid overloading electrical outlets.

e. Store flammable materials such as kerosene or gasoline in proper containers and in a safe area. If you spill a flammable liquid, wipe it up immediately.

f. Do not allow clutter to accumulate in rooms, closets, doorways, or traffic areas. Make sure no equipment or supplies block any fire exits.

g. When oxygen is in use, observe special precautions. Post a "No Smoking—Oxygen in Use" sign. Remove all smoking materials and matches from the room. Avoid the use of electrically operated equipment whenever possible. Do not use flammable liquids such as alcohol, nail polish, and oils. Avoid static electricity by using cotton blankets, sheets, and gowns.

STUDENT *Go to the workbook and complete the assignment sheet for 11:3, Observing Fire Safety. Then return and continue with the procedure.*

PROCEDURE

Observing Fire Safety   11:3

EQUIPMENT AND SUPPLIES

Fire alarm box, fire extinguishers

PROCEDURE

1. Read the information section on Observing Fire Safety.
2. Learn the four classes of fire extinguisher and know what kind of fire each type is used for.
3. Locate the nearest fire alarm box. Read the instructions on how to operate the alarm. Be sure you would be able to set off the alarm in case of a fire.

4. Locate any fire extinguishers in the laboratory area. Look for extinguishers in both the room and surrounding building. Identify each extinguisher and the kind of fire for which it is meant to be used.

5. Learn how to operate a fire extinguisher. Read the manufacturer's operating instructions carefully. Work with a practice extinguisher or do a mock demonstration.
   CAUTION: Do *not* discharge a real extinguisher in the laboratory.
   a. Check the extinguisher type to be sure it is the proper one to use for the mock fire (see figure 11-11A).
   b. Locate the lock or pin at the top handle. Release the lock following the manufacturer's instructions, then grasp the handle (see figure 11-11B).
      NOTE: During a mock demonstration, only pretend to release the lock.
   c. Hold the extinguisher firmly in an upright position.

Figure 11-11A Check the extinguisher type to make sure it is the correct one to use.

d. Stand approximately 6 to 10 feet from the near edge of the fire.

e. Aim the nozzle at the fire.

f. Discharge the extinguisher. Use a side-to-side motion. Spray toward the near edge of the fire.

CAUTION: Do not spray into the center of the fire.

g. Continue with the same motion until the fire is extinguished.

h. At all times, stay a safe distance from the fire to avoid personal injury.

CAUTION: Avoid contact with residues from chemical extinguishers.

i. After an extinguisher has been used, it must be recharged or replaced. Another usable extinguisher must be put in position if the extinguisher is removed.

6. Check the policy in your area for evacuating the laboratory area during a fire. Practice the method and know the locations of all exits.

NOTE: Remember to remain calm and avoid panic.

7. Replace all equipment used.

Figure 11-11B Release the pin, aim the nozzle at the near edge of the fire, and push the handle to discharge the extinguisher.

PRACTICE *Use the evaluation sheet for 11:3, Observing Fire Safety, to practice this procedure. When you feel you have mastered this skill, sign the sheet and give it to your instructor for further action.*

✔ *FINAL CHECKPOINT* Using the criteria listed on the evaluation sheet, your instructor will grade you on your performance.

PRACTICE *Study the safety regulations throughout Unit 11 in preparation for the safety examination.*

✔ *FINAL CHECKPOINT* Take the safety examination and obtain a passing grade to demonstrate your knowledge of safety.

UNIT *11* SUMMARY

Safety is the responsibility of every health care worker. It is essential that established safety standards be observed by everyone. This protects the worker, the employer, and the patient.

One important aspect of safety is the correct use of body mechanics. Body mechanics refer to the way the body moves and maintains balance while making the most efficient use of all its parts. Practicing basic principles of good body mechanics prevents strain and maintains muscle strength. In addition, correct body mechanics make lifting, pulling, and pushing easier.

Knowing and following basic safety standards is also important. In this unit, basic standards are listed in regard to the use of equipment and solutions, patient safety, and personal safety. It is important for everyone to learn and follow the established standards at all times.

An awareness of the causes and prevention of fires is essential. Every health care worker should be familiar with the types and use of fire extinguishers. In addition, every facility has a fire emergency plan. By following the fire emergency plan, knowing the location of fire extinguishers and exit doors, and remaining calm, the health care worker can help prevent loss of life or serious injury during a fire.

UNIT 11
SUGGESTED REFERENCES

Caldwell Esther, and Barbara R. Hegner, *Nursing Assistant: A Nursing Process Approach.* 7th ed. Albany, NY: Delmar Publishers, 1995.

Cooper, Marian G., and David E. Cooper. *The Medical Assistant.* 6th ed. New York, NY: McGraw-Hill, 1993.

Grant, Harvey. *Action Guide for Emergency Services.* 6th ed. Englewood Cliffs, NJ: Brady Communications, 1994.

UNIT 12

Infection Control

After completing this unit of study, you should be able to:

◆ Identify five classes of microorganisms by describing the characteristics of each class
◆ List the six components of the chain of infection
◆ Differentiate between antisepsis, disinfection, and sterilization
◆ Wash hands according to recommended aseptic technique
◆ Observe universal precautions while working in the laboratory or clinical area
◆ Wash, wrap, and autoclave instruments, linen, and equipment
◆ Operate an autoclave with accuracy and safety
◆ Follow basic principles on using chemicals for disinfection
◆ Demonstrate the use of boiling water for disinfection
◆ Clean instruments with an ultrasonic unit
◆ Open sterile packages without contaminating the contents
◆ Don sterile gloves without contaminating the gloves
◆ Prepare a sterile dressing tray without contaminating the supplies
◆ Change a sterile dressing without contaminating the materials
◆ Don and remove an isolation mask, gloves, and gown
◆ Relate specific basic tasks to the care of a patient in an isolation unit
◆ Define, pronounce, and spell all of the key terms

KEY TERMS

aerobic

anaerobic

antisepsis
(ant"-ih-sep´-sis)

asepsis
(a-sep´-sis)

autoclave

bacteria

boiling water

cavitation
(kav"-ih-tay´-shun)

chain of infection

chemical disinfection

clean

communicable disease

contaminated

disinfection

endogenous

exogenous

fungi
(fun´-guy)

isolation

microorganism
(my-crow-or´-gan-izm)

nonpathogens

nosocomial

opportunistic

pathogens
(path´-oh-jenz")

protective (reverse) isolation

protozoa
(pro-toe-zo´-ah)

rickettsiae
(rik-et´-z-ah)

sterile

sterile field

sterilization

ultrasonic

universal precautions

viruses

INFORMATION
12:1
Understanding the Principles of Infection Control

OBRA

Understanding the basic principles of infection control is essential for any health care worker in any field of health care. The principles described in this unit provide a basic knowledge of how disease is transmitted and the main ways to prevent disease transmission.

A **microorganism,** or microbe, is a small, living plant or animal that is not visible to the naked eye. It must be viewed under a microscope. Microorganisms are found everywhere in the environment, including on and in the human body. Many microorganisms are part of the normal flora of the body and are beneficial in maintaining certain body processes. These are called **nonpathogens.** Other microorganisms cause infection and disease and are called **pathogens,** or germs. At times, a microorganism that is beneficial in one body system can become pathogenic when it is present in another body system. For example, a bacteria called *Escherichia coli* (*E. coli*) is part of the natural flora of the large intestine. If *E. coli* enters the urinary system, however, it causes an infection.

There are several different classes of microorganisms. In each class, some of the microorganisms are pathogenic to humans. Some of the main classes include:

◆ Bacteria—These are simple, one-celled plants that multiply rapidly. They are classified by shape and arrangement. Cocci are round or spherical in shape (see figure 12-1). If cocci occur in pairs, they are diplococci. Diplococci bacteria cause diseases such as gonorrhea, meningitis, and pneumonia. If cocci occur in chains, they are streptococci. A common streptococcus causes a severe sore throat (strep throat) and rheumatic fever. If cocci occur in clusters or groups, they are staphylococci. These are the most common pyogenic (pus-producing) microorganisms. Staphylococci cause infections such as boils, wound infections, and toxic shock. Rod-shaped bacteria are called bacilli (see figure 12-2). They can occur singly, in pairs, or in chains. Many bacilli contain flagella, which are threadlike projec-

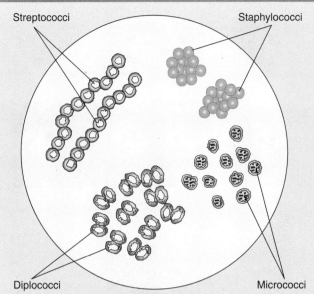

Figure 12-1 Kinds of cocci bacteria.

Figure 12-2 Bacilli bacteria.

tions that are similar to tails and allow the organisms to move. Bacilli also have the ability to form spores, or thick-walled capsules, when conditions for growth are poor. In the spore form, bacilli are extremely difficult to kill. Diseases caused by different types of bacilli include tuberculosis; tetanus; pertussis, or whooping cough; botulism; diphtheria; and typhoid. Bacteria that are spiral or corkscrew in shape are called spirilla (see figure 12-3). These include the comma-shaped vibrio and the corkscrew-shaped spirochete. Diseases caused by spirilla include syphilis and cholera.

◆ **Protozoa**—These are one-celled animals often found in decayed materials and contaminated water (see figure 12-4). Some protozoa are pathogenic and cause diseases such as malaria, amebic dysentery, trichomonas, and African sleeping sickness.

◆ **Fungi**—These are simple, plantlike organisms that live on dead organic matter. Yeasts and molds are two common fungi forms that can be pathogenic. They cause diseases such as ringworm, athlete's foot, histoplasmosis, and thrush (see figure 12-5).

◆ **Rickettsiae**—These are parasitic microorganisms, which means they cannot live outside the cells of another living organism.

Figure 12-3 Spirilla bacteria.

They are commonly found on fleas, lice, ticks, and mites and are transmitted to humans by the bites of these insects. Rickettsiae cause diseases such as typhus fever and Rocky Mountain spotted fever.

◆ **OBRA** **Viruses**—These are the smallest microorganisms, visible only using an electron microscope (see figure 12-6). They

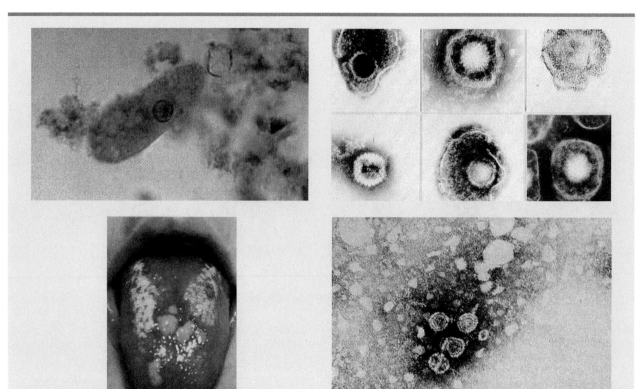

Figure 12-4 (Top) An intestinal protozoa, *Entamoeba coli. (Courtesy of the Centers for Disease Control, Atlanta, GA)*
Figure 12-5 (Bottom) The yeast (fungus) called thrush causes these characteristic white patches on the tongue.

Figure 12-6 (Top) Electron micrographs of the various types of herpes simplex virus. *(Courtesy of the Centers for Disease Control, Atlanta, GA)*
Figure 12-6 (Bottom) Electron micrograph of the hepatitis B virus. *(Courtesy of the Centers for Disease Control, Atlanta, GA)*

cannot reproduce unless they are inside another living cell. They are spread from human to human by blood and other body secretions. It is important to note that viruses are more difficult to kill because they are resistant to many disinfectants and are usually not affected by antibiotics. Viruses cause many diseases including the common cold, measles, mumps, chicken pox, herpes, warts, influenza, and polio. Two diseases of major concern to the health care worker are hepatitis B and acquired immune deficiency syndrome (AIDS). Hepatitis B, or serum hepatitis, is caused by the HBV virus and is transmitted by blood serum and other body secretions. It affects the liver and can lead to the destruction and scarring of liver cells. A vaccine has been developed to protect individuals from

this disease. The vaccine is expensive and involves a series of three injections. Under federal law, employers must provide the vaccination at no cost to any health care worker with occupational exposure to blood or other body secretions that may carry the HBV virus. An individual does have the right to refuse the vaccination, but a written record must be kept proving that the vaccine was offered. Acquired immune deficiency syndrome is caused by the human immunodeficiency virus (HIV) and suppresses the immune system. An individual with AIDS cannot fight off many cancers and infections that would not affect a healthy person. Presently there is no cure and no vaccine available, so it is important for the health care worker to take precautions to prevent the spread of this disease.

In order to grow and reproduce, microorganisms need certain things. Most microorganisms prefer a warm environment, and body temperature is ideal. Darkness is also preferred by most microorganisms, and many are killed quickly by sunlight. In addition, a source of food and moisture is needed. Some microorganisms, called aerobic organisms, require oxygen to live. Others, called anaerobic organisms, live and reproduce in the absence of oxygen. The human body is the ideal supplier of all of the requirements of microorganisms.

Pathogenic microorganisms cause infection and disease in different ways. Some pathogens produce poisons, called *toxins,* which harm the body. An example is the bacillus tetanus, which produces toxins that damage the central nervous system. Some pathogens cause an allergic reaction in the body, resulting in a runny nose, watery eyes, and sneezing. Other pathogens attack and destroy the living cells they invade. An example is the protozoa that causes malaria. It invades red blood cells and causes them to rupture.

Infections and diseases are also classified as endogenous, exogenous, nosocomial, or opportunistic. Endogenous means the infection or disease originates within the body. These include metabolic disorders, congenital abnormalities, tumors, and infections caused by microorganisms within the body. Exogenous means the infection or disease originates outside the body. Examples include pathogenic organisms that invade the body, radiation, chemical agents, trauma, electric shock, and temperature extremes. A nosocomial infection is one acquired by an individual in a health care facility such as a hospital or long-term care facility. Nosocomial infections are usually present in the facility and transmitted by health care workers to the patient. Many of the pathogens transmitted in this manner are antibiotic resistant and can cause serious and even life-threatening infections in patients. Two common examples are staphylococcus and pseudomonas. Infection-control programs are used in health care facilities to prevent and deal with nosocomial infections. Opportunistic infections are those that occur when the body defenses are weak. These diseases do not usually occur in individuals with intact immune systems. Examples include the development of Kaposi's sarcoma (a rare type of cancer) or *Pneumocystis carinii* pneumonia in individuals with AIDS.

In order for disease to occur and spread from one individual to another, certain conditions must be met. First, there must be a causative agent, or pathogen, such as a bacterium or virus. Second, the causative agent must find a reservoir where it can live. Some common reservoirs include the human body, animals, the environment, and fomites, or objects contaminated with infectious material that contains the pathogens. The pathogen must then have a portal of exit, or a way to escape from the reservoir in which it has been growing. In the human body, pathogens can leave the body through urine, feces, saliva, blood, tears, mucous discharge, sexual secretions, and draining wounds. When the pathogen leaves the reservoir, it must be transmitted to another reservoir or host where it can live. The pathogen can be transmitted in different ways. One way is by direct person-to-person contact (physical or sexual contact), or direct contact with a body secretion containing the pathogen. Contaminated hands are one of the most common sources of direct transmission. Another way is by indirect contact, when the pathogen is transmitted from contaminated substances such as food, air, soil, insects, feces, clothing, instruments, and equipment. Examples include touching contaminated equipment and spreading the pathogen on the hands, breathing in droplets carrying airborne infections, and being bitten by an insect carrying a pathogen. A portal of entry, or a way to enter a new reservoir or host, is also essential. Some ways pathogens can enter the body are through breaks in the skin, breaks in the mucous membrane, the respiratory tract, the digestive tract, the genitourinary tract, and the circulatory system. If the defense mechanisms of the body are intact and the immune system is functioning, a human can frequently fight off the causative agent and not contract the disease. Body defenses include the mucous membrane that lines the respiratory, digestive, and reproductive tracts and traps pathogens; cilia (tiny, hairlike structures) that line the respiratory tract and propel pathogens out of the body; coughing and sneezing; hydrochloric acid, which destroys pathogens in the stomach; tears in the eye, which contain bacteriocidal (killing bacteria) chemicals; fever; inflammation resulting in leukocytes, or white blood cells, destroying pathogens; and the immune response, where the body produces antibodies, protective proteins that combat pathogens. However, if large numbers of a pathogen invade the body, or if the body defenses are weak, the individual can contract the infection or disease. This individual is called a susceptible host, or a person likely to get an infection or disease. These factors—a causative agent, a reservoir, a portal of exit, a means of transmission, a portal of entry, and a susceptible host—form what is commonly called the chain of infection (see figure 12-7). If any part of the chain is eliminated, the spread of disease or infection will be stopped. A health care worker who is aware of this can follow practices to interrupt or break this chain and prevent the transmission of disease. It is important to remember that pathogens are everywhere and that preventing their transmission is a continuous process.

A major way to break the chain of infection is to use aseptic techniques while providing health care. Asepsis is defined as the absence of disease-producing microorganisms, or pathogens. Any object or area that may contain pathogens is considered to be contaminated. Aseptic techniques are directed toward maintaining cleanliness and eliminating or preventing contamination. Common aseptic techniques include handwashing, good personal hygiene, use of disposable gloves when contacting body secretions or contaminated objects, proper cleaning of instruments and equipment, and thorough cleaning of the environment.

Various levels of aseptic control are possible. These include:

◆ Antisepsis—Antiseptics prevent or inhibit growth of pathogenic organisms but are not effective against spores and viruses. They can usually be used on the skin. Common examples include alcohol and betadine.

◆ Disinfection—This is a process that destroys or kills pathogenic organisms. It is not always effective against spores and viruses. Boiling water and chemical disinfectants are used in this process. Disinfectants can irritate or damage the skin and are used mainly on objects, not people. Some common disinfectants are bleach solutions and zephirin.

◆ Sterilization—This is a process that destroys all microorganisms, both pathogenic and nonpathogenic, including spores and viruses. Steam under pressure, gas, radiation, and chemicals can be used to sterilize objects. An autoclave is the most common piece of equipment used for sterilization.

In the sections that follow, correct methods of aseptic techniques are described. It is important for the health care worker to know and use these methods in every aspect of providing health care in order to prevent the spread and transmission of disease.

STUDENT *Go to the workbook and complete the assignment sheet for 12:1, Understanding the Principles of Infection Control.*

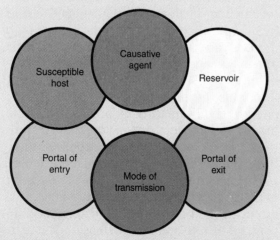

Figure 12-7 Note the components in the chain of infection.

INFORMATION
12:2 *Washing Hands*

OBRA Handwashing is a basic task required in any health occupation. The method described in this unit has been developed to ensure that a thorough cleansing occurs. This section provides information about the basic principles of handwashing.

An aseptic technique is a method followed to prevent the spread of germs or pathogens. Hand-washing is one way to practice aseptic technique.

The hands are a perfect media for the spread of pathogens. Thoroughly washing the hands helps prevent and control the spread of pathogens from one person to another. It also helps protect the health worker from disease and illness.

Handwashing should be performed before and after every procedure. In addition, if the hands become contaminated during a procedure, the hands should be washed again. If gloves are worn during a procedure, the hands should be washed immediately after removing the gloves.

The recommended method for handwashing is based on the following principles; they should be observed whenever hands are washed:

a. Soap is used as a cleansing agent because it aids in the removal of germs through its sudsy action and alkali content.

b. Warm water should be used. This is less damaging to the skin than hot water. It also creates a better lather with soap than does cold water.

c. Friction should be used in addition to soap and water. This action helps rub off pathogens from the surface of the skin.

d. All surfaces on the hands must be cleaned. This includes the palms, the backs/tops of the hands, and the areas between the fingers.

e. Fingertips should be pointed downward. The downward direction prevents water from getting on the forearms and then running down to contaminate the clean hands.

f. Dry paper towels should be used to turn the faucet on and off. This action prevents contamination of the hands from germs on the faucet. A dry towel should be used because pathogens can travel more readily through a wet towel.

Nails also harbor dirt and must be cleaned during the handwashing process. An orange/cuticle stick can be used. Care must be taken to use the blunt end of the stick because the pointed end can injure the nailbeds. A brush can also be used to clean the nails.

STUDENT *Go to the workbook and complete the assignment sheet for 12:2, Washing Hands. Then return and continue with the procedure.*

PROCEDURE
Washing Hands 12:2

EQUIPMENT AND SUPPLIES

Paper towels, running water, waste container, hand brush or orange/cuticle stick, soap

PROCEDURE

1. Turn the faucet on by holding a paper towel between your hand and the faucet (see figure 12-8A). Regulate the temperature of the water and let water flow over your hands.

   NOTE: Water should be warm and all surfaces on the hands must be cleaned.

   CAUTION: Hot water will burn your hands.

2. With your fingertips pointing downward, wet your hands.

Figure 12-8A Use a dry towel to turn the faucet on.

Figure 12-8B Point the finger-tips downward and use the palm of one hand to clean the back of the other hand.

Figure 12-8C Interlace the fingers to clean between the fingers.

Figure 12-8D The blunt end of an orange stick can be used to clean the nails.

Figure 12-8E A hand brush can also be used to clean the nails.

Figure 12-8F With the finger-tips pointing downward, rinse the hands thoroughly.

NOTE: Washing in a downward direction prevents water from getting on the forearms and then running back down to contaminate hands.

3. Use soap to get a lather on your hands.
4. Put the palms of your hands together and rub them back and forth several times.
5. Put the palm of one hand on the back of the other hand. Rub together several times. Repeat this after reversing position of hands (see figure 12-8B).
6. Interlace the fingers on both hands and rub them back and forth (see figure 12-8C).
   NOTE: Steps 3 through 6 ensure that all parts of both hands are clean.
7. Clean the nails with an orange/cuticle stick and/or hand brush (see figures 12-8D and E).
   ⊘ *CAUTION:* Use the blunt end of orange/cuticle stick to avoid injury.
8. Rinse your hands, keeping fingertips pointed downward (see figure 12-8F).

9. Dry hands thoroughly, from tips of fingers to wrist.
10. Use a dry paper towel to turn off the faucet.
    ⊘ *CAUTION:* Wet towels allow passage of pathogens.
11. Discard all used towels in the wastecan. Leave the area neat and clean.

PRACTICE *Go to the workbook and use the evaluation sheet for 12:2, Washing Hands, to practice this procedure. When you feel you have mastered this skill, sign the sheet and give it to your instructor for further action.*

✔ *Final Checkpoint* Using the criteria listed on the evaluation sheet, your instructor will grade you on your performance.

INFORMATION
12:3 *Observing Universal Precautions*

In order to prevent the spread of pathogens and disease, the chain of infection must be broken. The universal precautions discussed in this unit are an important way health care workers can break this chain.

One of the main ways that pathogens are spread is by blood and body fluids. Two pathogens of major concern are the hepatitis B virus (HBV) and the human immunodeficiency virus (HIV), which causes AIDS. Consequently, extreme care must be taken at all times when an area, object, or person is contaminated with blood or body fluids. In 1991, the Occupational Safety and Health Administration (OSHA) established regulations that must be followed by all health care facilities. The employer faces civil penalties if the regulations are not implemented by the employer and followed by the employees. These regulations require all health care facility employers to:

◆ Determine all employees who have occupational exposure to blood or potentially infectious materials such as semen, vaginal secretions, and other body fluids.
◆ Provide hepatitis B vaccine free of charge to all employees who have occupational exposure, and obtain a written release form signed by any employee who does not want the vaccine.
◆ Provide personal protective equipment (PPE) such as gloves, gowns, lab coats, masks, and face shields in appropriate sizes and in accessible locations.
◆ Provide adequate handwashing facilities and supplies.
◆ Ensure that the worksite is maintained in a clean and sanitary condition, follow measures for immediate decontamination of any surface that comes in contact with blood or infectious materials, and dispose of infectious waste correctly.
◆ Enforce rules of no eating, drinking, smoking, applying cosmetics or lip balm, handling contact lenses, and mouth pipetting or suctioning in any area that can be potentially contaminated by blood or other body fluids.
◆ Provide appropriate containers that are color coded (fluorescent orange or orange-red) and labeled for contaminated sharps (needles, scalpels) and other infectious wastes.
◆ Post signs at the entrance to work areas where there is occupational exposure.
◆ Provide a confidential medical evaluation and follow-up for any employee who has an exposure incident. Examples might include an accidental needle stick or the splashing of blood or body fluids on the skin, eyes, or mucous membranes.
◆ Provide training about the regulations to all employees at no cost during working hours, and provide additional education as needed when procedures or working conditions are changed or modified.

In addition, employers must make sure that every employee uses universal precautions at all times to prevent contact with blood or other potentially infectious materials. Universal precautions (see figure 12-9) are rules developed by the Centers for Disease Control (CDC) and the Federal Drug Administration (FDA). According to universal precautions, every body fluid should be considered a potentially infectious material, and all patients should be considered potential sources of infection. By following universal precautions, health care workers can protect themselves and patients from exposure.

A major precaution is to wash your hands before and after contact with any patient. If your hands or other skin surfaces are contaminated with blood or other body fluids, they should be washed immediately and thoroughly with soap and water. Hands should always be washed immediately after removal of gloves.

Gloves (see figure 12-10) should be worn whenever contact with blood and body fluids, mucous membranes, or nonintact skin is possible; when handling items or surfaces soiled with blood or body fluids; when performing any

Universal Blood/Body Fluid Precautions

VISITORS: Ask nurse for instructions

GLOVE

Before touching blood, body fluids, mucous membranes, non-intact skin or performing venipuncture. Change gloves after contact with each patient.

WASH

Wash hands immediately after gloves are removed. Wash hands and other skin surfaces immediately if contaminated with blood or other body fluids.

GOWN/APRON

For procedures likely to generate splashes of blood or other body fluids.

MASK EYE PROTECTION

Masks and protective eyewear or face shields for procedures likely to generate splashes of blood or other body fluids.

SHARPS

Dispose of needles with syringes and other sharp items in puncture-resistant container near point-of-use.

DO NOT RECAP BY HAND

Do not recap needles or otherwise manipulate by hand before disposal.

RESUSCITATION

Mouthpieces or resuscitator bags should be available to minimize need for emergency mouth-to-mouth resuscitation.

WASTE/LINEN

Waste and soiled linen should be handled in accordance with hospital policy and local law.

1. Health-care workers who have exudative lesions or weeping dermatitis should refrain from all direct patient care.
2. Pregnant health-care workers should be especially familiar with and strictly adhere to precautions to minimize the risk of HIV transmission to the infant.
3. Blood spills should be cleaned up promptly with an approved chemical germicide or appropriately diluted sodium hypochlorite (bleach).

Figure 12-9 Universal precautions must be observed while working with all patients.

Figure 12-10 Gloves should be worn whenever contact with blood, body fluids, mucous membranes, or nonintact skin is possible.

invasive (entering the body) procedure; and when performing venipuncture or blood tests. Gloves should be changed after contact with each patient, and hands should be washed immediately after removal of gloves. Care must be taken while removing gloves to avoid contamination of the skin. Gloves should not be washed or disinfected for reuse because washing may allow penetration of liquids through undetected holes, and disinfecting agents may cause deterioration of gloves.

Gowns or aprons should be worn during any procedure that is likely to cause splashing of blood or other body fluids. This helps prevent contamination of clothing or uniforms. Contaminated gowns or aprons should be handled according to agency policy and local and state laws.

Masks and protective eyewear or face shields (see figure 12-11) should be worn during procedures that may produce droplets of blood or body fluids. Examples include irrigation of wounds, suctioning, dental procedures, delivery of a baby, and surgical procedures. This prevents exposure of the mucous membranes of the mouth, nose, and eyes to any pathogens.

To avoid accidental cuts or punctures, extreme care should be taken while handling sharp objects. Needles should never be bent or broken after use. They should be left uncapped and attached to the syringe and placed in a puncture-resistant sharps container (see figure 12-12). Surgical blades and other sharp objects should also be discarded in the sharps container. The containers should not be emptied or reused. Federal, state, and local laws establish regulations for the disposal of sharps containers. In some areas, the filled container is placed in a special oven and melted. The material remaining is packaged as infectious waste and

Figure 12-12 All needles and sharp objects should be discarded immediately in a puncture-resistant sharps container.

Figure 12-11 Gloves, a gown, a mask, and protective eyewear should be worn during any procedure that may produce droplets or cause splashing of blood or body fluids.

disposed of according to legal requirements for infectious waste.

Spills or splashes of blood and/or body fluids should be wiped up immediately (see figure 12-13). Gloves should be worn while wiping up the area. The area should then be cleaned with a disinfectant solution such as a 10-percent bleach solution. In addition, any contaminated instruments or equipment should be cleaned and disinfected immediately.

Whenever possible, mouthpieces or resuscitation devices should be used to avoid the need for mouth-to-mouth resuscitation. These devices should be placed in convenient locations and be readily accessible for use.

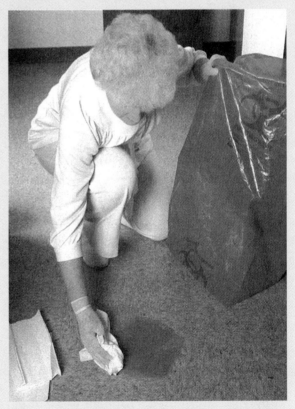

Figure 12-13 Gloves must be worn while wiping up any spills of blood or body fluids.

Figure 12-14 All infectious wastes must be placed in special infectious waste or biohazardous material bags.

Figure 12-15 The health care worker must know the requirements for disposal of waste materials and dispose of wastes in the proper containers.

To dispose of waste and soiled linen, wear gloves and follow the agency policy developed according to law. Infectious wastes such as contaminated dressings, gloves, and body tissues must be placed in special infectious waste or biohazardous material bags (see figure 12-14) according to law. These bags are then autoclaved prior to disposal. Other trash is frequently placed in plastic bags and incinerated. The health care worker must dispose of waste in the proper container (see figure 12-15) and know the requirements for disposal. Soiled linen should be placed in laundry bags to pre-

vent any contamination. Linen soiled with blood, body fluids, or excretions is usually soaked in a disinfectant prior to being laundered. Gloves must be worn while handling any contaminated linen, and any bag containing contaminated linen should be clearly labeled and color coded.

Report any cut, injury, needle stick, or splashing of blood or body fluids immediately. Follow agency policy to deal with the injury or contamination.

Universal precautions must be followed at all times by all health care workers. By observing these precautions, health care workers can help break the chain of infection and protect themselves, their patients, and all other individuals.

STUDENT   *Go to the workbook and complete the assignment sheet for 12:3, Observing Universal Precautions. Then return and continue with the procedure.*

PROCEDURE

Observing Universal Precautions
12:3

EQUIPMENT AND SUPPLIES

Disposable gloves, infectious waste bags, needle and syringe, sharps container, gown or apron, masks, protective eyewear, resuscitation devices

NOTE: This procedure will help you learn universal precautions. It is important for you to observe these precautions at all times while working in the laboratory or clinical area.

PROCEDURE

1. Assemble equipment.
2. Review the precautions in the information section for Observing Universal Precautions. Note points that are not clear, and ask your instructor for an explanation.
3. Practice handwashing according to Procedure 12:2. Identify at least four times that hands must be washed according to universal precautions.

4. Name four instances when gloves must be worn to observe universal precautions. Put on a pair of disposable gloves. Practice removing the gloves without contaminating the skin. With a gloved hand, grasp the cuff of the glove on the opposite hand, handling only the outside of the glove (see figure 12-16A). Pull the glove down and turn it inside out while removing it. Take care not to touch the skin with the gloved hand. Using the ungloved hand, slip the fingers under the cuff of the glove on the opposite hand (see figure 12-16B). Touching only the inside of the glove and taking care not to touch the skin, pull the glove down and turn it inside out while removing it. Place the gloves in the proper waste container. Wash your hands immediately.
5. Practice putting on a gown or apron. State when a gown or apron is to be worn. To remove the gown or apron, touch only the inside. Fold the contaminated gown or apron so the outside is folded inward. Roll it into a bundle and place it in a laundry bag.
   CAUTION: If a gown is contaminated, gloves should be worn while removing the gown.
   NOTE: Folding the gown and rolling it prevents transmission of pathogens.
6. Practice putting on a mask and protective eyewear. To remove the mask, handle it by the

Figure 12-16A To remove the first glove, use a gloved hand to grasp the outside of the glove on the opposite hand. Pull the glove down and turn it inside out while removing it.

Figure 12-16B To remove the second glove, slip the fingers of the ungloved hand inside the cuff of the glove. Touch only the inside of the glove while pulling it down and turning it inside out.

ties only. Clean and disinfect protective eye-wear after use.

7. Practice proper disposal of sharps. Uncap a needle attached to a syringe, taking care not to stick yourself with the needle. Place the entire needle and syringe in a sharps container. State the rules regarding disposal of the sharps container.

8. Spill a small amount of water on a counter. Pretend that it is blood. Put on gloves and use disposable towels or gauze to wipe up the spill. Put the contaminated towels or gauze in an infectious waste bag. Use clean disposable towels or gauze to wipe the area thoroughly with a disinfectant agent. Put the towels or gauze in the infectious waste bag, remove your gloves, and wash your hands.

9. Practice handling an infectious waste bag. Fold down the top edge of the bag to form a cuff at the top of the bag. Wear gloves to close the bag after contaminated wastes have been placed in it. Put your hands under the folded cuff (see figure 12-17A) and gently expel excess air from the bag. Twist the top of the bag shut and fold down the top edges to seal the bag. Secure the fold with tape or a tie according to agency policy (see figure 12-17B).

10. Examine mouthpieces and resuscitation devices that can be used in place of mouth-to-mouth resuscitation. You may be taught to use these devices when you learn cardiopulmonary resuscitation (CPR).

11. Discuss the following situations with another student and determine which universal precautions should be observed:

   ◆ A patient has an open sore on the skin and pus is seeping from the area. You are going to bathe the patient.
   ◆ You are cleaning a tray of instruments that contains a disposable surgical blade and needle with syringe.
   ◆ A tube of blood drops to the floor and breaks, spilling the blood on the floor.
   ◆ Drainage from dressings on an infected wound has soiled the linen on the bed you are changing.
   ◆ You work in a dental office and are assisting a dentist while a tooth is being extracted (removed).

12. Replace all equipment used.

Figure 12-17A To close an infectious waste bag, wear gloves and place your hands under the cuff to gently expel excess air.

Figure 12-17B After folding down the top edge of the infectious waste bag, tie or tape it securely.

PRACTICE *Go to the workbook and use the evaluation sheet for 12:3, Observing Universal Precautions. When you feel you have mastered this skill, sign the sheet and give it to your instructor for further action.*

✔ *Final Checkpoint* Using the criteria listed on the evaluation sheet, your instructor will grade you on your performance.

INFORMATION

12:4 Sterilizing with an Autoclave

Sterilization of instruments and equipment is essential in preventing the spread of infection. In any of the health fields, you may be responsible for proper sterilization. The following basic principles relate to sterilization methods. The autoclave is the safest, most efficient sterilization method.

An autoclave is a piece of equipment that uses steam under pressure or gas to sterilize equipment and supplies (see figure 12-18). It is the most efficient method of sterilizing most articles, and it will destroy all microorganisms, both pathogenic and nonpathogenic, including spores and viruses.

Autoclaves are available in various sizes and types. Offices and health clinics usually have smaller units, and hospitals or surgical areas have large floor model units. A pressure cooker can be used in home situations.

Before any equipment or supplies are sterilized in an autoclave, they must be prepared properly. All items must be washed thoroughly and then rinsed. Oily substances can often be removed with alcohol or ether. Any residue left on articles will tend to bake and stick to the article during the autoclaving process.

Items that are to remain sterile must be wrapped before they are autoclaved. A wide variety of wraps are available. The wrap must be a material that will allow for the penetration of steam during the autoclaving process. Samples of wraps include muslin, autoclave paper, special plastic or paper bags, and autoclave containers (see figure 12-19).

Autoclave indicators are used to ensure that articles have been sterilized (see figure 12-20). Examples of indicators include autoclave tape, sensitivity marks on bags or wraps, and indicator capsules. The indicator is usually placed on or near the article when the article is put into the autoclave. The indicator will change appearance during the autoclaving process due to time and temperature, which leads to sterilization. Learn how to recognize that an article is sterile by reading the directions provided with indicators.

The autoclave must be loaded correctly in order for all parts of an article to be sterilized. Steam builds at the top of the chamber and moves downward. As it moves down, it pushes

Figure 12-18 An autoclave uses steam under pressure to sterilize items.

Figure 12-19 Special plastic or paper autoclave bags can be used to sterilize instruments.

Figure 12-20 Autoclave indicators change color to show that sterilization has occurred. The strips below each package show how the indicators looked before sterilization.

ARTICLES	TIME 250° TO 254° (121° TO 123°C)
Glassware: empty, inverted	15 minutes
Instruments: metal in covered or open, padded or unpadded tray	
Needles, unwrapped	
Syringes: unassembled, unwrapped	
Flasked solutions, 75–250 mL	
Instruments, metal combined with other materials in covered and/or padded tray	
Instruments wrapped in double-thickness muslin	20 minutes
Rubber gloves, catheters, drains, tubing, etc., unwrapped or wrapped in muslin or paper	
Dressings wrapped in paper or muslin (small packs only)	
Flasked solutions, 500–1,000mL	
Needles, individually packaged in glass tubes or paper	
Syringes: unassembled, individually packed in muslin or paper	30 minutes
Sutures: silk, cotton, or nylon; wrapped in paper or muslin	
Treatment trays wrapped in muslin or paper	

Figure 12-21 The length of time required to sterilize different items varies.

cool, dry air out of the bottom of the chamber. Therefore, materials must be placed so the steam can penetrate along the natural planes between the packages of articles in the autoclave. Place the articles in such a way that there is space between all pieces. Packages should be placed on the sides, not flat. Jars, basins, and cans should be placed on their sides, not flat, so that steam can enter and air can flow out. No articles should come in contact with the sides, top, or door of the autoclave.

The length of time and amount of pressure required to sterilize different items varies (see figure 12-21). *It is important to check the directions that come with the autoclave.* Because different types of articles require different times and pressures, it is important to separate loads so that all articles sterilized at one time require the same time and pressure. For example, rubber tubings usually require a relatively short period of time and can be damaged by long exposure. Certain instruments and needles require a longer period of time to ensure sterilization; so, items of this type should not be sterilized in the same load as are rubber tubings.

Wet surfaces permit rapid infiltration of organisms, so it is important that all items are thoroughly dry before being removed from the autoclave. The length of time for drying varies. Follow the manufacturer's instructions.

Sterilized items must be stored in clean, dustproof areas. Items usually remain sterile for 30 days after autoclaving. However, if the wraps loosen or tear, if they become wet, or if any chance of contamination occurs, the items should be rewrapped and autoclaved again. *NOTE:* At the end of the 30-day sterile period—providing that the wrap has not loosened, been torn, or gotten wet—remove the old autoclave tape from the package, replace with a new, dated tape, and resterilize according to correct procedure.

Some autoclaves are equipped with a special door that allows the autoclave to be used as a dry-heat sterilizer. Dry heat involves the use of a high temperature for a long period of time. The temperature is usually a minimum of 320°F to 350°F (160°C to 177°C). The minimum time is usually 60 minutes. Dry-heat sterilization is a good method for sterilizing instruments that may corrode, such as knife blades, or items that would be destroyed by the moisture in steam sterilization, such as powders. Dry heat should never be used on soft rubber goods because the heat will destroy the rubber. An oven can be used for dry-heat sterilization in home situations.

Procedures 12:4A and 12:4B, following, describe wrapping articles for autoclaving and au-

toclaving techniques. These procedures vary in different agencies and areas, but the same principles apply. In some facilities, many supplies are purchased as sterile, disposable items; needles and syringes are purchased in sterilized wraps, used once, and then destroyed. In other facilities, however, special treatment trays are sterilized and used more than one time.

It is important that you follow the directions specific to the autoclave with which you are working, and the agency policy for sterile supplies. Careless autoclaving permits the transmission of disease-producing organisms. Infection control is everyone's responsibility.

STUDENT *Go to the workbook and complete the assignment sheet for 12:4, Sterilizing with an Autoclave. Then return and continue with the procedures.*

PROCEDURE

Wrapping Items for Autoclaving 12:4A

EQUIPMENT AND SUPPLIES

Items to wrap: instrument, towel, bowl; autoclave wrap: paper, muslin, plastic or paper bag; autoclave tape or indicator; disposable or utility gloves; pen or autoclave marker; masking tape (if autoclave tape is not used)

PROCEDURE

1. Assemble equipment.
2. Wash hands.
3. Sanitize the items to be sterilized. Instruments, bowls, and similar items should be cleaned thoroughly in soapy water. The items should then be rinsed well in cool water to remove any soapy residue. If stubborn stains

are present, it may be necessary to soak the items.

NOTE: If the items to be autoclaved are contaminated with blood, body fluids, or tissues, gloves should be worn while cleaning the items. Frequently, heavy-duty utility gloves are used for this procedure.

NOTE: Check the teeth on serrated (notched like a saw) instruments. Scrub with a brush as necessary.

4. To prepare linen for wrapping, check first to make sure it is clean and dry. Fold the linen in half lengthwise. If it is very wide, fold lengthwise again. Fanfold or accordian pleat the linen from end to end until a compact package is formed (see figure 12-22A). All folds should be the same size. Fold back one corner on the top fold (see figure 12-22B). This provides a piece to grab when opening the linen.

NOTE: Fanfolding linens allows for easy handling after sterilization.

5. Select the correct wrap for the item. Make sure the wrap is large enough to enclose the item to be wrapped.

NOTE: Double-thickness muslin, disposable paper wraps, and plastic or paper bags are the most common wraps.

Figure 12-22A Fanfold clean, dry linen so all of the folds are the same size. *(Photo by Michael Dzaman)*

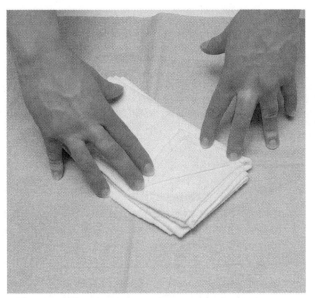

Figure 12-22B Fold back one corner on the top fold of the linen. *(Photo by Michael Dzaman)*

6. With the wrap positioned at a diagonal angle and one corner pointing toward you, place the item to be sterilized in the center of the wrap (see figure 12-23A).
   NOTE: Make sure that hinged instruments are open so the steam can sterilize all edges.
7. Fold up bottom corner to center (see figure 12-23B). Double back a small corner (see figure 12-23C).
8. Fold the right corner over. Make sure the edges are sealed and that there are no air pockets. Bring back a small corner (see figure 12-23D).
   🛑 *CAUTION:* Any open areas at corners will allow pathogens to enter.
9. Fold in the left corner. Again, watch for and avoid open edges. Bring back a small corner (see figure 12-23E).
10. Bring the final corner up and over the top of the package. Check the two edges to be sure they are sealed and tight. Tuck this under the pocket created by the previous folds. Leave a small corner exposed so it can be used when unwrapping the package (see figure 12-23F).
    NOTE: This is frequently called an "envelope" wrap, because the final corner is tucked into the wrap similar to the way the flap is tucked into an envelope.
11. Secure with autoclave or pressure-sensitive indicator tape.

NOTE: If regular masking tape is used, attach an autoclave indicator to reflect when contents are sterilized.

12. Label the package by marking the tape with the date and contents. Some health care agencies may require you to put your initials on the label.
    NOTE: For certain items, the type or size of item should be noted, for example, curved hemostat or mosquito hemostat, hand towel or bath towel, or small bowl or large bowl.
    NOTE: Contents will not be sterile after 30 days, so the date of sterilization must be noted on the package.
13. Check the package. It should be firm enough for handling but loose enough for proper circulation of steam.
14. To use a plastic or paper autoclave bag (refer back to figure 12-19), select or cut the correct size for the item to be sterilized. Place the clean item inside the bag. Double fold the open end(s) and tape or secure with autoclave tape. Check the package to make sure it is secure.
    NOTE: In some agencies, the ends are sealed with heat prior to autoclaving.
    NOTE: If the bag has an autoclave indicator, regular masking tape can be used to seal the ends.
15. Replace all equipment used.
16. Wash hands.

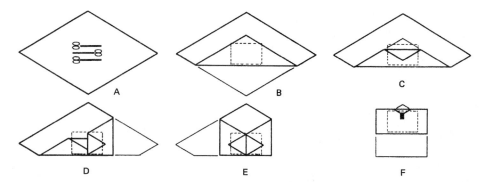

Figure 12-23A-F To wrap items for autoclaving, **(A)** place the items in the center of the wrap, **(B)** fold the bottom corner in to the center, **(C)** fold back a tab, **(D)** fold in the right corner and fold back a tab, **(E)** fold in the left corner and fold back a tab, and **(F)** bring the final corner up and over the top of the pack and tuck it in, leaving a small corner exposed.

PRACTICE   *Go to the workbook and use the evaluation sheet for 12:4A, Wrapping Items for Autoclaving, to practice this procedure. When you feel you have mastered this skill, sign the sheet and give it to your instructor for further action.*

✔ *Final Checkpoint*   Using the criteria listed on the evaluation sheet, your instructor will grade you on your performance.

PROCEDURE

Loading and Operating an Autoclave   *12:4B*

NOTE: Follow the operating instructions for your autoclave. The basic principles of loading apply to all autoclaves. Basic controls for one autoclave are shown in figure 12-24.

EQUIPMENT AND SUPPLIES

Autoclave, distilled water, small pitcher or measuring cup, items wrapped or prepared for autoclaving, time chart for autoclave, 12:4 Information section

PROCEDURE

Review the Information section for 12:4, Sterilizing with an Autoclave. Then proceed with the following activities. It is suggested that you read through the procedure first, checking against the diagram. Then practice with an autoclave.

1. Assemble equipment.
2. Wash and dry hands thoroughly.
3. Check the three-prong plug and the electrical cord. If either is damaged or prongs are missing, do not use the autoclave. If no problems are present, plug the cord into a wall outlet.
4. Use distilled water to fill the reservoir to within $2\frac{1}{2}$ inches below the opening or to the level indicated on the autoclave.
    NOTE: Distilled water prevents the collection of mineral deposits and prolongs the life and effectiveness of the autoclave.
5. Check the pressure gauge to make sure it is at zero.
    ! *CAUTION:* Never open the door unless the pressure is zero.
6. Open the safety door by following the manufacturer's instructions. Some door handles require an upward and inward pressure; others require a side-pressure technique.
7. Load the autoclave. Make sure all articles have been prepared correctly. Check for autoclave indicators, secure wraps, and correct labels. Separate loads so all items require the same time, temperature, and pressure. Place

Figure 12-24 Autoclave control valves vary, but most contain the same basic controls.

Figure 12-25 Bowls or basins should be placed on their sides in the autoclave so air and steam can flow in and out of the container: **(Top)** shows incorrect placement, while **(Bottom)** shows correct placement.

packages on their sides. Place bowls or basins on their sides so air and steam can flow in and out of the container (see figure 12-25). Make sure there is space between the packages so the steam can circulate.

NOTE: Check to make sure no large packages block the steam flow to smaller packages. Place large packages on the bottom.

❗ *CAUTION:* Make sure no item comes in contact with the sides, top, or door of the autoclave chamber.

8. Follow the instructions for filling the chamber with the correct amount of water. Most autoclaves have a "Fill" setting on the control. Allow water to enter the chamber until the water covers the fill plate inside the chamber.

9. When the correct amount of water is in the chamber, follow the instructions for stopping the flow of water. In many autoclaves, turning the control valve to "Sterilize" stops the flow of water from the reservoir.

10. Check the load in the chamber to be sure it is properly spaced. The chamber can also be loaded at this point, if this has not been done previously.

11. Close and lock the door.

❗ *CAUTION:* Be sure the door is securely locked; check by pulling slightly.

12. Read the time chart for the specific time and temperature required for sterilization of items that were placed in the autoclave.

13. After referring to the chart provided with the autoclave or reviewing figure 12-21, set the control valves to allow the temperature and pressure to increase in the autoclave.

14. When the desired temperature has been reached, set the controls to maintain the desired temperature during the sterilization process. Follow the manufacturer's instructions.

15. Based on the information in the time chart, set the timer to the correct time.

NOTE: Many autoclaves require you to rotate the timer past 10 (minutes) before setting the time.

16. Check the pressure and temperature gauges at intervals to make sure they remain as originally set.

NOTE: Most autoclaves automatically shut-off when pressure reaches 35.

17. When the required time has passed, set the controls so the autoclave will vent the steam from the chamber.

18. Put on safety glasses.

❗ *CAUTION: Never* open the door without glasses. The escaping steam can burn the eyes.

19. Check the pressure gauge. When it is at zero, open the door about $1/2$ inch to permit thorough drying of contents.

⚠ *CAUTION:* Do not open the door until pressure is zero.

20. After the autoclaved items are dry, remove and store them in a dust-free area.

⚠ *CAUTION:* Handle supplies and equipment carefully. They may be hot.

21. If there are additional loads to run, leave the main valve in the vent position. This will keep the autoclave ready for immediate use.

22. If this is the final load, turn the autoclave off. Unplug the cord from the wall outlet; do not pull on the cord.

23. Replace all equipment used.

24. Wash hands.

PRACTICE *Go to the workbook and use the evaluation sheet for 12:4B, Loading and Operating an Autoclave, to practice this procedure. When you feel you have mastered this skill, sign the sheet and give it to your instructor for further action.*

✔ *Final Checkpoint* Using the criteria listed on the evaluation sheet, your instructor will grade you on your performance.

INFORMATION
12:5 Using Chemicals for Disinfection

Many health fields require the use of chemicals for aseptic control. Certain points that must be observed while using the chemicals are discussed in the following information.

Chemicals are frequently used for aseptic control. Most chemicals do not kill spores and viruses; therefore, chemicals are not a method of sterilization. Because sterilization does not occur, chemical disinfection is the appropriate term (rather than cold sterilization, a term sometimes used).

Chemicals are used to disinfect instruments that do not penetrate body tissue. Many dental instruments, percussion hammers, scissors, and similar items are examples. In addition, chemicals are used to disinfect thermometers and other items that would be destroyed by the high heat used in the autoclave.

Proper cleaning of all instruments or articles is essential. Particles or debris on items may contaminate the chemicals and reduce their effectiveness. In addition, all items must be rinsed thoroughly because the presence of soap can also reduce the effectiveness of chemicals. The articles should be dry before being placed in the disinfectant in order to keep the chemical at its most effective strength.

Some chemical solutions used as disinfectants are 90-percent isopropyl alcohol, formaldehyde-alcohol, 2-percent phenolic germicide, 10-percent bleach solution, Lysol, and benzalkonium (zephiran). The manufacturer's directions should be read completely before using any solution. Some solutions must be mixed before use. The directions will also specify the recommended time for the most thorough disinfection.

Chemical solutions can cause rust to form on certain instruments, so antirust tablets or solutions are frequently added to the chemicals. Again, it is important to read the directions provided with the tablets or solution. If improperly used, antirust substances may cause a chemical reaction with a solution and reduce the effectiveness of the chemical disinfectant.

The chemical disinfectant should completely cover the article. This is the only way to be sure that all parts of the article will be disinfected.

The container used for chemical disinfection should be large enough to accommodate the items. In addition, the items should be separate so each one will come in contact with the chemical. A tight-fitting lid should be placed on the container while the articles are in the solution.

Before removing items from solutions, health workers should wash their hands. Sterile pick-ups or transfer forceps may be used to remove the instruments from the solution. The instruments are placed on a sterile or clean towel to dry, and then stored in a drawer or dust-free closet.

Solutions should be changed frequently. Some solutions can be used over a period of time, but others should be discarded after one use. Follow the manufacturer's instructions. However, any time contamination occurs or dirt is present in the solution, discard it. A fresh solution must be used.

STUDENT *Go to the workbook and complete the assignment sheet for 12:5, Using Chemicals for Disinfection. Then return and continue with the procedure.*

PROCEDURE

Using Chemicals for Disinfection   *12:5*

EQUIPMENT AND SUPPLIES

Chemicals, container with tight-fitting lid, basin, soap, water, instruments, brush, sterile pick-ups or transfer forceps, sterile towel, disposable gloves

PROCEDURE

1. Assemble equipment.
2. Wash hands.
3. Wash all instruments or equipment thoroughly. Use warm soapy water. Use the brush on serrated edges of instruments.
    NOTE: Wear gloves if any of the instruments or equipment are contaminated with blood or body fluids. Heavy-duty utility gloves are frequently used for this procedure.
4. Rinse in cool water to remove soapy residue. Dry all instruments or equipment thoroughly.
   NOTE: Water on the instruments or equipment will dilute the chemical disinfectant.
5. Check container. Make sure lid fits securely.
   NOTE: A loose cover will permit entrance of pathogens.
6. Place instruments in the container. Make sure there is a space between instruments. Leave hinged edges open so the solution can flow between the surfaces.
7. Carefully read instructions about the chemical solution. Some solutions must be diluted. Check the manufacturer's recommended soaking time.

⊘ *CAUTION:* Reread instructions to be sure solution is safe to use on instruments.
NOTE: An antirust substance must be added to some solutions.

8. Pour solution into the container. Make sure that all instruments are covered (see figure 12-26).
   NOTE: Read label three times: before pouring, while pouring, and after pouring.
   ⊘ *CAUTION:* Avoid splashing the chemical on your skin. Improper handling of chemicals can cause burns and/or injuries.
9. Leave the instruments in the solution for the length of time recommended by the manufacturer.
   NOTE: Twenty to thirty minutes is the usual soaking time.
10. Wash hands.

Figure 12-26 Pour the chemical disinfectant into the container until all instruments are covered with solution.

11. When instruments have soaked the correct amount of time, use sterile pick-ups or transfer forceps to remove the instruments from the solution. Place them on a sterile towel to dry. A second sterile towel is sometimes used to cover the instruments while they are drying. Store the instruments in special drawers or containers or dust-free closets.
    NOTE: Some contamination occurs when instruments are exposed to the air. In some cases, such as with external instruments, this minimal contamination will not affect usage.
12. Replace all equipment used.
13. Wash hands.

PRACTICE *Go to the workbook and use the evaluation sheet for 12:5, Using Chemicals for Disinfection, to practice this procedure. When you feel you have mastered this skill, sign the sheet and give it to your instructor for further action.*

✔ *Final Checkpoint* Using the criteria listed on the evaluation sheet, your instructor will grade you on your performance.

INFORMATION
12:6 *Using Boiling Water for Disinfection*

Using boiling water for aseptic control is not common. However, it is still used in some health agencies and in home care situations. This section provides the main facts regarding this method of aseptic control.

Boiling water is an aseptic method used when an autoclave is not available or when total sterilization is not required. This method does not kill spores and viruses; therefore, it disinfects but does not sterilize. In a home care setting, where instruments/supplies are used for one person only, it can be a satisfactory method.

Boiling-water units, sometimes called "office sterilizers," are available in a variety of types and sizes. Most units use the same principles. A pot with a tight-fitting lid can be used in a home.

Before any item is placed in the boiling-water unit, it must be thoroughly washed and rinsed. Particles or debris left on articles will interfere with complete, thorough disinfection.

Items should be completely immersed in the boiling water to ensure that all parts are disinfected.

Most manufacturers of units recommend using distilled water. This prevents the buildup of mineral deposits. The water level should be based on the manufacturer's recommendation, but all instruments must be completely submerged in the water.

Water tends to rust instruments, so antirust tablets or solutions are frequently added. It is important to read the directions provided with the tablets or solution to determine the correct amount to use.

Instruments are usually boiled for 15 to 30 minutes. The water must be brought to a full boil (212°F, or 100°C) before timing starts.

It is best to remove instruments from the unit while they are hot. This allows for rapid drying and helps prevent rust. Instruments should be placed on a sterile or clean towel. When they are dry, they may be stored in dust-proof drawers or cabinets. Instruments can also be placed in sterile wraps for storage.

STUDENT *Go to the workbook and complete the assignment sheet for 12:6, Using Boiling Water for Disinfection. Then return and continue with the procedure.*

PROCEDURE

Using Boiling Water for Disinfection 12:6

Figure 12-27 Make sure all instruments are submerged in the water for boiling-water disinfection.

EQUIPMENT AND SUPPLIES

Boiling-water unit or pot, basin with soap and water, brush, instruments, distilled water, sterile pick-ups or transfer forceps, sterile towel, sterile wrap, disposable gloves

PROCEDURE

1. Assemble equipment.
2. Wash hands.
3. Wash all instruments or equipment thoroughly in soap and water. Use the brush on serrated edges of instruments. Rinse thoroughly in cool water to remove soapy residue.

   NOTE: Wear gloves if any of the instruments or equipment are contaminated with blood or body fluids. Heavy-duty utility gloves are frequently used for this procedure.
4. Fill the boiling-water unit/pot one-half full or to the level recommended by manufacturer. Use distilled water to avoid mineral deposits. Add antirust tablet or solution, if indicated.
5. Place the instruments in the unit. Make sure there is space between all instruments. Leave serrated edges and hinged edges open.

   NOTE: Be sure the water level is high enough to cover the instruments (see figure 12-27). Boiling water must come in contact with all surfaces of the instruments.
6. Close the unit. Turn it on. Let the water come to a boil.
7. When the water starts boiling, begin to time the process. Most instruments are boiled for 15 to 30 minutes from the time the water begins to boil.

   CAUTION: Do not start timing until water boils, or reaches 212°F (100°C). Pathogens will not be killed at lower temperatures.
8. When the time period is over, use sterile pick-ups or transfer forceps to remove the instruments. Place the instruments on a double thickness of sterile towel.

   NOTE: Do not contaminate the instruments. Avoid touching any clothing, surfaces, or other items.
9. After the instruments are dry, wrap them in sterile wraps as previously taught, or store in dust-free drawers or cabinets.

   NOTE: The method used depends on agency policy.

   NOTE: Instruments not used to penetrate the body are usually stored in drawers or cabinets.
10. Clean and replace all equipment.
11. Wash hands.

PRACTICE *Go to the workbook and use the evaluation sheet for 12:6, Using Boiling Water for Disinfection, to practice this procedure. When you feel you have mastered this skill, sign the sheet and give it to your instructor for further action.*

✔ **Final Checkpoint** Using the criteria listed on the evaluation sheet, your instructor will grade you on your performance.

INFORMATION

12:7 *Cleaning with an Ultrasonic Unit*

Ultrasonic units are used in many dental and medical offices and other health agencies to efficiently clean a large variety of instruments prior to sterilizing them. The following information explains operation of the unit.

Ultrasonic cleaning is used on a large variety of instruments and items in health care agencies. An ultrasonic unit uses sound waves to clean. When the unit is turned on, the sound waves produce millions of microscopic bubbles in a cleaning solution. When the bubbles strike the items being cleaned, they explode, a process known as cavitation, and drive the cleaning solution onto the article. Accumulated dirt and residue is easily and gently removed from the article.

Ultrasonic cleaning is not sterilization because spores and viruses remain on the articles. If sterilization is desired, other methods must be used after the ultrasonic cleaning.

Only ultrasonic solutions should be used in the unit. Different solutions are available for different materials. A general, all-purpose cleaning solution is usually used in the permanent tank and to clean many items. There are other specific solutions for alginate, plaster and stone removal, and tartar removal. The solution chart provided with the ultrasonic unit will state which solution should be used. It is important to read labels carefully before using any solutions. Some solutions must be diluted before use. Some can be used only on specific materials. All solutions are toxic. They can also cause skin irritation, so contact with the skin and eyes should be avoided. Solutions should be discarded when they become cloudy or contaminated, or if cleaning results are poor.

The permanent tank of the ultrasonic unit (figure 12-28) should contain a solution at all times. A general, all-purpose cleaning solution is used most of the time. Glass beakers or auxiliary pans can then be placed in the permanent tank. The items to be cleaned and the proper cleaning solution are then put in the beakers or

Figure 12-28 Parts of an ultrasonic cleaning unit.

pans. The bottoms of the beakers or pans must always be positioned below the level of the solution present in the permanent tank. In this way, cavitation can be transmitted from the main tank and through the solution to the items being cleaned in the beakers or pans. Never run the ultrasonic unit unless solutions are in both containers. In addition, the items being cleaned must be submerged in the cleaning solution.

Many different items can be cleaned in an ultrasonic unit. Examples include instruments, impression trays, glass products, and most jewelry. Do not use the ultrasonic unit on jewelry with pearls or pasted stones. The sound waves can destroy the pearls or the paste holding the stones. Prior to cleaning, most of the dirt or particles should be brushed off the items being cleaned. It is better to clean a few articles at a time and avoid overloading the unit. If items are close together, the process of cavitation is poor because the bubbles cannot strike all parts of the items being cleaned.

The glass beakers used in the ultrasonic unit are made of a type of glass that allows the passage of sound waves. After continual use, the sound waves etch the bottom of the beakers. A white, opaque coating forms. The beakers must be discarded and replaced when this occurs. After each use, the beakers should be washed with soap and water and rinsed thoroughly to remove any soapy residue. They must be dry before being filled with solution because water in the beaker can dilute the solution.

The permanent tank of the unit must be drained and cleaned at intervals based on tank use or appearance of the solution in the tank. A drain valve on the side of the tank is opened to allow the solution to drain. The tank is then wiped with a damp cloth or disinfectant.

Another damp cloth or disinfectant is used to wipe off the outside of the unit. Never submerge the unit in water to clean it. After cleaning, a fresh solution should be placed in the permanent tank.

Read the manufacturer's instructions carefully before using any ultrasonic unit. Most manufacturers provide cleaning charts that state the type of solution and time required for a variety of cleaning problems. Each time an item is cleaned in an ultrasonic unit, the chart should be used to determine the correct cleaning solution and time required.

STUDENT Go to the workbook and complete the assignment sheet for 12:7, *Cleaning with an Ultrasonic Unit. Then return and continue with the procedure.*

PROCEDURE

Cleaning with an Ultrasonic Unit 12:7

EQUIPMENT AND SUPPLIES

Ultrasonic unit, permanent tank with solution, beakers or auxiliary pans with covers, beaker bands, cleaning solutions, transfer forceps or pickups, paper towels, brush, soap, water for rinsing, articles for cleaning, solution chart

PROCEDURE

1. Assemble all equipment.
2. Wash hands.
3. Use a brush and soap and water to remove any large particles of dirt from articles to be cleaned. Rinse articles thoroughly.
   NOTE: Rinsing is important because soap may interact with the cleaning solution.
4. Check the permanent tank to be sure it has enough cleaning solution. An all-purpose cleaning solution is usually used in this tank.

(!) *CAUTION:* Never run the unit without solution in the permanent tank.
   NOTE: Many solutions must be diluted before use; if new solution is needed, read the instructions on the bottle.
5. Pour the proper cleaning solution into the auxiliary pans or beakers.
   NOTE: Use the cleaning chart to determine which solution to use.

(!) *CAUTION:* Read label before using.
   CAUTION: Handle solutions carefully. Avoid contact with skin and eyes.
6. Place the beakers or auxiliary pans into the permanent tank (see figure 12-29). Use beaker positioning covers and beaker bands. Beaker bands are large bands that circle the beakers to hold them in position and keep them from hitting the bottom of the permanent tank.
7. Check to be sure that the bottoms of the beakers or pans are below the level of solution in the permanent tank.
   NOTE: In order for sonic waves to flow through solutions in beakers or pans, the two solution levels must overlap.
8. Place articles to be cleaned in the beakers or pans. Be sure the solution completely covers the articles. Do not get solution on your hands.

Figure 12-29 The auxiliary basket **(top)** can be used to clean larger items in an ultrasonic unit. Glass beakers **(right)** can be used to clean smaller items in an ultrasonic unit.

NOTE: Remember that pearls or pasted stones cannot be cleaned in an ultrasonic unit.

9. Turn the timer past 5 (minutes) and then set the proper cleaning time. Use the cleaning chart to determine the correct amount of time required for the items. Most articles are cleaned in 2 to 5 minutes.

10. Check that the unit is working. You should see a series of bubbles in both solutions. This is called cavitation.

   ! *CAUTION:* Do not get too close. Solution can spray into your face and eyes. Use beaker lids to prevent spray.

11. When the timer stops, cleaning is complete. Use transfer forceps or pick-ups to lift articles from the pans or beakers. Place the articles on paper towels. Then rinse articles thoroughly under running water.

   ! *CAUTION:* Avoid contact with skin. Solutions are toxic.

12. Allow articles to air dry or dry them with paper towels. Inspect the articles for cleanliness. If they are not clean, repeat the process.

13. Periodically change solutions in the permanent tank and auxiliary containers. Do this when solutions become cloudy or cleaning has not been effective. To clean the permanent tank, place a container under the side drain to collect the solution. Then open the valve and drain solution from the tank. Wash the inside with a damp cloth or disinfectant. To clean the auxiliary pans or beakers, discard the solution. (It can be poured down the sink, but allow water to run for a time after disposing of the solution.) Then wash the containers and rinse thoroughly.

   NOTE: If the bottoms of beakers are etched and white, the beakers must be discarded and replaced.

14. Clean and replace all equipment used. Make sure all beakers are covered with lids.

15. Wash hands.

PRACTICE Go to the workbook and use the evaluation sheet for 12:7, Cleaning with an Ultrasonic Unit, to practice this procedure. When you feel you have mastered this skill, sign the sheet and give it to your instructor for further action.

✔ *Final Checkpoint* Using the criteria listed on the evaluation sheet, your instructor will grade you on your performance.

INFORMATION
12:8 *Using Sterile Techniques*

Many procedures require the use of sterile techniques to protect the patient from further infection. *Surgical asepsis* refers to procedures that keep an object or area free from living organisms. The main facts are presented here.

Sterile means "free from all organisms," including spores and viruses. **Contaminated** means that organisms and pathogens are present. While working with sterile supplies, it is important that correct techniques be followed to maintain sterility and avoid contamination. It is also important that you are able to recognize sterile surfaces and contaminated surfaces.

A clean, uncluttered working area is required when working with sterile supplies. If other objects are in the way, it is easy to contaminate sterile articles. If sterile articles touch the skin or any part of your clothing, they are no longer sterile. Because any area below the waist is considered contaminated, sterile articles must be held away from and in front of the body and above the waist.

Once a **sterile field** has been set up (for example, a sterile towel has been placed on a tray), never reach across the top of the field. Microorganisms can drop from your arm or clothing and contaminate the field. Always reach in from either side to place additional articles on the field. Never turn your back to a sterile field.

The 2-inch border around the sterile field (towel-covered tray) is considered contaminated. Therefore, 2 inches around the outside of the field must not be used when sterile articles are placed on the sterile field.

Various techniques can be used to remove articles from sterile wraps, depending on the article being unwrapped. Some common techniques are the drop, mitten, and transfer-forceps techniques:

◆ *Drop technique*: for gauze pads, dressings, small items. The wrapper is partially opened and then held upside down over the sterile field. The item drops out of the wrapper and onto the sterile field (see figure 12-30A). It is important to keep fingers back so the article does not touch the skin as it falls out of the wrapper. It is also important to avoid touching the inside of the wrapper.

◆ *Mitten technique*: for bowls, drapes, linen, and other similar items. The wrapper is opened and its loose ends are grasped around the wrist with the opposite hand (see figure 12-30B). In this way, a mitten is formed around the hand that is still holding the item (for example, a bowl). With the mitten hand, the item can be placed on the sterile tray.

◆ *Transfer forceps*: for cotton balls, small items, or articles that cannot be removed by the drop or mitten techniques. Either sterile gloves or sterile transfer forceps (pick-ups) are used. Sterile transfer forceps or pick-ups are removed from their container of disinfectant solution and used to grasp the article from the opened package. Remove the item

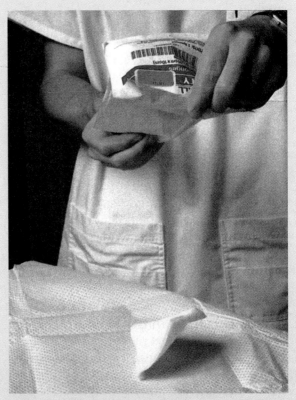

Figure 12-30A Sterile items can be dropped from the wrapper onto the sterile field.

Figure 12-30B By using the wrap as a mitten, sterile supplies can be placed on a sterile field. *(Photo by Michael Dzaman)*

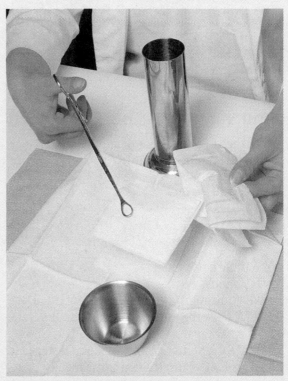

Figure 12-30C Sterile transfer forceps or pick-ups can be used to grasp sterile items and place them on a sterile field. *(Photo by Michael Dzaman)*

from the opened, sterile wrap and place it on the sterile field (see figure 12-30C). It is important to keep the transfer forceps pointed in a downward direction. If they are pointed upward, the solution will flow back to the handle, become contaminated, and return to contaminate the sterile tips when they are being used to pick up items. In addition, care must be taken not to touch the sides of the forceps container while removing or inserting the transfer forceps. Also, before using the transfer forceps, carefully shake them to get rid of excess disinfectant solution.

Organisms and pathogens travel quickly through a wet surface, so the sterile field must be kept dry. If a sterile towel or article gets wet, contamination has occurred. It is very important to use care when pouring solutions into sterile bowls or using solutions around a sterile field.

Make sure your sterile tray is open and you are ready to do the sterile procedure *before* putting the sterile gloves on your hands. Sterile gloves are considered sterile on the outside and

contaminated on the inside (side against the skin). Once they have been placed on the hands, it is important to hold the hands away from the body and above the waist to avoid contamination. You must handle only sterile objects while wearing sterile gloves.

If at any time during a procedure there is any suspicion that you have contaminated any article, start over. Never take a chance on using contaminated equipment or supplies.

A wide variety of commercially prepared sterile supplies is available. Packaged units are often set up for special procedures, such as changing dressings. Many agencies use these units instead of setting up special trays. Observe all sterile principles while using these units and read any directions provided with the units.

STUDENT *Go to the workbook and complete the assignment sheet for 12:8, Using Sterile Techniques. Then return and continue with the procedures.*

PROCEDURE

Opening Sterile Packages   12:8A

EQUIPMENT AND SUPPLIES

Sterile package of equipment or supplies, a table or other flat surface, sterile field (tray with sterile towel)

PROCEDURE

1. Assemble equipment.
2. Wash hands.
3. Take equipment to the area where it will be used. Check the autoclave indicator and date on the package.
   NOTE: Contents are not considered sterile if 30 days have elapsed since autoclaving.
4. Pick up the package with the tab or sealed edge pointing toward you. If the item is small, it can be held in the hand while being un-wrapped. If it is large, place it on a table or other flat surface.
5. Loosen the wrapper fastener (usually tape).
6. Check to be sure the package is away from your body. If it is on a table, make sure it is not close to other objects.
   NOTE: Avoid possible contamination by keeping sterile supplies away from other objects.
7. Open the distal (furthest) flap of the wrapper by grasping the outside of the wrapper and pulling it away from you (see figure 12-31A).
   🛑 *CAUTION:* Do not reach across the top of the package. Reach around the package to open it.
8. With one hand, raise a side flap and pull later-ally (sideways) away from the package (see figure 12-31B).
   🛑 *CAUTION:* Do *not* touch the inside of the wrapper at any time.
9. With the opposite hand, open the other side flap by pulling the tab to the side (see figure 12-31C).
   NOTE: Always reach in from the side. Never reach across the top of the sterile field or across any opened edges.

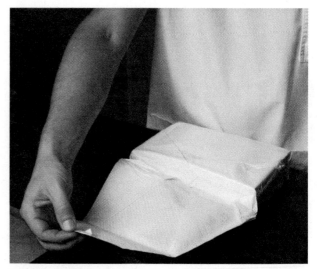

Figure 12-31A To open a sterile package, open the top flap away from you, handling only the outside of the wrap.

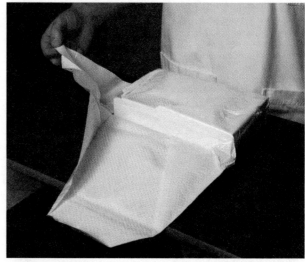

Figure 12-31B Open one side by pulling the wrap out to the side.

10. Open the proximal (closest) flap by lifting the flap up and toward you. Then drop it over the front of your hand (or the table), see figure 12-31D.
    🛑 *CAUTION:* Be careful not to touch the in-side of the package or the contents of the package.
11. Transfer the contents of the sterile package using one of the following techniques:
    a. Drop: Separate the ends of the wrap and pull apart gently (see figure 12-32). Avoid touching the inside of the wrap. Secure the loose ends of the wrap and hold the pack-

Figure 12-31C Open the opposite side by pulling the wrap out to the opposite side.

Figure 12-31D Open the side nearest to you by pulling back on the wrap.

Figure 12-32 Separate the ends of the wrap and pull the edges apart gently without touching the contents.

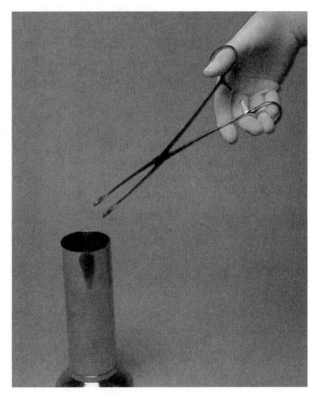

Figure 12-33 Remove the transfer or pick-up forceps without touching the sides of the container and point them in a downward direction.

age upside down over the sterile field. Allow the contents to drop onto the sterile tray.

b. Mitten: Grasp the contents securely by holding on to the outside of the wrapper as you unwrap it. With your free hand, gather the loose edges of the wrapper together and hold them securely around your wrist. This can be compared to making a mitten of the wrapper (with the sterile equipment on the outside of the mitten). Place the item on the sterile tray or hand it to someone who is wearing sterile gloves.

c. Transfer forceps: Remove forceps from their sterile container, taking care not to touch the side of the container with the forceps (see figure 12-33). Hold the forceps pointed downward. Shake them to remove excess disinfectant solution. Take care not to touch anything with the forceps. Use the forceps to grasp the item in the package and then place the item on the sterile tray.

NOTE: The method of transfer depends on the sterile item being transferred.

NOTE: If at any time during the procedure there is any suspicion that you have contaminated any article, start over. Never take a chance on using equipment for a sterile procedure if there is any possibility that the equipment is contaminated.

12. Replace all equipment used.
13. Wash hands.

PRACTICE *Go to the workbook and use the evaluation sheet for 12:8A, Opening Sterile Packages, to practice this procedure. When you feel you have mastered this skill, sign the sheet and give it to your instructor for further action.*

✔ *Final Checkpoint* Using the criteria listed on the evaluation sheet, your instructor will grade you on your performance.

PROCEDURE

Preparing a Sterile Dressing Tray 12:8B

EQUIPMENT AND SUPPLIES

Tray, sterile towels, sterile basin, sterile cotton balls or gauze sponges, sterile dressings (different sizes), antiseptic solution, forceps in disinfectant solution

PROCEDURE

1. Assemble all equipment.
2. Wash hands.
3. Check the date and autoclave indicator for sterility. If more than 30 days have elapsed, use another package with a more recent date. Put the unsterile package aside for re-sterilization.

4. Place the tray on a flat surface or a Mayo stand.
   NOTE: Make sure the work area is clean and dry and there is sufficient room to work.
5. Open the package that contains the sterile towel. Be sure it is held away from your body. Place the wrapper on a surface away from the tray or work area. Touch only the outside of the towel. Pick up the towel at its outer edge. Allow it to open by releasing the fanfolds. Place the towel with the outer side (side you have touched) on the tray. The untouched, or sterile, side will be facing up. Holding onto the outside edges of the towel, fanfold the back of the towel so the towel can be used later to cover the supplies.
   ⊘ *CAUTION:* Do not reach across the top of the towel. Reach in from either side.
   NOTE: If you are setting up a relatively large work area, one towel may not be large enough when fanfolded to cover the supplies. In such a case, you will need a second sterile towel (later) to cover your sterile field.
   ⊘ *CAUTION:* At all times, make sure that you do *not* touch the sterile side of the towel. Avoid letting the towel come in contact with your uniform, other objects, or contaminated areas.
6. Correctly unwrap the package containing the sterile basin. Place the basin on the tray. Do not place it close to the edge of the towel.
   NOTE: A 2-inch border around the outside edges of the towel is considered to be contaminated. No equipment should come in contact with this border.
   ⊘ *CAUTION:* Make sure that the wrapper does *not* touch the towel while placing the basin in position.
7. Unwrap the package containing the sterile cotton balls or gauze sponges. Use a dropping motion to place them in the basin. Do not touch the basin with the wrapper.
8. Unwrap the package containing the larger dressing. Use the sterile forceps to remove the dressing from the package and place it on the tray. Make sure the dressing is not too close to the edge of the towel.
   NOTE: The larger, outside dressing is placed on the tray first (before other dressings). In this way, the supplies will be in the order of use. For example, gauze dressings placed directly on the skin will be on top of the pile,

and a thick abdominal pad used on top of the gauze pads will be on the bottom of the pile.
NOTE: The forceps must be lifted straight up out of the container and must *not* touch the side of the container. Keep the tips pointed down and above the waist at all times. Shake off excess disinfectant solution.

9. Unwrap the inner dressings correctly. Use the sterile forceps to place them on top of the other dressings on the sterile towel, or use a drop technique.
NOTE: Dressings are now in a pile; the dressing that will be used first is on the top of the pile.
NOTE: The number and type of dressings is determined by checking the patient being treated.

10. Open the bottle containing the correct antiseptic solution. Place the cap on the table, with the inside of the cap facing up. Pour a small amount of the solution into the sink to clean the lip of the bottle. Then hold the bottle over the basin and pour a sufficient amount of solution into the basin (see figure 12-34).
CAUTION: Make sure that no part of the bottle touches the basin or the sterile tray. Pour carefully to avoid splashing. If the tray gets wet, the entire tray will be contaminated, and you must begin again.

11. Check the tray to make sure all needed equipment is on it.

12. Pick up the fanfolded edge of the towel by placing one hand on each side edge of the towel on the underside, or contaminated side. Do not touch the sterile side. Keep your hands and arms to the side of the tray, and bring the towel forward to cover the supplies.
NOTE: A second sterile towel may be used to cover the supplies if the table or sterile field area is too large to be covered by the one fanfolded towel.
CAUTION: Never reach across the top of the sterile tray.

13. Once the sterile tray is ready, never allow it out of your sight. Take it to the patient area and use it immediately. If you need more equipment, you must take the tray with you. This is the only way to be completely positive that the tray does not become contaminated.

14. Replace equipment.

15. Wash hands.

PRACTICE Go to the workbook and use the evaluation sheet for 12:8B, Preparing a Sterile Dressing Tray, to practice this procedure. When you feel you have mastered this skill, sign the sheet and give it to your instructor for further action.

✔ *Final Checkpoint* Using the criteria listed on the evaluation sheet, your instructor will grade you on your performance.

PROCEDURE

Donning and Removing Sterile Gloves
12:8C

EQUIPMENT AND SUPPLIES

Sterile gloves, powder (if necessary)

PROCEDURE

1. Assemble equipment and take it to the area where it is to be used. Check the date and/or

Figure 12-34 Avoid splashing the solution onto the sterile field while pouring it into the basin. *(Photo by Michael Dzaman)*

Figure 12-35A Open the package of gloves, taking care not to touch the inside of the inner wrapper.

Figure 12-35B Pick up the first glove by grasping the glove on the top edge of the folded-down cuff.

Figure 12-35C Hold the glove securely by the cuff and slip the opposite hand into the glove.

Figure 12-35D Slip the gloved fingers under the cuff of the second glove to lift it from the package, and insert the other hand into the glove.

Figure 12-35E Adjust the gloves into position, taking care not to touch the skin with the gloved hands.

autoclave indicator on the package to be sure gloves are still sterile. If they are not, put the package aside for re-sterilization and select a package with a current sterilization date.

2. Remove rings. Wash hands. Dry hands thoroughly.

3. Open the package of gloves, taking care not to touch the inside of the inner wrapper. The inner wrapper contains the gloves. Gently open it (see figure 12-35A). The folded cuffs will be nearest you.

   CAUTION: If you touch the *inside* of the package (where the gloves are), get a new package and start again.

4. If a powder packet is in the package, lift the packet out without touching the gloves. Do *not* hold the powder over the gloves. Hold it over a waste container or sink and open the packet. Sprinkle the powder on your hands and then rub your hands together to distribute the powder.

NOTE: Most sterile gloves are prepowdered on the inside. If they are, this step is not necessary.

5. The glove for the right hand will be on the right side of the package. With the thumb and forefinger of the left hand pick up the top edge of the folded-down cuff (inside of glove). Remove the glove carefully (see figure 12-35B).

⬣ *CAUTION:* Do *not* touch the outside of the glove. This is sterile. Only the part that will be next to the skin can be touched. Remember, unsterile touches unsterile and sterile touches sterile.

NOTE: Left-handed people may remove the left glove first.

6. Hold the glove by the inside cuff and slip the fingers and thumb of your right hand into the glove. Pull it on carefully (see figure 12-35C).

NOTE: Hold the glove away from the body. Pull gently to avoid tearing the glove.

7. Insert your gloved right hand under the cuff (outside) of the left glove and remove the left glove from the package (see figure 12-35D). Do not touch any other area with your gloved right hand while removing the left glove from the package.

⬣ *CAUTION:* If contamination occurs, discard the gloves and start again.

8. Holding your gloved right hand under the cuff of the left glove, insert your left hand in the left glove. Keep the thumb of your gloved right hand tucked in to avoid possible contamination.

9. Turn the cuffs up by manipulating only the sterile surface of the gloves (sterile touches sterile). Go up under the folded cuffs, pull out slightly, and turn cuffs over and up (see figure 12-35E.) Do not touch the inside of the gloves or the skin with your gloved hand.

⬣ *CAUTION:* If contamination occurs, start again with a new pair of gloves.

10. Do not touch anything that is not sterile once the gloves are in place. Gloves are applied for the purpose of performing procedures requiring sterile technique. During any procedure, they become contaminated with organisms related to the patient's condition, for example, wound drainage or blood and other body discharges. Even a clean, dry wound may contaminate gloves.

NOTE: Gloved hands should remain in position above the waist. Do *not* allow them to fall below waist.

11. After the procedure requiring sterile gloves is completed, dispose of all contaminated supplies before removing gloves.

NOTE: This reduces the danger of cross-infection caused by handling contaminated supplies without glove protection.

12. To remove the gloves, use one gloved hand to grasp the other glove by the outside of the cuff. Taking care not to touch the skin, remove the glove by pulling it down over the hand. It will be wrong side out when removed.

NOTE: This prevents contamination of your hands by organisms picked up during performance of the procedure. Now you must consider the outside of the gloves contaminated, and the area inside, next to your skin, clean.

13. Insert your bare fingers on the inside of the second glove. Remove the glove by pulling it down gently, taking care not to touch the outside of the glove with your bare fingers. It will be wrong side out when removed.

⬣ *CAUTION:* Avoid touching your uniform or any other object with the contaminated gloves.

14. Put the contaminated gloves in an infectious waste container immediately after removal.

NOTE: Most sterile gloves are disposable. If not, gloves should be placed in a container of disinfectant solution to soak. Soaking prevents contamination and helps keep substances from drying and sticking to the gloves.

15. Wash your hands immediately and thoroughly after removing gloves.

16. Once the gloves have been removed, do not handle any contaminated equipment or supplies such as soiled dressings or drainage basins. Protect yourself.

17. Replace equipment if necessary.

18. Wash hands thoroughly.

PRACTICE *Go to the workbook and use the evaluation sheet for 12:8C, Donning and Removing Sterile Gloves, to practice this procedure. When you feel you have mastered this skill, sign the sheet and give it to your instructor for further action.*

Final Checkpoint Using the criteria listed on the evaluation sheet, your instructor will grade you on your performance.

PROCEDURE

Changing a Sterile Dressing 12:8D

EQUIPMENT AND SUPPLIES

Sterile tray with basin, solution, gauze sponges and pads (or a prepared sterile dressing package); sterile gloves; adhesive or nonallergic tape; disposable gloves; infectious waste bag

PROCEDURE

1. Check doctor's written orders or obtain orders from immediate supervisor.
   NOTE: Dressings should *not* be changed without orders.
   NOTE: The policy of your agency will determine how you obtain orders for procedures.
2. Assemble equipment. Check autoclave indicator and date on all equipment. If more than 30 days have elapsed, use another package with a more recent date. Put the unsterile package aside for resterilization.
3. Wash hands thoroughly.
4. Prepare a sterile tray as previously taught (in Procedure 12:8B) or obtain a commercially prepared sterile dressing package.
   NOTE: Prepared packages are used in some agencies.
   CAUTION: Never let the tray out of your sight once it has been prepared.
5. Take all necessary equipment to the patient area. Place it where it will be convenient for use yet free from possible contamination by other equipment, for example, an uncluttered bedside tray or stand.
6. Introduce yourself. Identify the patient. Explain the procedure. Close the door and/or windows to avoid drafts and flow of organisms into the room.

7. Screen the unit or draw curtains to provide privacy for the patient. If the patient is in a bed, elevate the bed to a comfortable working height and lower the siderail. Expose the body area needing the dressing change. Use sheets or drapes as necessary to prevent unnecessary exposure of the patient.
8. Fold down a 2- to 3-inch cuff on the top of the infectious waste bag. Position it in a convenient location. Tear off the tape you will need later to secure the clean dressing. Place it in an area where it will be available for easy access.
9. Put on disposable, nonsterile gloves. Gently but firmly remove the tape from the soiled dressing. Discard it in the infectious waste bag. Hold the skin taut and then lift the dressing carefully, taking care not to pull on any surgical drains. Note the type, color, and amount of drainage on the dressing. Discard dressing in the infectious waste bag.
   NOTE: Surgical drains are placed in some surgical incisions to aid the removal of secretions. Care must be taken to avoid moving the drains when the dressing is removed.
10. Check the incision site. Observe the type and amount of remaining drainage, color of drainage, and degree of healing.
    CAUTION: Report any unusual observations immediately to your supervisor. Examples are bright-red blood, pain, faintness, pus, swelling, or abnormal discharges.
11. Remove disposable gloves and place in infectious waste bag. Immediately wash your hands.
    CAUTION: Nonsterile disposable gloves should be worn while removing dressings to avoid contamination of the hands or skin by blood or body discharge.
12. Fanfold the towel back to uncover the sterile tray.
    CAUTION: Handle only the contaminated (outside) side of the towel. The side in contact with the tray's contents is the sterile side.
    NOTE: If a prepared package is used, open it at this time.
13. Don sterile gloves as previously taught in Procedure 12:8C.
14. Using thumb and forefinger, pick up a gauze sponge from the basin. Squeeze it slightly to remove any excess solution. Warn the patient that the solution may be cool.

15. Cleanse the wound. Use a circular motion (see figure 12-36).

    NOTE: Begin near the center of the wound and move outward or away from the wound. Make an ever-widening circle. Discard the wet gauze sponge after use. Never go back over the same area with the same gauze sponge. Repeat this procedure until the area is clean, using a new gauze sponge each time.

16. Do not cleanse directly over the wound unless there is a great deal of drainage or it is specifically ordered by the physician. If this is to be done, use sterile gauze and wipe with a single stroke from the top to the bottom. Discard the soiled gauze. Repeat as necessary, using a new sterile gauze sponge each time.

17. The wound is now ready for clean dressings. Lift the sterile dressings from the tray and place them lightly on the wound. Make sure they are centered over the wound.

    NOTE: The inner dressing is usually made up of 4-by -4-inch gauze sponges.

18. Apply outer dressings until the wound is sufficiently protected.

    NOTE: Heavier dressings such as abdominal pads are usually used.

    NOTE: The number and size of dressings needed to dress the wound will depend on the amount of drainage and the size of the wound.

19. Remove the sterile gloves as previously taught. Discard them in the infectious waste bag. Immediately wash your hands.

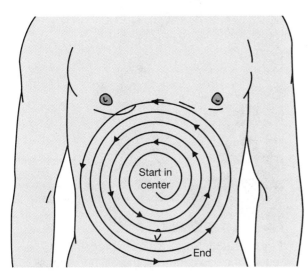

Figure 12-36 Use a circular motion to clean the wound, starting at the center of the wound and moving in an outward direction.

Figure 12-37 Tape should be applied so that it runs opposite to body action or movement. *(Photo by Michael Dzaman)*

20. Place the precut tape over the dressing at the proper angle. Check to make sure that the dressing is secure and the ends are closed.

    NOTE: Tape should be applied so it runs opposite from body action or movement (see figure 12-37). It should be the correct width for the dressing. It should be long enough to support the dressing, but it should not be too long because it will irritate the patient's skin.

21. Check to be sure the patient is comfortable and that safety precautions have been observed before leaving the area.

22. Put on disposable, nonsterile gloves. Clean and replace all equipment used. Tie or tape the infectious waste bag securely. Dispose of it according to agency policy.

    NOTE: Disposable, nonsterile gloves should be worn to provide a protective barrier while cleaning equipment or supplies that may be contaminated by blood or body fluids.

23. Remove disposable gloves. Wash hands thoroughly. Protect yourself from possible contamination.

24. Record the following information on the patient's chart or agency form: date, time, dressing change, amount and type of drainage, and any other pertinent information, or tell this information to your immediate supervisor.

    Example: 1/8/—, 9:00 A.M. Dressing changed on right abdominal area. Small amount of thick, light-yellow discharge noted on dressings. No swelling or inflammation apparent at incision site. Sterile dressing applied. Your signature and title.

    NOTE: Report any unusual observations immediately.

INFORMATION
12.9 *Maintaining Isolation*

OBRA In health occupations, you will deal with many different diseases/disorders. Some diseases are communicable and require isolation. A communicable disease is caused by a pathogenic organism that can be easily transmitted to others. This section introduces you to isolation principles and procedures.

Isolation is a method or technique of caring for patients who have communicable diseases. Examples of communicable diseases are tuberculosis, wound infections, and pertussis (whooping cough). Universal precautions, discussed in Information Section 12:3, do not eliminate the need for specific isolation precautions. Universal precautions are used on all patients. Isolation techniques are used to provide extra protection against specific diseases or pathogens to prevent their spread.

Communicable diseases are spread in many ways. Some examples include direct contact with the patient; contact with dirty linen, equipment, and/or supplies; and contact with blood and body excretions such as urine, feces, droplets (from sneezing, coughing, or spitting), and discharges from wounds. Isolation techniques are used to limit contact with pathogenic organisms. These techniques help prevent the spread of the disease to other people and protect patients, their families, and health care providers.

The type of isolation used depends on the causative organism of the disease, the way the organism is transmitted, and whether or not the pathogen is antibiotic resistant (not affected by antibiotics). Some isolation precautions require the use of gowns, gloves, and masks (see figure 12-38), while others only require the use of a mask.

Two terms are extensively used in isolation: *contaminated* and *clean*. These words refer to the presence of organisms on objects.

a. Contaminated, or dirty, means that objects contain disease-producing organisms. These objects must not be touched, unless the health worker is protected by gloves, gown, and other required items.
NOTE: The outside of the gown, protective gloves, mask, and waist ties are considered contaminated.

b. Clean means that objects or parts of objects do *not* contain disease-producing organisms and therefore have minimal chance of spreading the disease. Every effort must be made to prevent contamination of these objects or parts of objects.

Figure 12-38 Some isolation precautions require the use of gowns, gloves, and a mask, while others only require the use of a mask.

NOTE: The insides of the gown and gloves are clean, as are the neckband, its ties, and the mask ties.

The Centers for Disease Control (CDC) in conjunction with the National Center for Infectious Diseases (NCID) and the Hospital Infection Control Practices Advisory Committee (HICPAC) has recommended four main classifications of precautions that should be followed: standard, airborne, droplet, and contact. Health care facilities are provided with a list of infections/conditions that shows the type and duration of precautions needed for each specific disease. In this way, facilities can follow the guidelines to determine the type of isolation that should be used along with the specific precautions that must be followed.

Standard precautions, also called universal precautions (discussed in Information Section 12:3), are used on all patients. In addition, a patient should be placed in a private room if the patient contaminates the environment or does not (or cannot be expected to) assist in maintaining appropriate hygiene. Every health care worker must be well informed about universal or standard precautions and follow the recommendations for the use of gloves, masks, gowns, and face masks when conditions indicate their use.

Airborne precautions are used for patients known or suspected to be infected with pathogens transmitted by airborne droplet nuclei, small particles of evaporated droplets that contain microorganisms and remain suspended in the air. Examples of diseases requiring these isolation precautions are measles, varicella (chicken pox), tuberculosis, and herpes zoster (varicella-zoster). In addition to using standard or universal precautions, several other precautions are required. The patient should be placed in a private room, and the door should be kept closed. Air in the room should be discharged to outdoor air or filtered before being circulated to other areas. Each person who enters the room must wear respiratory protection in the form of a mask. People susceptible to measles or chicken pox should not enter the room. If at all possible, the patient should not be moved from the room. If transport is essential, however, the patient should wear a surgical mask during transport to minimize the release of droplets into the air.

Droplet precautions must be followed for a patient known or suspected to be infected with pathogens transmitted by large-particle droplets expelled during coughing, sneezing, or talking. Examples of diseases requiring these isolation precautions include *Haemophilus influenzae* meningitis and pneumonia; *Neisseria* meningitis and pneumonia; multidrug-resistant *Streptococcus* meningitis, pneumonia, sinusitis, and otitis media; diphtheria; *Mycoplasma* pneumonia; pertussis; adenovirus; mumps; and severe viral influenza. In addition to using standard or universal precautions, the patient should be placed in a private room. If a private room is not available and the patient cannot be placed in a room with a patient who has the same infection, a distance of at least 3 feet should separate the infected patient and other patients or visitors. Masks must be worn when working within three feet of the patient, and the use of masks anywhere in the room is strongly recommended. If transport or movement of the patient is essential, the patient should wear a surgical mask.

Contact precautions must be followed for any patients known or suspected to be infected with epidemiologically (capable of spreading rapidly from person to person, an epidemic) important microorganisms that can be transmitted by either direct or indirect contact. Examples of diseases requiring these precautions include any gastrointestinal, respiratory, skin, or wound infections caused by multidrug-resistant organisms; diapered or incontinent patients with enterohemorrhagic *E. coli*, *Shigella*, hepatitis A, or rotavirus; viral or hemorrhagic conjunctivitis or fevers; and any skin infections that are highly contagious or that may occur on dry skin, such as diphtheria, herpes simplex virus, impetigo, pediculosis, scabies, and staphylococcal infections. In addition to using standard or universal precautions, the patient should be placed in a private room or, if a private room is not available, in a room with a patient who has an active infection caused by the same organism. Gloves should be worn when entering the room. Gloves should be changed after having contact with any material that may contain high concentrations of the microorganism, such as wound drainage or fecal material. Gloves should be removed before leaving the room, and the hands should be washed with an antimicrobial agent. A gown should be worn in the room if there is any chance of contact with the patient, environmental surfaces, or items in the room. The gown should be removed before leaving the room and care should be taken to ensure that clothing is not contaminated after gown removal. Movement and transport of the patient from the room should be for essential purposes only. The room and items in it should receive daily cleaning and disinfection as needed. If possible, patient-care equipment (bedside commode, stethoscope, sphygmomanometer, thermometer) should be left in the room and used only for the patient. If this is not possible, all equipment must be cleaned and disinfected before being used on another patient.

Protective or reverse isolation refers to methods used to protect certain patients from organisms present in the environment. Protective isolation is used mainly for immunocompromised patients, or patients whose body defenses are not capable of protecting them from infections and disease. Examples of patients requiring this protection are patients whose immune systems have been depressed prior to receiving transplants (such as bone marrow transplants), severely burned patients, or patients whose immune systems have failed. Precautions vary depending on the patient's condition. The patient is usually placed in a room that has been cleaned and disinfected. Frequent disinfection occurs while the patient occupies the room. Many facilities require anyone entering the room to wear clean or sterile gowns, gloves, and masks. All equipment or supplies brought into the room are clean, disinfected, and/or sterile. Special filters may be used to purify air that enters the room. Every effort is made to protect the patient from microorganisms that cause infection or disease.

Exact procedures for maintaining isolation vary from one facility to another. The procedures used depend on the type of units provided for isolation patients, and on the kind of supplies or special isolation equipment available. Most facilities convert a regular patient room into an isolation room, but some facilities use special, two-room isolation units. Some facilities use disposable supplies like gloves, gowns, treatment packages, and other items for their patients in isolation. Therefore, it is essential that you learn the isolation procedure followed by your agency. However, the basic principles for maintaining isolation are the same regardless of the facility. Therefore, if you know these basic principles, you will be able to adjust to any setting.

STUDENT Go to the workbook and complete the assignment sheet for 12:9, Maintaining Isolation. Then return and continue with the procedures.

PROCEDURE

Donning and Removing Isolation Garments 12:9A

NOTE: The following procedure deals with contact isolation. For other types of isolation, follow only the steps that apply.

EQUIPMENT AND SUPPLIES

Isolation gown, surgical mask, gloves, small plastic bag, linen cart or container, plastic-lined waste can, paper towels, sink with running water

PROCEDURE

1. Assemble equipment.
   NOTE: In many agencies, clean isolation garments and supplies are kept available on a

cart outside the isolation unit, or in the outer room of a two-room unit. A waste container should be positioned just inside the door.

2. Wash hands.
3. Remove rings and place them in your pocket or pin them to your uniform.
4. Remove your watch and place it in a small plastic bag or centered on a clean paper towel. If placed on a towel, handle only the bottom part of the towel; do not touch the top.
   NOTE: The watch will be taken into the room and placed on the bedside stand for taking vital signs. Because it cannot be sterilized, it must be kept clean.
   NOTE: In some agencies, a plastic-covered watch is left in the isolation room.
5. Put on the mask. Secure it under your chin. Make sure to cover your mouth and nose. Handle the mask as little as possible. Tie the mask securely behind your head and neck. Tie the top ties first and the bottom ties second.
   NOTE: The tie bands on the mask are considered clean. The mask is considered contaminated.
   NOTE: The mask is considered to be contaminated after 30 minutes in isolation or anytime it gets wet. If you remain in isolation longer than 30 minutes, or if the mask gets wet, you must wash your hands, remove and discard the old mask, wash your hands again, and put on a clean mask.
6. If uniform sleeves are long, roll them up above the elbows before putting on the gown.
7. Lift the gown by placing your hands inside the shoulders (see figure 12-39A).
   NOTE: The inside of the gown and the ties at the neck are considered clean.
   NOTE: Most agencies use disposable gowns that are discarded after use.
8. Work your arms into the sleeves of the gown by gentle twisting. Take care not to touch your face with the sleeves of the gown.
9. Place your hands *inside* the neckband, adjust until it is in position, and then tie the bands at the back of your neck (see figure 12-39B).
10. Reach behind and fold the edges of the gown over so that the uniform is completely covered. Tie the waistbands (see figure 12-39C). Some waistbands are long enough to wrap around your body before tying.

Figure 12-39A After tying the mask in place, put on the gown by placing your hands inside the shoulders.

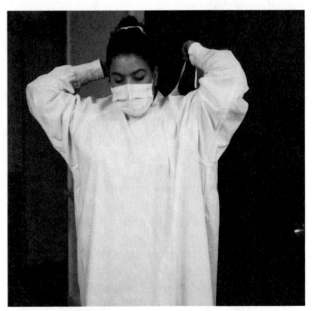

Figure 12-39B Slip your fingers inside the neckband to tie the gown at the neck.

11. If gloves are to be worn, put them on. Make sure that the cuff of the glove comes over the top of the cuff of the gown. In this way, there are no open areas for entrance of organisms.
12. You are now ready to enter the isolation room. Double check to be sure you have all equipment and supplies that you will need for patient care before you enter the room.

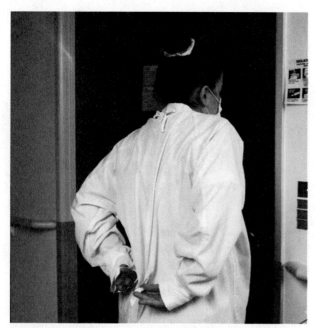

Figure 12-39C Overlap the back edges of the gown so your uniform is completely covered before tying the waist ties.

13. When patient care is complete, you will be ready to remove isolation garments. In a two-room isolation unit, go to the outer room. In a one-room unit, remove garments while you are standing close to the inside of the door. Take care to avoid touching the room's contaminated articles.

14. Untie the waist ties. Loosen the gown at the waist.
NOTE: The waist ties are considered contaminated.

15. If gloves are worn, remove the first glove by grasping the outside of the cuff with the opposite gloved hand. Pull the glove over the hand so that the glove is inside out. Remove the second glove by placing the bare hand inside the cuff. Pull the glove off so it is inside out. Place the disposable gloves in the proper waste container.
NOTE: Almost all gloves worn in isolation are disposable. If nondisposable gloves are used and are to be sterilized, a basin for soaking should be inside the isolation room.

16. To avoid unnecessary transmission of organisms, use paper towels to turn on the water faucet. Wash and dry your hands thoroughly. When they are dry, use a clean, dry paper towel to turn off the faucet.

⚠ CAUTION: Organisms travel rapidly through wet towels.

17. Untie the mask. Holding the mask by the ties only, drop it into the waste container.
NOTE: The ties of the mask are considered clean. Do not touch any other part of the mask because it is considered contaminated.

18. Untie the neck ties. Loosen the gown at the shoulders, handling only the inside of the gown.
NOTE: The neck ties are considered clean.

19. Slip the fingers of one hand inside the opposite cuff. Do *not* touch the outside. Pull the sleeve well down over the hand (see figure 12-40A).

⚠ CAUTION: The outside of the gown is considered contaminated and should not be touched.

20. Using the gown-covered hand, pull the sleeve down over the opposite hand (see figure 12-40B).

21. Ease your arms and hands out of the gown. Keep the gown in front of your body and keep your hands away from the outside of the gown. Use as gentle a motion as possible.
NOTE: Excessive flapping of the gown will spread organisms.

22. With your hands inside the gown at the shoulders, bring the shoulders together and turn the gown so that it is inside out (see figure 12-40C). In this manner, the outside of the con-taminated gown is on the inside. Fold the gown in half and then roll it together. Place it in the linen hamper. If the gown is disposable, place it in the waste container.
NOTE: Avoid excess motion during this procedure because motion causes the spread of organisms.

23. Wash hands thoroughly. Use dry, clean paper towels to operate the faucets.

24. Touch only the inside of the plastic bag to remove your watch. Discard the bag in the waste container. If the watch is on a paper towel, handle only the "clean," top portion (if necessary). Discard the towel in the waste container.

25. Use a clean paper towel to open the door. Discard the towel in the waste container before leaving the room.

⚠ CAUTION: The inside of the door is considered contaminated.
NOTE: The waste container should be positioned just inside the door of the room.

Figure 12-40A To remove the gown, slip the fingers of one hand under the cuff of the opposite arm to pull the gown down over the opposite hand.

Figure 12-40B Using the gown-covered hand, grasp the outside of gown on the opposite arm and pull the gown down over the hand.

Figure 12-40C With your hands inside the gown at the shoulders, bring the shoulders together and turn the gown so that it is inside out, with the contaminated side on the inside.

26. After leaving the isolation room, wash hands thoroughly. This will help prevent spread of the disease. It also protects you from the illness.

PRACTICE *Go to the workbook and use the evaluation sheet for 12:9A, Donning and Removing Isolation Garments, to practice this procedure. When you feel you have mastered this skill, sign the sheet and give it to your instructor for further action.*

✔ *Final Checkpoint* Using the criteria listed on the evaluation sheet, your instructor will grade you on your performance.

PROCEDURE

Working in a Hospital Isolation Unit   OBRA   *12:9B*

EQUIPMENT AND SUPPLIES

Clothes hamper, two laundry bags, two trays, dishes, cups, bowls, waste container lined with a plastic bag, infectious waste bags, bags, tape, pencil, pen, paper

PROCEDURE

1. Assemble all equipment.
    NOTE: Any equipment or supplies to be used in the isolation room must be assembled prior to entering the room.
2. Wash hands.
3. Put on appropriate isolation garments as previously instructed.
4. Tape paper to the outside of the isolation door. This will be used to record vital signs.
5. Enter the isolation room. Take all needed equipment into the room.
6. Introduce yourself. Greet and identify patient. Provide patient care as needed.

NOTE: All care is provided in a routine manner. However, isolation garments must be worn as ordered.

7. To record vital signs:
   a. Take vital signs using the watch in the plastic bag. (If the watch is not in a plastic bag, hold it with the bottom part of a paper towel.) Use other equipment in the room as needed.
   b. Open the door touching only the inside, or contaminated side.
   c. Using a pencil, record the vital signs on the paper taped to the door. Do *not* touch the outside of the door at any time.
      NOTE: The pencil remains in the room because it is contaminated.

8. To transfer food into the isolation unit:
   a. Transfer of food requires two people; one person must stay outside the unit and one inside.
   b. The person inside the isolation unit picks up the empty tray in the room and opens door, touching only the inside of the door.
   c. The person outside hands in the cups, bowls, and plates of food.
   d. When transfering food, the two people should handle the opposite sides of the dishes. In this manner, one person will not touch the other person.
   e. Glasses should be held near the top by the transfer person on the outside. The transfer person on the inside should receive the glasses by holding them on the bottom.

9. To dispose of leftover food or waste:
   a. Liquids can be poured down the sink or flushed down the toilet.
   b. Soft foods such as mashed potatoes or cooked vegetables can be flushed down the toilet.
   c. Hard particles of food, such as bone, should be placed in the plastic-lined trash container.
   d. Disposable utensils or dishes should be placed in the plastic-lined trash container.
   e. Metal utensils should be washed and kept in the isolation room to be used as needed for other meals. These utensils, however, are contaminated. When they are removed from the isolation room, they must be disinfected or double bagged and labeled before being sent for decontamination and reprocessing.

10. To transfer soiled linen from the unit, two people are required:
    a. All dirty linen should be folded and rolled.
    b. Place linen in the linen hamper.
    c. Person outside the unit should cuff the top of a clean laundry bag and hold it. Hands should be kept on the inside of the bag's cuff to avoid contamination.
    d. Person in isolation should seal the isolation bag. The bag is then placed inside the outer bag, which is being held by the person outside.
    e. Outer bag should be folded over at the top and taped by the person outside. The bag should then be labeled as "ISOLATION LINEN."
    f. At all times, no direct contact should occur between the two people transferring linen.
       NOTE: Many agencies use special isolation linen bags. Hot water dissolves the bags during the washing process. Therefore, no other personnel handle the contaminated linen after it leaves the isolation unit.

11. To transfer trash from the isolation unit, two people are required:
    a. Any trash in the isolation room should be in plastic bags. Any trash or disposable items contaminated with blood or body secretions should be placed in infectious waste bags.
    b. When the bag is full, expel excess air by pushing gently on the bag.
    c. Tie a knot at the top of the bag to seal it or fold the top edge twice and tape it securely.
    d. Place this bag inside a cuffed bag held by a "clean" person outside the unit.
    e. The outside person then ties the outer bag securely or tapes the outer bag shut, and labels it "ISOLATION."
    f. The double-bagged trash should then be burned. Double-bagged infectious waste is autoclaved prior to incineration or disposal as infectious waste according to legal requirements.
    g. At all times, direct contact between the two people transferring trash must be avoided.

12. To transfer equipment from the isolation unit two people are required:

a. Thoroughly clean all equipment in the unit.
b. After cleaning, place equipment in a plastic bag or special isolation bag. Label the bag with the contents and the word "ISOLATION."
c. After folding the bag down twice at the top, tape the bag shut.
d. A second person outside the isolation room should hold a second, cuffed bag.
e. The person in isolation places the sealed, contaminated bag inside the bag being held outside the unit. The person in isolation should have no direct contact with the clean bag.
f. The person outside the unit turns down the top of the outside bag twice and securely tapes the bag. The outside person then labels the bag with the word "isolation" and the contents, for example, "ISOLATION DISHES."
g. The double-bagged material is then sent to Central Supply or another designated area for sterilization and/or decontamination.
13. The isolation unit must be kept clean and neat at all times. Equipment no longer needed should be transferred out of the unit following the previous procedures.
14. Before leaving an isolation room, ask the patients whether a urinal or bedpan is needed. This will save time and energy by reducing the need to return to complete patient care shortly after leaving. Also, prior to leaving, check all safety and comfort points to make sure patient care is complete.
15. Remove isolation garments as previously instructed (in Procedure 12:9A).
16. Wash hands thoroughly.

PRACTICE *Go to the workbook and use the evaluation sheet for 12:9B, Working in a Hospital Isolation Unit, to practice this procedure. When you feel you have mastered this skill, sign the sheet and give it to your instructor for further action.*

✔ *Final Checkpoint* Using the criteria listed on the evaluation sheet, your instructor will grade you on your performance.

UNIT *12* SUMMARY

Understanding the basic principles of infection control is essential for any health care worker in any health care field. Disease is caused by a wide variety of pathogens, or germs. An understanding of the types of pathogens, methods of transmission, and the chain of infection allows health care workers to take precautions to prevent the spread of disease.

Asepsis is defined as "the absence of disease-producing microorganisms, or pathogens." Various levels of aseptic control are possible. Antisepsis refers to methods that prevent or inhibit the growth of pathogenic organisms. Proper handwashing and using an ultrasonic unit to clean instruments and supplies are examples. Disinfection is a process that destroys or kills pathogenic organisms, but is not always effective against spores and viruses. Boiling water and chemical disinfectants are used for this purpose. Sterilization is a process that destroys all microorganisms, including spores and viruses. The use of an autoclave is an example. Instruments and equipment are properly prepared, and then processed in the autoclave to achieve sterilization.

Following the universal precautions established by the Centers for Disease Control helps prevent the spread of pathogens by way of blood and body fluids. The universal precautions provide guidelines for handwashing; wearing gloves; using gowns, masks, and protective eyewear, when splashing is likely; proper handling and disposal of contaminated sharp objects; proper disposal of contaminated waste; and proper methods to wipe up spills of blood and/or body fluids. Every health care worker must be familiar with and follow the recommended universal precautions while working with all patients.

Sterile techniques are used in specific procedures, such as the changing of dressings. Health care workers must learn and follow sterile techniques when they are required to perform these procedures.

Isolation techniques are used for patients who have communicable diseases, or diseases that are easily transmitted from one person to another. An awareness of the major types of isolation presented in this unit will help the health care worker prevent the transmission of communicable diseases.

Infection control must be followed when performing any and every health care procedure. By learning and following the principles discussed in this unit, health care workers will protect themselves, patients, and others from disease.

——— UNIT 12 ———
SUGGESTED REFERENCES

Burhoe, Steven. *Bloodborne Pathogens: An Overview of OSHA's Standards.* Columbia, MO: Instructional Materials Laboratory, 1992.

Chasteen, Joseph E. *Essentials of Clinical Dental Assisting.* 4th ed. St. Louis, MO: C. V. Mosby, 1989.

Cooper, Marian G., and David E. Cooper. *The Medical Assistant.* 7th ed. New York, NY: McGraw-Hill, 1993.

Fong, Elizabeth, and Lynne Grover Lakomia. *Microbiology for Health Careers.* 5th ed. Albany, NY: Delmar Publishers, 1994.

Hegner, Barbara, and Esther Caldwell. *Nursing Assistant: A Nursing Process Approach.* 7th ed. Albany, NY: Delmar Publishers, 1995.

Keir, Lucille, Connie Krebs, and Barbara A. Wise. *Medical Assisting: Administrative and Clinical Competencies.* 3rd ed. Albany, NY: Delmar Publishers, 1993.

Long, Barbara C., and Wilma J. Phipps. *Medical Surgical Nursing.* 3rd ed. St. Louis, MO: C. V. Mosby, 1993.

National Safety Council. *Bloodborne Pathogens.* Boston, MA: Jones and Bartlett, 1993.

Palmer, Darwin, Sue Palmer, and Jeanne Giddens. *The Infection Control Book.* St. Louis, MO: Mosby, 1995.

Schaffer, Susan, Laurel Garzon, and Denise Korniewicz. *Pocket Guide to Infection Control.* St. Louis, MO: Mosby, 1995.

Schwarzrock, Shirley, and James R. Jenson. *Effective Dental Assisting.* 7th ed. Dubuque, IA: Wm. C. Brown, 1991.

U.S. Department of Health and Human Services. "Guidelines for Isolation Precautions in Hospitals." *Federal Register.* Vol. 59, No. 214, November 7, 1994.

For information on federal recommendations, contact the Centers for Disease Control, Atlanta, Georgia 30333.

Descriptive literature supplied with equipment such as autoclave, boiling water units, ultrasonic cleaners.

UNIT 13

Vital Signs

UNIT OBJECTIVES

After completing this unit of study, you should be able to:

- List the four main vital signs
- Convert Fahrenheit temperatures to Celsius, or Celsius to Fahrenheit
- Read a clinical thermometer to the nearest two-tenths of a degree
- Measure and record oral temperature accurately
- Measure and record rectal temperature accurately
- Measure and record axillary temperature accurately
- Measure and record tympanic temperature accurately
- Measure and record radial pulse to an accuracy within ± 2 beats per minute
- Count and record respirations to an accuracy within ± 1 respiration per minute
- Measure and record apical pulse to an accuracy within ± 2 beats per minute
- Measure and record blood pressure to an accuracy within ± 2 mm of actual mercury reading
- State the normal range for oral temperature, axillary temperature, rectal temperature, pulse, respirations, systolic pressure, and diastolic pressure
- Define, pronounce, and spell all of the key terms

KEY TERMS

apical pulse
(ape´-ih-kal)

apnea
(ap´-knee˝-ah)

aural

axillary

blood pressure

bradycardia
(bray˝-dee-car´-dee-ah)

character

Cheyne-Stokes
(chain´ stokes˝)

diastolic
(die˝-ah-stall´-ik)

dyspnea
(dis(p)´-knee˝-ah)

fever

homeostasis
(home˝-ee-oh-stay´-sis)

hyperthermia
(high-pur-therm´-ee-ah)

hypothermia
(high-po-therm´-ee-ah)

oral

pulse

pulse deficit

rale (rawl)

rate

rectal

respirations

rhythm

sphygmomanometer
(sfig˝-moh-ma-nam´-eh-ter)

stethoscope
(steth´-uh-scope)

systolic (sis˝-tall´-ik)

tachycardia
(tack˝-eh-car´-dee-ah)

temperature

thermometers

tympanic

vital signs

volume

INFORMATION
13:1 Measuring and Recording Vital Signs

Vital signs are important indicators of health states of the body. This unit discusses all of the vital signs in detail. The basic information that follows serves as an introduction for this topic.

Vital signs are defined as various determinations that provide information about the basic body conditions of the patient. The four main vital signs are temperature, pulse, respirations, and blood pressure. As a health care worker, it will be your responsibility to measure and record the vital signs of patients. However, it is not in your realm of duties to reveal this information to the patient. The physician will decide if the patient should be given this information. It is essential that vital signs be accurate. They are often the first indication of a disease or abnormality in the patient.

1/2 Temperature is a measurement of the balance between heat lost and heat produced by the body. It can be taken orally, rectally, axillary, and aurally. A low or high reading can indicate disease. Most temperatures are measured on a thermometer that has a Fahrenheit scale. However, some health care facilities are now measuring temperature on a Celsius scale. A comparison of the two scales is shown in figure 13-1. At times, it may be necessary to convert Fahrenheit temperatures to Celsius, or Celsius to Fahrenheit. The formulas for the conversion are as follows:

a. To convert Fahrenheit (F) temperatures to Celsius (C) temperatures, subtract 32 from the Fahrenheit temperature and then multiply the result by 5/9, or 0.5556. For example, to convert a Fahrenheit temperature of 212 to Celsius, subtract 32 from 212 to get 180. Then multiply 180 by 5/9, or 0.5556, to get the Celsius temperature of 100.0.

b. To convert Celsius (C) temperatures to Fahrenheit (F) temperatures, multiply the Celsius temperature by 9/5, or 1.8, and then add 32 to the total. For example, to convert a Celsius temperature of 37 to Fahrenheit, multiply 37 by 9/5, or 1.8, to get 66.6. Then add 32 to 66.6 to get the Fahrenheit temperature of 98.6.

Pulse is the pressure of the blood felt against the wall of an artery as the heart contracts and relaxes, or beats. The rate, rhythm, and volume are recorded. Rate refers to the number of beats per minute, rhythm refers to regularity, and volume refers to strength. The

Figure 13-1 Normal oral body temperature on Fahrenheit and Celsius thermometers.

pulse is usually taken over the radial artery, although it may be felt over any superficial artery that has a bone behind it. Any abnormality can indicate disease.

Respirations reflect the breathing rate of the patient. In addition to the respiration count, the rhythm (regularity) and character (type) of respirations are noted. Abnormal respirations usually indicate that a health problem or disease is present.

Blood pressure is the force exerted by the heart against the arterial walls when the heart contracts or relaxes. Two readings (systolic and diastolic) are noted to show the greatest pressure and the least pressure. Both are very important. Abnormal blood pressure is often the first indication of disease.

Another vital sign is the **apical pulse.** This pulse is taken with a stethoscope at the apex of the heart. The actual heartbeat is heard and counted. At times, because of illness, hardening of the arteries, a weak or very rapid radial pulse, or doctor's orders, you will be required to take an apical pulse. Also, because infants and small children have a very rapid radial pulse that is difficult to count, apical pulses are usually taken.

C If you note any abnormality or change in any vital sign, it is your responsibility to report this immediately to your supervisor. If you have difficulty obtaining a correct reading, ask another individual to check the patient. Never guess, or report an inaccurate reading.

STUDENT Go to the workbook and complete the assignment sheet for 13:1, Measuring and Recording Vital Signs.

INFORMATION

13:2 *Measuring and Recording Temperature*

OBRA Body temperature is one of the main vital signs. This section provides the basic guidelines for taking and recording temperature.

Temperature is defined as "the balance between heat lost and heat produced by the body." Heat is lost through perspiration, respiration, and excretion (urine and feces). Heat is produced by the metabolism of food, and muscle and gland activity. A constant state of fluid balance, known as **homeostasis,** is the

ideal health state in the human body. The rates of chemical reactions in the body are regulated by body temperature. Therefore, if body temperature is too high or low, the body's fluid balance is affected.

The normal range for body temperature is 97° to 100° Fahrenheit, or 36.1° to 37.8° Celsius (sometimes called centigrade). However, variations in body temperature can occur, as noted in the following information:

a. Individuals have different body temperatures. Some people have accelerated body processes and, thus, usually have higher temperatures. Others have slower body processes and, thus, lower temperatures.

b. Time of day also affects body temperature. Body temperature is usually lower in the morning, after the body has rested. It is higher in the evening, after muscular activity and daily food intake have taken place.

c. Parts of the body where temperatures are taken lead to variations.

(1) Oral temperatures are taken in the mouth. The clinical thermometer is left in place for 3 to 5 minutes. The normal oral temperature is 98.6°F (37°C), with a range of 97.6° to 99.6°F (36.5° to 37.5°C). This is usually the most common, convenient, and comfortable method of obtaining a temperature.

(2) Rectal temperatures are taken via the rectum. The clinical thermometer is left in place for 3 to 5 minutes. This is an internal measurement and is the most accurate of all methods. Normal temperature is 99.6°F (37.6°C), with a range of 98.6° to 100.6°F (37° to 38.1°C).

(3) An axillary temperature is taken in the armpit, under the upper arm. The arm is held close to the body, and the thermometer is inserted between the two folds of skin. A groin temperature is taken between the two folds of skin formed by the inner part of the thigh and the lower abdomen. Both axillary and groin are external temperatures and, thus, less accurate. The clinical thermometer is held in place for 10 minutes. Normal axillary or groin temperature is 97.6°F (36.4°C), with a range of 96.6° to 98.6°F (36° to 37°C).

(4) An aural temperature is taken with a special thermometer that is placed in the ear or auditory canal. The thermometer detects and measures the thermal, infrared energy radiating from the tympanic membrane, or eardrum. Because this provides a measurement of body core temperature, there is no normal range. Instead, the temperature is calculated by the thermometer into an equivalent of one of four usual settings: equal mode, oral equivalent, rectal equivalent, or core equivalent. The equal mode provides no offset and is recommended for newborns, for whom axillary temperature is often taken. The oral equivalent is calculated with an offset; this mode is used for adults and children over 3 years of age, for whom oral readings are commonly used. The rectal mode is calculated with an offset and is used mainly for infants up to 3 years of age, for whom rectal temperatures are commonly taken. When the rectal mode is used on adults, the temperature may read higher than average. The core equivalent is calculated with an offset and measures core body temperatures such as those found in the bladder or pulmonary artery. The core equivalent mode should only be used where adult "core" temperatures are commonly used and should not be used for routine vital sign measurements. Most aural thermometers record temperature in less than 2 seconds; so this is a fast and convenient method for obtaining temperature.

d. Factors that lead to increased body temperature include illness, infection, exercise, excitement, and high temperatures in the environment.

e. Factors that lead to decreased body temperature include starvation or fasting, sleep, decreased muscle activity, exposure to cold temperatures in the environment, and certain diseases.

Very low or high body temperatures are indicative of abnormal conditions. Hypothermia is a low body temperature, below 95°F (35°C) measured rectally. It can be caused by prolonged exposure to cold. Death usually occurs if body temperature drops below 93°F (33.9°C) for a period of time. A fever is an elevated body temperature, usually above 101°F (38.3°C) measured rectally. Fevers are usually caused by infection or injury. Hyperthermia occurs when the body temperature exceeds 104°F (40°C) measured rectally. It can be caused by prolonged exposure to hot temperatures, brain damage, and serious infections. Immediate actions must be taken to lower body temperature, because temperatures above 106°F (41.1°C) can quickly lead to convulsions and death.

Clinical thermometers are used to record temperatures. A clinical thermometer consists

Bulb with mercury

Stem with calibrations

Oral thermometer

Security thermometer

Rectal thermometer

Figure 13-2 Types of clinical thermometers

of a slender glass tube containing mercury, which expands when exposed to heat. There are different types of clinical thermometers (see figure 13-2). The glass oral thermometer has a long, slender bulb or a blue tip. A security oral thermometer has a shorter, rounder bulb and is usually marked with a blue tip. A rectal thermometer has a short, stubby, rounded bulb and may be marked with a red tip. In addition, some clinical thermometers have the word "oral" or "rectal" written on their stems.

Electronic thermometers are also used in many facilities. This type of thermometer registers the temperature on a viewer in a few seconds (see figure 13-3). Electronic thermometers can be used to take oral, rectal, axillary, and/or groin temperatures. Most facilities have electronic thermometers with blue probes for oral use and red probes for axillary or rectal use. To prevent cross contamination, a disposable cover is placed over the thermometer probe before the temperature is taken. By changing the disposable cover after each use, one unit can be used on many patients. Tympanic thermometers are specialized electronic thermometers that record the aural temperature in the ear. A disposable plastic cover is placed on the ear probe. By inserting the probe into the auditory canal and pushing a scan button, the temperature is recorded on the screen within 1 to 2 seconds. It is important to read and follow instructions while using this thermometer in order to obtain an accurate reading.

Plastic or paper thermometers are used in some health care facilities (see figure 13-4). These thermometers contain special chemical dots or strips that change color when exposed to specific temperatures. They are used once and discarded.

Figure 13-3 An electronic thermometer registers the temperature in easy-to-read numbers on a viewer. *(Photo courtesy of IVAC Corporation, San Diego, CA)*

Figure 13-4 Plastic disposable thermometers have chemical dots that change color to register body temperature. The matrix shown reads 101°F.

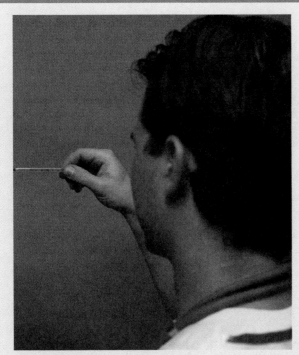

Figure 13-5 Hold the thermometer at eye level to find the solid column of mercury.

Electronic and tympanic thermometers are easy to read because they have digital displays. Reading a glass clinical thermometer is a procedure that must be practiced. Hold it at eye level and find the solid column of mercury (see figure 13-5). Read the thermometer at the point where the mercury line ends. Each long line on a thermometer is read as one degree. An exception to this is the long line for 98.6°F (37°C), which is the normal oral body temperature. Each short line represents .2 (two-tenths) of a degree. Temperature is always recorded to the next nearest two-tenths of a degree. In figure 13-6, the mercury line ends at 98.6°F. Top figures explain the markings for each line.

C To record the temperature, write 98⁶ instead of 98.6. This reduces the possibility of making an error in reading. For example, a temperature of 100.2 could easily be read as 102. By writing 100², the chance of error decreases. If a temperature is taken orally, it is not necessary to indicate that it is an oral reading. If it is taken rectally, place an (R) beside the recording. If it is taken in the axillary area, place an (Ax) beside the recording. If it is taken tympanically (aurally), place a (T) beside the recording. For example:

◆ 98⁶ is an oral reading
◆ 99⁶ (R) is a rectal reading
◆ 97⁶ (Ax) is an axillary reading
◆ 98⁶ (T) is an aural reading

Eating, drinking hot or cold liquids, and/or smoking can alter the temperature in the mouth. It is important to make sure the patient has *not* had anything to eat or drink, or has *not* smoked for at least 15 minutes prior to taking the patient's temperature. If the patient has done any of these things, explain why you cannot take the temperature and that you will return to do so.

Thermometers must be cleaned thoroughly after use. The procedure used varies with different agencies. In some agencies, the glass thermometer is washed and rinsed. Cool water is used to prevent breakage and to avoid destroying the column of mercury. The thermometer is then soaked in a disinfectant solution (frequently 70-percent alcohol) for a minimum of 30 minutes before it is used again. Other agen-

Figure 13-6 Each line on a thermometer equals two-tenths of a degree, so the thermometer shown reads 98.6°F.

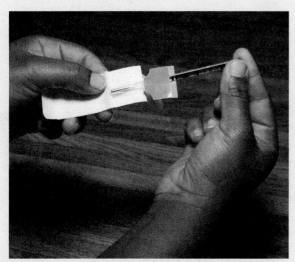

Figure 13-7 A clinical thermometer can be covered with a paper or plastic sheath that is discarded after each use.

cies cover the glass thermometer with a paper/plastic sheath that is discarded after use (see figure 13-7). The probe on electronic thermometers is covered with a plastic sheath that is discarded after each use. These covers prevent the thermometers from coming into contact with each patient's mouth or skin and prevent transmission of germs. Follow your agency's policy for cleaning and care of thermometers.

Remember that it is not your duty to tell the patient the temperature reading. That is the physician's responsibility.

STUDENT *Go to the workbook and complete the assignment sheet for 13:2, Measuring and Recording Temperature. Then return and continue with the procedures.*

PROCEDURE

Cleaning the Thermometer

OBRA

13:2A

EQUIPMENT AND SUPPLIES

Thermometers, soapy cotton balls, small trash bag or waste can, running water, soaking basin with 70-percent alcohol, alcohol sponges or cotton balls, dry cotton balls or gauze pads, thermometer holder

PROCEDURE

1. Assemble equipment.
2. Wash hands.
3. After using the thermometer, use a soapy cotton ball or gauze pad to wipe the thermometer once from the top toward the tip or bulb (see figure 13-8A). Discard the soiled cotton ball in trash bag or wastecan.
   NOTE: Rotate the thermometer while wiping it to clean all sides and parts.
4. With the bulb pointed downward, hold the thermometer by the stem and rinse the thermometer in cool water.

⚠ *CAUTION:* Hot water will break the thermometer or destroy the mercury column.
5. Shake the thermometer down to 96°F (35.6°C).
⚠ *CAUTION:* Hold the thermometer securely between your thumb and index finger. Use a snapping motion of the wrist. Avoid countertops, tables, and other surfaces.
6. Place the thermometer in a small basin or container filled with disinfectant solution (usually 70-percent alcohol). Make sure the thermometer is completely covered by the solution (see figure 13-8B).

Figure 13-8A After each use, use a soapy cotton ball or gauze to wipe the thermometer in a circular motion from the stem to the bulb.

Figure 13-8B Soak the thermometer in a disinfectant solution for a minimum of 30 minutes.

NOTE: Thirty minutes is usually the minimum time recommended for soaking.

7. Use soap and water to clean the container or thermometer holder. Rinse and dry. Place a clean, dry cotton ball in the bottom to prevent breakage. If several thermometers are to be kept in a flat container, place a piece of sterile or clean gauze in the container.

8. After 30 minutes, remove the thermometer from the soaking solution and use an alcohol cotton ball or alcohol sponge to wipe it from the stem toward the bulb. This removes any sediment from the thermometer.

9. Rinse the thermometer in cool water. Examine it carefully for any signs of breakage. Discard any broken thermometers.

10. Read the thermometer to be sure it reads 96° F (35.6°C) or lower. Place it in the clean container. It is now ready for use.
    NOTE: Many health care agencies fill the container or thermometer holder with a disinfectant, usually 70-percent alcohol.

11. Replace all equipment used.

12. Wash hands.
    NOTE: This procedure may vary according to agency policy.

PRACTICE *Go to the workbook and use the evaluation sheet for 13:2A, Cleaning the Thermometer, to practice this procedure. When you feel you have mastered this skill, sign the sheet and give it to your instructor for further action.*

✔ *Final Checkpoint* Using the criteria listed on the evaluation sheet, your instructor will grade you on your performance.

PROCEDURE

Measuring and Recording Oral Temperature
OBRA
13:2B

EQUIPMENT AND SUPPLIES

Oral thermometer, holder with disinfectant solution, tissues or dry cotton balls, container for used tissues, watch with second hand, soapy cotton balls, notepaper, pencil/pen

PROCEDURE

1. Assemble equipment.
2. Wash hands.
3. Introduce yourself. Identify the patient. Explain the procedure.
4. Position the patient comfortably. Ask the patient if he/she has eaten, has had hot or cold fluids, or has smoked in the past 15 minutes.
   NOTE: Eating, drinking liquids, or smoking can affect the temperature in the mouth. Wait at least 15 minutes if the patient says "yes" to your question.
5. Remove the clean thermometer by the upper end. Use a clean tissue or dry cotton ball to wipe the thermometer from stem to bulb.
   NOTE: If the thermometer was soaking in a disinfectant, rinse first in cool water.
   ⚠ *CAUTION:* Hold the thermometer securely to avoid breaking.
6. Read the thermometer to be sure it reads 96°F (35.6°C) or lower. Check carefully for chips or breaks.
   ⚠ *CAUTION:* Never use a cracked thermometer because it may injure the patient.
   NOTE: If a plastic sheath is used, place it on the thermometer after checking for damage.

7. Insert the bulb under the patient's tongue, toward the side of the mouth (see figure 13-9). Ask the patient to hold it in place with the lips, and caution against biting it.
   NOTE: Check to be sure patient's mouth is closed.
8. Leave the thermometer in place for 3 to 5 minutes.
   NOTE: Some agencies require that the thermometer be left in place for 8 minutes. Follow your agency's policy.
9. Remove the thermometer. Hold it by the stem and use a tissue or cotton ball to wipe toward bulb.
   NOTE: If a plastic sheath was used to cover the thermometer, there is no need to wipe the thermometer. Simply remove the sheath, taking care not to touch the part that was in the patient's mouth.
   CAUTION: Do *not* hold the bulb end. This could alter the reading because of the warmth of your hand.
10. Read the thermometer. Record the reading on notepaper.

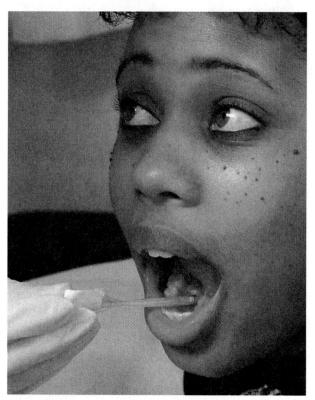

Figure 13-9 Insert the bulb of the thermometer under the patient's tongue (sublingually).

NOTE: Recheck the reading and your notation for accuracy.
NOTE: If the reading is less than 97°F, reinsert the thermometer in the patient's mouth for 1 to 2 minutes.
11. Clean the thermometer as instructed. Shake down to 96°F (35.6°C) or lower for next use.
12. Check the patient for comfort and safety before leaving.
13. Replace all equipment.
14. Wash hands.
15. Record required information on the patient's chart or agency form, for example, date and time, T 98⁶, your signature and title. Report any abnormal reading to your supervisor immediately.

PRACTICE *Go to the workbook and use the evaluation sheet for 13:2B, Measuring and Recording Oral Temperature, to practice this procedure. When you feel you have mastered this skill, sign the sheet and give it to your instructor for further action.*

✔ *Final Checkpoint* Using the criteria listed on the evaluation sheet, your instructor will grade you on your performance.

PROCEDURE

Measuring and Recording Rectal Temperature

OBRA

13:2C

EQUIPMENT AND SUPPLIES

Rectal thermometer, lubricant, tissues/cotton balls, waste bag or container, watch with second hand, paper, pencil/pen, soapy cotton ball, disposable gloves

NOTE: A manikin is frequently used to practice this procedure.

PROCEDURE

1. Assemble equipment.
2. Wash hands and put on gloves.

3. Introduce yourself. Identify the patient. Explain the procedure. Screen unit, draw curtains, or close door to provide privacy for the patient.

4. Remove rectal thermometer from its container. If the thermometer was soaking in a disinfectant, hold it by the stem end and rinse in cool water. Use a dry tissue/cotton ball to wipe from stem to bulb. Check that the thermometer reads 96°F (35.6°C) or lower. Check condition of thermometer.

   ⊘ *CAUTION:* Breaks in a thermometer can injure the patient. Never use a cracked thermometer.

5. Place a small amount of lubricant on the tissue. Roll the bulb end of the thermometer in the lubricant to coat it. Leave the lubricated thermometer on the tissue until the patient is properly positioned.

6. Turn the patient on his or her side. If possible, use Sims's position. Infants are usually placed on their backs, with legs raised and held securely, or on their abdomens (see figure 13-10).

7. Fold back covers just enough to expose the anal area.
   NOTE: Avoid exposing the patient unnecessarily.

8. With one hand, raise the upper buttock gently. With the other hand, insert the lubricated thermometer approximately 1 to 1½ inches (1 inch for an infant) into the rectum. Tell the patient what you are doing.
   NOTE: At times, rotating the thermometer slightly will make it easier to insert.

   ⊘ *CAUTION:* Never force the thermometer. It can break. If you are unable to insert it, obtain assistance.

9. Replace the covers. Keep your hand on the thermometer the entire time it is in place.

   ⊘ *CAUTION: Never* let go of the thermometer. It could slide further into the rectum or break.

10. Hold the thermometer in place for 3 to 5 minutes.

11. Remove the thermometer gently. Tell the patient what you are doing.

12. Use a tissue to remove excess lubricant from the thermometer. Wipe from stem to bulb. Hold by the stem area only. Discard the tissue into a waste container.

13. Read and record. Recheck your reading for accuracy. Remember to place an (R) next to

Figure 13-10 The infant can be positioned on the back or abdomen for a rectal temperature.

the recording to indicate a rectal temperature was taken.

14. Reposition the patient. Observe all safety checkpoints before leaving the patient.

15. Clean the thermometer as instructed in Procedure 13:2A, Cleaning the Thermometer.

16. Replace all equipment.

17. Remove gloves and wash hands.

18. Ⓒ Record required information on the patient's chart or agency form, for example, date and time, T 99⁶ (R), your signature and title. Report any abnormal reading immediately to your supervisor.

PRACTICE *Go to the workbook and use the evaluation sheet for 13:2C, Measuring and Recording Rectal Temperature, to practice this procedure. When you feel you have mastered this skill, sign the sheet and give it to your instructor for further action.*

✔ *Final Checkpoint* Using the criteria listed on the evaluation sheet, your instructor will grade you on your performance.

PROCEDURE

Measuring and Recording Axillary Temperature 13:2D **OBRA**

EQUIPMENT AND SUPPLIES

Oral thermometer, tissues/cotton balls, towel, waste container, watch with second hand, paper, pencil/pen, soapy cotton ball

PROCEDURE

1. Assemble equipment.
2. Wash hands.
3. Introduce yourself. Identify the patient. Explain the procedure.
4. Remove oral thermometer from its container. Use a tissue to wipe from stem to bulb. Check thermometer for damaged areas. Read the thermometer to be sure it reads below 96°F (36.5°C).
5. Expose the axilla and use a towel to pat the armpit dry.
   NOTE: Moisture can alter a temperature reading. Do not rub area hard because this too can alter the reading.
6. Raise the patient's arm and place the bulb end of the thermometer in the hollow of the axilla (see figure 13-11). Bring the arm over the chest and rest the hand on the opposite shoulder.
   NOTE: This position holds the thermometer in place.

Figure 13-11 To take an axillary temperature, insert the bulb end of the thermometer in the hollow of the axilla or armpit.

7. Leave the thermometer in place for 10 minutes.
8. Remove the thermometer. Wipe from stem to bulb to remove moisture. Hold by the stem end only.
   ❗ *CAUTION:* Holding the bulb end will change the reading.
9. Read and record. Check your reading for accuracy. Remember to mark (Ax) by the recording to indicate axillary temperature.
10. Reposition the patient. Be sure to check for safety and comfort before leaving.
11. Clean the thermometer as instructed.
12. Replace all equipment used.
13. Wash hands.
14. Record required information on the patient's chart or agency form, for example, date and time, T 97⁶ (Ax), your signature and title. Report any abnormal reading immediately to your supervisor.

PRACTICE *Go to the workbook and use the evaluation sheet for 13:2D, Measuring and Recording Axillary Temperature, to practice this procedure. When you feel you have mastered this skill, sign the sheet and give it to your instructor for further action.*

✔ *Final Checkpoint* Using the criteria listed on the evaluation sheet, your instructor will grade you on your performance.

PROCEDURE

Measuring and Recording Tympanic Temperature

OBRA

13:2E

EQUIPMENT AND SUPPLIES

Tympanic thermometer, probe cover, paper, pencil/pen, container for soiled probe cover

PROCEDURE

1. Assemble equipment.
   NOTE: Read the operating instructions so you understand exactly how the thermometer must be used.
2. Wash hands.
3. Introduce yourself. Identify the patient. Explain the procedure.
4. Remove the thermometer from its base. Set the thermometer on the proper mode according to operating instructions. The equal mode is usually used for newborn infants, the rectal mode for children under 3 years of age, and the oral mode for children over 3 years of age and all adults. In areas where core body temperatures are recorded, such as critical care units, the core mode may be used.
5. Install a probe cover according to instructions. This will usually activate the thermometer, showing the mode selected and the word *ready*, indicating the thermometer is ready for use.
   ⚠ *CAUTION:* Do not use the thermometer until *ready* is displayed because inaccurate readings will result.
6. Position the patient. Infants under 1 year of age should be positioned lying flat with the head turned for easy access to the ear. Small children can be held on the parent's lap, with the head held against the parent's chest for support. Adults that can cooperate and hold the head steady can either sit or lie flat. Patients in bed should have the head turned to the side, and stabilized against the pillow.

7. Hold the thermometer in your right hand to take a temperature in the right ear, and in your left hand to take a temperature in the left ear. With your other hand, pull the ear pinna (external lobe) up and back on any child over 1 year of age and on adults. Pull the ear pinna straight back for infants under 1 year of age.
   NOTE: Pulling the pinna correctly straightens the auditory canal so the probe tip will point directly at the tympanic membrane.
8. Insert the covered probe into the ear canal as far as possible to seal the canal (see figure 13-12).
9. Hold the thermometer steady and press the scan or activation button. Hold it for the required amount of time, usually 1 to 2 seconds.
10. Remove the thermometer from the patient's ear. Read and record the temperature. Place a (T) by the recording to indicate tympanic temperature.
    NOTE: The temperature will remain on the screen until the probe cover is removed.
    ⚠ *CAUTION:* If the temperature reading is low or does not appear to be accurate, change the probe cover and repeat the procedure. The opposite ear can be used for comparison.
11. Press the eject button on the thermometer to discard the probe cover into a waste container.
12. Return the thermometer to its base.
13. Reposition the patient. Observe all safety checkpoints before leaving the patient.

Figure 13-12 Insert the covered probe of the tympanic thermometer into the ear canal as far as possible to seal the canal.

14. Wash hands.
15. Record required information on the patient's chart or agency form, for example, date and time, T 98 (T), your signature and title. Report any abnormal reading immediately to your supervisor.

PRACTICE *Go to the workbook and use the evaluation sheet for 13:2E, Measuring and Recording Tympanic Temperature, to practice this procedure. When you feel you have mastered this skill, sign the sheet and give it to your instructor for further action.*

✔ *Final Checkpoint* Using the criteria listed on the evaluation sheet, your instructor will grade you on your performance.

PROCEDURE

Measuring Temperature with an Electronic Thermometer

OBRA

13:2F

EQUIPMENT AND SUPPLIES

Electronic thermometer with probe, sheath (probe cover), paper, pen/pencil, container for soiled sheath

PROCEDURE

1. Assemble equipment.
   NOTE: Read the operating instructions for the electronic thermometer so you understand how the particular model operates.
2. Wash hands.
3. Introduce yourself. Identify the patient. Explain the procedure.
4. Position the patient comfortably and correctly.
   NOTE: For an oral temperature, ask the patient if he/she has eaten, has had hot or cold fluids, or has smoked in the past 15 minutes.

Wait at least 15 minutes if the patient answers "yes."
   NOTE: For a rectal temperature, position the patient in Sims's position if possible.
5. If the probe has to be connected to the thermometer unit, insert the probe into the correct receptacle. If the thermometer has an "on" or "activate" button, push the button to turn the thermometer on.
6. Cover the probe with the sheath or probe cover.
   NOTE: For a rectal temperature, the sheath must be lubricated.
7. Insert the covered probe into the desired location. Most probes are heavy, so it is usually necessary to hold the probe in position (see figure 13-13A).
   ⚠ *CAUTION:* Hold on to the probe at all times for a rectal temperature.
8. When the unit signals that the temperature has been recorded, remove the probe.
   NOTE: Many electronic thermometers have an audible "beep." Others indicate that temperature has been recorded when the numbers stop flashing and become stationary.
9. Read and record the temperature. Recheck your reading for accuracy.
   NOTE: Remember to place an (R) next to rectal readings or an (Ax) next to axillary readings.
10. Without touching the sheath, remove it from the probe (see figure 13-13B). Many thermometers have a button you push to remove

Figure 13-13A While taking a temperature, hold the probe of the electronic thermometer in place.

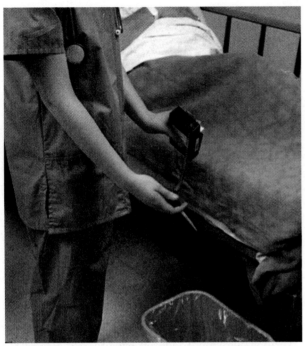

Figure 13-13B Discard the probe cover in the proper waste container without touching the cover.

the sheath. Discard the sheath in a bag or other waste container.

11. Reposition the patient. Observe all safety checkpoints before leaving the patient.

12. Return the probe to the correct storage position in the thermometer unit. Turn the unit off if this is necessary. Place the unit in the charging stand if the model has a charging unit.

13. Replace all equipment.

14. Wash hands.

15. Record required information on the patient's
C chart or agency form, for example, date and time, T 98⁸, your signature and title. Report any abnormal reading immediately to your supervisor.

PRACTICE *Go to the workbook and use the evaluation sheet for 13:2F, Measuring Temperature with an Electronic Thermometer, to practice this procedure. When you feel you have mastered this skill, sign the sheet and give it to your instructor for further action.*

✔ *Final Checkpoint* Using the criteria listed on the evaluation sheet, your instructor will grade you on your performance.

INFORMATION
13:3 *Measuring and Recording Pulse*

OBRA Pulse is a vital sign that you will be required to take. There are certain facts you must know when you take this measurement. This section provides the main information.

Pulse is defined as "the pressure of the blood pushing against the wall of an artery as the heart beats and rests." In other words, it is a throbbing of the arteries that is caused by the contractions of the heart. The pulse is more easily felt in arteries that lie fairly close to the skin and can be pressed against a bone by the fingers.

The pulse can be felt at different arterial sites on the body. Some of the major sites are shown in figure 13-14 and include:

a. temporal—at the side of the forehead
b. carotid—at the neck
c. brachial—inner aspect of forearm at the antecubital space (crease of the elbow)
d. radial—at the inner aspect of the wrist, above the thumb
e. femoral—at the inner aspect of the upper thigh
f. popliteal—behind the knee
g. dorsalis pedis—at the top of the foot arch
NOTE: Pulse is usually taken over the radial artery.

Pulse rate is measured as the number of beats per minute. Pulse rates vary among individuals, depending on age, sex, and body size:

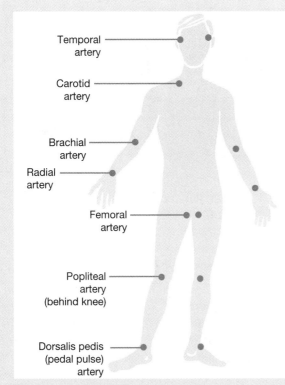

Temporal
artery

Carotid
artery

Brachial
artery

Radial
artery

Femoral
artery

Popliteal
artery
(behind knee)

Dorsalis pedis
(pedal pulse)
artery

Figure 13-14 Major pulse sites.

- Adults have a general range of 60 to 90 beats per minute.
- Adult men: 60 to 70 beats per minute.
- Adult women: 65 to 80 beats per minute.
- Children aged over 7: 70 to 90 beats per minute.

- Children aged from 1 to 7: range of 80 to 110 beats per minute.
- Infants: 90 to 160 beats per minute.
- Rates under 60 beats per minute are usually known as bradycardia.
- Rates over 100 beats per minute (except in children) are usually known as tachycardia.

NOTE: Any variations or extremes in pulse rates should be reported immediately.

Rhythm of the pulse is also noted. Rhythm refers to the regularity of the pulse, or the spacing of the beats. It is described as *regular* or *irregular.*

Volume, or the strength or intensity of the pulse, is also noted. It is described by words such as *strong, weak, thready,* or *bounding.*

Various factors will change pulse rate. Increased, or accelerated, rates can be caused by exercise, stimulant drugs, excitement, fever, shock, nervous tension, and other similar factors. Decreased, or slower, rates can be caused by sleep, depressant drugs, heart disease, coma, and other similar factors.

Remember that it is the physician's responsibility to tell the patient about pulse rate.

STUDENT Go to the workbook and complete the assignment sheet for 13:3, Measuring and Recording Pulse. Then return and continue with the procedure.

PROCEDURE

Measuring and Recording Radial Pulse

OBRA

13:3

EQUIPMENT AND SUPPLIES

Watch with second hand,
paper,
pencil/pen

PROCEDURE

1. Assemble equipment.
2. Wash hands.
3. Introduce yourself. Identify the patient. Explain the procedure.
4. Place the patient in a comfortable position, with the arm supported and the palm of the hand turned downward.

NOTE: If the forearm rests on the chest, it will be easier to count respirations after taking the pulse.

5. With the tips of your first two or three fingers, locate the pulse on the thumb side of the patient's wrist (see figure 13-15).
   NOTE: Do not use your thumb; use your fingers. The thumb contains a pulse that you may confuse with the patient's pulse.

6. When the pulse is felt, exert slight pressure and start counting. Use the second hand of the watch and count for 1 full minute.
   NOTE: In some agencies, the pulse is counted for 30 seconds and the final number multiplied by 2. To detect irregularities, it is better to count for 1 full minute.

7. While counting the pulse, also note the volume (character or strength) and the rhythm (regularity).

8. Record the following information: date, time, rate, rhythm, and volume. Follow your agency's policy for recording.

9. Check the patient before leaving. Observe all safety precautions to protect the patient.

10. Replace all equipment used.

11. Wash hands.

12. Record all required information on the patient's chart or agency form, for example, date, time, P 82 strong and regular, your signature and title. Report any unusual observations immediately to your supervisor.

Figure 13-15 To count a radial pulse, put the tips of two or three fingers on the thumb side of the patient's wrist.

PRACTICE *Go to the workbook and use the evaluation sheet for 13:3, Measuring and Recording Radial Pulse, to practice this procedure. When you feel you have mastered this skill, sign the sheet and give it to your instructor for further action.*

✔ *Final Checkpoint* Using the criteria listed on the evaluation sheet, your instructor will grade you on your performance.

INFORMATION
13:4 Measuring and Recording Respirations

OBRA Respirations are another vital sign that you must observe, count, and record correctly. This section provides the main points you must note when counting and recording the quality of respirations.

 Respiration is the process of taking in oxygen (O_2) and expelling carbon dioxide (CO_2) from the lungs and respiratory tract. One respiration consists of one inspiration (breathing in) and one expiration (breathing out).

The normal rate for respirations in adults is 14 to 18 breaths per minute, although wider ranges may be observed (12 to 20 breaths per minute). Respirations above 25 per minute are said to be *accelerated*. In children, respirations are slightly faster than those for adults and average 16 to 25 per minute. In infants, the rate may be 30 to 50 per minute.

In addition to rate, the character and rhythm of respirations should be noted. **Character** refers to the depth and quality of respirations. Words used to describe character include *deep, shallow, labored, difficult, stertorous* (abnormal sounds like snoring), and *moist*. Rhythm refers to the regularity of respirations, or equal spacing between breaths. It is described as *regular* or *irregular*.

The following terminology is used to describe abnormal respirations:

- **dyspnea**—difficult or labored breathing.
- **apnea**—absence of respirations.
- **Cheyne-Stokes** respirations—periods of dyspnea followed by periods of apnea; frequently noted in the dying patient.

◆ **rales**—bubbling or noisy sounds caused by fluids or mucus in the air passages.

Respirations must be counted in such a way that the patient is unaware of the procedure. Because respirations are partially under voluntary control, patients may breathe more quickly or more slowly when they become aware of the fact that respirations are being counted. Do not tell the patient you are counting respirations. Also, leave your hand on the pulse site while counting respirations. The pa-

tient will think you are still counting pulse and will not be likely to alter the respiratory rate.

Do not reveal any information regarding respirations to the patient. This is the physician's responsibility.

STUDENT *Go to the workbook and complete the assignment sheet for 13:4, Measuring and Recording Respirations. Then return and continue with the procedure.*

PROCEDURE

Measuring and Recording Respirations

OBRA

13:4

Figure 13-16 Positioning the patient's hand on his or her chest makes it easier to count pulse and respiration.

EQUIPMENT AND SUPPLIES

Watch with second hand, paper, pen/pencil

PROCEDURE

1. Assemble equipment.
2. Wash hands.
3. Introduce yourself. Identify the patient.
4. After the pulse rate has been counted, leave your hand in position on the pulse site and count the number of times the chest rises and falls during one minute (see figure 13-16).
   NOTE: This is done so the patient is not aware that respirations are being counted. If patients are aware, they can alter rate of breathing.
5. Count each expiration and inspiration as one respiration.
6. Note the depth (character) and rhythm (regularity) of the respirations.
7. Record the following information: date, time, rate, character, and rhythm.
8. Check the patient before leaving the area.
9. Replace all equipment.
10. Wash hands.
11. Record all required information on the patient's chart or agency form, for example,

C date, time, R 16 deep and regular (or even), your signature and title. Report any unusual observations immediately to your supervisor.

PRACTICE *Go to the workbook and use the evaluation sheet for 13:4, Measuring and Recording Respirations, to practice this procedure. When you feel you have mastered this skill, sign the sheet and give it to your instructor for further action.*

✔ *Final Checkpoint* Using the criteria listed on the evaluation sheet, your instructor will grade you on your performance.

INFORMATION

13:5 Graphing TPR

C In some agencies, you may be required to chart temperature, pulse, and respirations (TPR) on graphic records. This section provides basic information about these records.

Graphic sheets are special records used for recording temperature, pulse, and respirations. The forms vary in different health care facilities, but all contain the same basic information. The graphic chart presents a visual diagram of variations in a patient's vital signs. The progress is easier to follow than a list of numbers that give the same information. Graphic charts are used most often in hospitals and long-term-care facilities. However, similar records may be kept in medical offices or other health care facilities. Patients are sometimes taught how to maintain these records.

Some charts make use of color coding. For example, temperature is recorded in blue ink, pulse is recorded in red ink, and respirations are recorded in green ink. Other agencies use blue ink for 7 A.M. to 7 P.M. (days) and red ink for 7 P.M. to 7 A.M. (nights). Follow the policy of your institution.

Factors that affect vital signs are often included on the graph. Examples include surgery, medications that lower temperature (such as aspirin), and antibiotics.

The graph is a medical record, so it must be neat, legible, and accurate. Double check all information recorded on the graph. If an error occurs, it should be crossed out carefully with red ink and initialed. Correct information should then be inserted on the graph.

STUDENT *Read the complete procedure for 13:5, Graphing TPR. Then go back and start doing the procedure. Your assignment will follow the procedure.*

PROCEDURE

Graphing TPR 13:5 **C**

EQUIPMENT AND SUPPLIES

Blank TPR graphic sheets in the workbook, information section and its TPR example graph, assignment sheets on graphing in the workbook, pen, ruler

PROCEDURE

1. Assemble equipment.
2. Examine the sample graphic sheet (see figure 13-17). This will vary, depending on the agency. However, most graphic sheets contain time blocks across the top and number blocks for TPRs on the side. Note areas for recording temperature, pulse, and respirations. Refer to the example while completing the procedure steps.
3. Using a blank graphic sheet, fill in patient information in the spaces provided at the top. Write last name first in most cases. Be sure patient identification, hospital, and room number are accurate.
   NOTE: Forms vary. Follow directions as they apply to your form.
4. Fill in the dates in the spaces provided after DATE.
   NOTE: A graphic chart provides a day-to-day visual representation of the variations in a patient's TPRs.
5. If your chart calls for DAY IN HOSPITAL below the dates, enter *Adm.* under the first date. This stands for day of admission. The second date would then be day *1*, or first full day in the hospital. The third date would be day *2*, and so forth.
6. Some graphs contain a third line, DAYS P.O. or PP, which means days post-op (after surgery) or postpartum (after delivery of a baby). The day of surgery would be shown as *O.R.* or *Surgery.* The next day would be day *1*, or first day after surgery. The day of delivery of a baby is shown as *Del.*, with the next day as day *1*, or first day after delivery. Numbers

GRAPHIC CHART

Family Name DOE	First Name JOHN	Attending Physician DR. JOHN JONES						Room No. 238	Hosp. No. 142-555	

Date	2/1/9_	2/2/9_	2/3/9_	2/4/9_	2/5/9_	2/6/9_	2/7/9_	2/8/9_
Day in Hospital	ADM	1	2	3	4	5	6	7
Day P.O. or P.P.			O.R.	1	2	3	4	5

Temperature / Pulse / Respiration graph with notations: ADMITTED, ASPIRIN GRX, SURGERY, R (rectal) and AX (axillary) markers.

Blood Pressure	128/74	136/78	130/76	130/74				
Fluid Intake			1850cc.					
Urine			1545cc.					
Defecation	✓		✓					
Weight	158							

Figure 13-17 A sample graphic sheet. *(Courtesy of Physician's Record Company, Berwyn, IL)*

continue in sequence for each following day.

7. Go to the Assignment Sheet #1. Note the TPRs. On the graphic sheet, find the correct *date and time column*. Move down the column until the correct temperature number is found on the side of the chart. Mark this with a dot (•) in the box. Do the same for the pulse and respirations.

CAUTION: Double check your notations. Be sure they are accurate.

CHECKPOINT: Your instructor will check your notations.

8. Repeat step 7 for the next TPR. Check to be sure you are in the correct time column. Mark the dots clearly under the time column and at the correct temperature measurement, pulse rate, or respiration rate.

9. Use a straight paper edge or ruler to connect the dots for temperature. Do the same with the dots for pulse and, finally, with the dots for respiration.

NOTE: A ruler makes the line straight and neat, and the readings are more legible.

10. Continue to graph the remaining TPRs from Assignment Sheet #1. Double check all entries for accuracy. Use a ruler to connect all dots for each of the vital signs.

11. Any drug that might alter or change temperature or other vital signs is usually noted on the graph in the time column closest to the time when the drug was first given. Turn the paper sideways and write the name of the drug in the correct time column. Aspirin is often recorded in this column because it lowers

temperature. A rapid drop in body temperature would be readily explained by the word *aspirin* in the time column. Antibiotics and medications that alter heart rate are also noted in many cases.

12. Other events in a patient's hospitalization are also recorded in the time column. Examples include surgery and discharge. In some hospitals, if the patient is placed in isolation, this is also noted on the graph.

13. Blood pressure, weight, height, defecation (bowel movements), and other similar information is often recorded in special areas at the bottom of the graphic record. Record any information required in the correct areas on your form.

14. Recheck your graph for neatness, accuracy, and completeness of information.

PRACTICE *Go to the workbook and complete Assignment Sheet #1 for Graphing TPR. Give it to your instructor for grading. Note all changes. Then complete Assignment Sheet #2 for graphing TPR in the workbook. Repeat this process by completing Graphing TPR assignments #3 to 5 until you have mastered graphic records.*

✔ *Final Checkpoint* Your instructor will grade you on this skill according to the accuracy of the completed assignments.

INFORMATION
13:6 *Measuring and Recording Apical Pulse*

At times, you will be required to take an apical pulse. This section provides basic information on this topic.

An apical pulse is a pulse count taken with a stethoscope and at the apex of the heart. A stethoscope is an instrument used to listen to internal body sounds. The actual heartbeat is heard and counted. The stethoscope amplifies the sounds so they are easier to hear. Parts of the stethoscope include the earpieces, tubing, and bell or thin, flexible disk called a *diaphragm.* The tips of the earpieces should be bent forward when they are placed in the ears. The earpieces should fit snugly but should not cause pain or discomfort. To prevent the spread of microorganisms, the earpieces and bell/diaphragm of the stethoscope should be cleaned with a disinfectant such as alcohol before and after every use.

Usually, a physician orders an apical pulse. It is frequently ordered for patients with irregular heart beats, hardening of the arteries, or weak or rapid radial pulses. Because children and infants have very rapid radial pulse counts,

apical pulse counts are usually taken (see figure 13-18). It is generally easier to count a rapid pulse while listening to it (through a stethoscope) than by feeling it with your fingers.

It is important that you protect the patient's privacy when counting an apical pulse. Avoid exposing the patient during this procedure.

Two separate heart sounds are heard while listening to the heartbeat. The sounds resemble a "lubb-dupp." Each lubb-dupp counts as one heartbeat. The sounds are

Figure 13-18 An apical pulse is frequently taken on infants and small children because their pulses are more rapid.

caused by the closing of the heart valves as blood flows through the chambers of the heart. Any abnormal sounds or beats should be reported immediately to your supervisor.

1/2 A **pulse deficit** is a condition that occurs with some heart conditions. In some cases, the heart is weak and does not pump enough blood to produce a pulse. In other cases, the heart beats too fast (tachycardia), and there is not enough time for the heart to fill with blood; therefore, the heart does not produce a pulse during each beat. In such cases, the apical pulse rate is higher than are the pulse rates at other pulse sites on the body. For the most accurate determination of a pulse deficit, one person should check the apical pulse while a second person checks another pulse site, usually the radial pulse (see figure 13-19). If this is not possible, one person should first check the apical pulse and then immediately check the radial pulse. Then, subtract the rate of the radial pulse from the rate of the apical pulse. The difference is the pulse deficit.

No information regarding the apical pulse should be given to the patient. It is the physician's responsibility to tell the patient about apical pulse.

Figure 13-19 To determine a pulse deficit, one person should count an apical pulse while another person is counting a radial pulse.

STUDENT *Go to the workbook and complete the assignment sheet for 13:6, Measuring and Recording Apical Pulse. Then return and continue with the procedure.*

PROCEDURE

Measuring and Recording Apical Pulse 13:6

EQUIPMENT AND SUPPLIES

Stethoscope, watch with second hand, paper, pencil/pen, alcohol gauze sponges or swab

PROCEDURE

1. Assemble equipment. Use alcohol to wipe the earpieces and the bell/diaphragm of the stethoscope.
2. Wash hands.

3. Introduce yourself. Identify the patient and explain the procedure. If the patient is an infant or child, explain the procedure to the parent(s).
   NOTE: It is usually best to say, "I am going to listen to your heartbeat." Some patients do not know what an apical pulse is.
4. Close the door to the room. Screen the unit or draw curtains around the bed to provide privacy.
5. Uncover the left side of the patient's chest. The stethoscope must be placed directly against the skin.
6. Place the stethoscope tips in your ears. Locate the apex of the heart, 2 to 3 inches to the left of the breastbone below the left nipple. Place the bell/diaphragm over the apical region and listen for heart sounds.
   ! *CAUTION:* Be sure the tips of the stethoscope are facing forward before placing them in your ears.

7. Count the apical pulse for 1 full minute. Note the rate, rhythm, and volume.
   NOTE: Remember to count each lubb-dupp as one beat.
8. If you doubt your count, recheck your count for another minute.
9. Record your reading. Note date, time, rate, rhythm, and volume. Chart according to the agency policy. Some use an *A* and others use an *A.P.* to denote apical pulse.
   NOTE: If both a radial and apical pulse are taken, it may be recorded as A82/R82. If a pulse deficit exists, it should be noted. For example, with A80/R64, there is a pulse deficit of 16 (that is, 80 – 64 = 16). This would be recorded as A80/R64 Pulse deficit: 16.
10. Check all safety and comfort points before leaving the patient.
11. Use an alcohol swab to clean the earpieces and the bell/diaphragm of the stethoscope. Replace all equipment.
12. Wash hands.
13. Record all required information on the patient's chart or agency form. For example: date, time, AP 86 strong and regular, your signature and title. If any abnormalities or changes were observed, note and report these immediately.

PRACTICE *Go to the workbook and use the evaluation sheet for 13:6, Measuring and Recording Apical Pulse, to practice this procedure. When you feel you have mastered this skill, sign the sheet and give it to your instructor for further action.*

✔ *Final Checkpoint* Using the criteria listed on the evaluation sheet, your instructor will grade you on your performance.

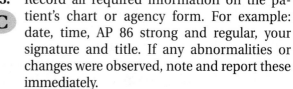

INFORMATION
13:7 *Measuring and Recording Blood Pressure*

Blood pressure (BP) is one of the vital signs you will be required to take. It is important that your recording be accurate and that you understand what the blood pressure reading means. This section provides basic information on this topic.

Blood pressure (BP) is a measurement of the pressure that the blood exerts on the walls of the arteries during the various stages of heart activity. Blood pressure is read in millimeters (mm) of mercury (Hg) on an instrument known as a sphygmomanometer.

There are two types of blood pressure measurements: systolic and diastolic. Systolic pressure occurs in the walls of the arteries when the heart is contracting and pushing blood into the arteries.
a. A normal systolic reading is 120 millimeters mercury (120 mm Hg).
b. Normal range for systolic readings is from 100 to 140 mm Hg.

Diastolic pressure is the constant pressure in the walls of the arteries when the heart is at rest, or between contractions. Blood has moved into the capillaries and veins, so the volume of blood in the arteries has decreased.
a. A normal diastolic reading is 80 mm Hg.
b. Normal range for diastolic readings is from 60 to 90 mm Hg.

Various factors can influence blood pressure readings. Some of these factors are:
a. force of the heartbeat
b. resistance of the arterial system
c. elasticity of the arteries
d. volume of the blood in the arteries

Many other factors can also influence blood pressure readings. These factors can cause blood pressure to be high or low. Some examples are as follows:
a. factors that may increase blood pressure:
   (1) excitement, anxiety, nervous tension
   (2) stimulant drugs
   (3) exercise and eating
b. factors that may decrease blood pressure:
   (1) rest or sleep
   (2) depressant drugs
   (3) shock
   (4) excessive loss of blood

c. factors that may cause miscellaneous readings:
   (1) lying down
   (2) sitting position
   (3) standing position

Blood pressure is recorded as a fraction. The systolic reading is the top number, or numerator. The diastolic reading is the bottom number, or denominator. For example, a systolic reading of 120 and a diastolic reading of 80 is recorded as 120/80.

Two main types of sphygmomanometers are used to obtain blood pressure readings. The mercury sphygmomanometer has a long column of mercury (see figure 13-20A). Each mark on the gauge represents 2 mm Hg. The mercury sphygmomanometer must always be placed on a flat, level surface or mounted on a wall (see figure 13-20B). If it is calibrated correctly, the level of mercury should be at zero when viewed at eye level. The aneroid sphygmomanometer does not have a mercury column (see figure 13-21). However, it is calibrated in mm Hg. Each line represents 2 mm Hg pressure. It is important for you to learn to use both types of sphygmomanometers.

In order to obtain accurate blood pressure readings, it is important to observe several factors. The American Heart Association (AHA) recommends that the patient sit quietly for at least 5 minutes before blood pressure is taken.

Figure 13-20A The gauge on a mercury sphygmomanometer has a column of mercury.

Figure 13-20B A mercury sphygmomanometer must be placed on a flat, level surface.

Figure 13-21A The gauge on an aneroid sphygmomanometer does not contain a column of mercury.

Figure 13-21B An aneroid sphygmomanometer has a gauge that attaches to the cuff. *(Courtesy of Omron Marshall Products, Inc)*

The AHA also recommends that two separate readings be taken and averaged, with a minimum wait of 30 seconds between readings.

The size and placement of the sphygmomanometer cuff is also important (see figure 13-22). The cuff contains a rubber bladder that fills with air to apply pressure to the arteries. Cuffs that are too wide or too narrow give inaccurate readings. To ensure the greatest degree of accuracy, the width of the cuff should be approximately the same as the diameter of the patient's arm. The patient should be seated or lying comfortably and have the forearm supported on a flat surface. The area of the arm covered by the cuff should be at heart level. The arm must be free of any constrictive clothing. The deflated cuff should be placed on the arm with the center of the bladder in the cuff directly over the brachial artery, and the lower edge of the cuff 1 to $1^1/_2$ inches above the antecubital area (bend of the elbow).

A final point relating to accuracy is placement of the stethoscope bell/diaphragm. The bell/diaphragm should be placed directly over the brachial artery at the antecubital area and held securely but with as little pressure as possible.

C As a health care worker, a major responsibility is accuracy in taking and record-

Figure 13-22 It is important to use the correct size cuff because cuffs that are too wide or too narrow will result in inaccurate readings.

ing blood pressure. You should *not* discuss the reading with the patient. This is the responsibility of the physician because the information may cause a personal reaction that can affect the treatment. Only the physician should determine whether an abnormal blood pressure is indication for treatment.

STUDENT *Go to the workbook and complete the assignment sheets for 13:7, Measuring and Recording Blood Pressure, Reading a Mercury Sphygmomanometer, and Reading an Aneroid Sphygmomanometer. Then return and continue with the procedure.*

PROCEDURE

Measuring and Recording Blood Pressure

13:7

EQUIPMENT AND SUPPLIES

Stethoscope, sphygmomanometer, alcohol swab or cotton balls, paper, pencil/pen

PROCEDURE

1. Assemble equipment. Use an alcohol cotton ball or swab to clean the earpieces and bell/diaphragm of the stethoscope.
2. Wash hands.
3. Introduce yourself. Identify the patient. Explain the procedure.
   NOTE: If possible, allow the patient to sit quietly for 5 minutes before taking the blood pressure.
   NOTE: Reassure the patient as needed. Nervous tension and excitement can alter or elevate blood pressure.
4. Roll up the patient's sleeve to approximately 5 inches above the elbow. Position the arm so that it is supported and comfortable. The palm should be up.
   NOTE: If the sleeve constricts the arm, remove the garment. The arm must be bare and unconstricted for an accurate reading.
5. Wrap the deflated cuff around the upper arm 1 to 1$^1/_2$ inches above the elbow and over the brachial artery. The center of the bladder inside the cuff should be over the brachial artery. If the cuff has velcro material above the tubing, it should be uppermost rather than against the skin. (Some cuffs have velcro instead of hooks to fasten.)
   CAUTION: Do not pull the cuff too tight. Cuff should be smooth and even.
6. Determine the palpatory systolic pressure (see figure 13-23A). To do this, find the radial pulse and keep your fingers on it. Inflate the cuff until the radial pulse disappears. Inflate the cuff 30 mm Hg above this point. Slowly release the pressure on the cuff while watch-

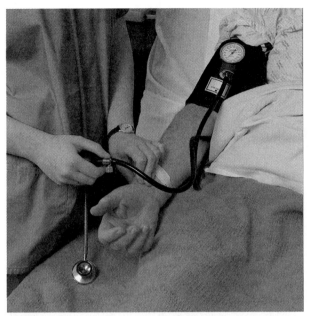

Figure 13-23A Determine the palpatory systolic pressure by checking the radial pulse as you inflate the cuff.

ing the gauge. When the pulse is felt again, note the reading on the gauge. This is the palpatory systolic pressure.

7. Deflate the cuff completely. Ask the patient to raise the arm and flex the fingers to promote blood flow. Wait 30 to 60 seconds to allow blood flow to resume completely.
8. Use your fingertips to locate the brachial artery (see figure 13-23B). The brachial artery is located on the inner part of the arm at the antecubital space (area where the elbow bends). Place the stethoscope over the artery (see figure 13-23C). Do not use your thumb to hold the stethoscope in place. Put the earpieces in your ears.
   NOTE: Earpieces should be pointed forward.
9. Check to make sure the tubings are separate and not tangled together.
10. Gently close the valve on the rubber bulb by turning it in a clockwise direction. Inflate the cuff to 30 mm Hg above the palpatory systolic pressure.
    NOTE: Make sure the sphygmomanometer gauge is at eye level.
11. Open the bulb valve slowly and let the air escape gradually.
12. When the first sound is heard, note the reading on the manometer. This is the systolic pressure.

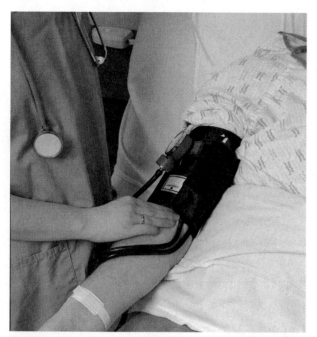

Figure 13-23B Locate the brachial artery on the inner part of the arm at the antecubital space.

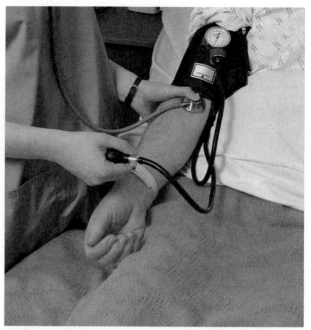

Figure 13-23C Place the stethoscope over the brachial artery as you listen for the blood pressure sounds.

13. Continue to release the air until there is an abrupt change of the sound, usually soft or muffled. Note the reading on the manometer. Continue to release the air until the sound changes again, becoming first faint and then no longer heard. Note the reading on the manometer. The point at which the first change in sound occurs is the diastolic pressure in children. The diastolic pressure in adults is the point at which the sound becomes very faint or stops.
    NOTE: If you still hear sound, continue to the zero mark. Record both readings (the change of sound and the zero reading). For a systolic of 122 and a continued diastolic of 78, this can be written as 122/78/0.
14. When the sound ceases, rapidly deflate the cuff.
15. If you need to repeat the procedure to recheck your reading, completely deflate the cuff, wait 1 minute, and repeat the procedure. Ask the patient to raise the arm and flex the fingers to promote blood flow.
    ⊘ *CAUTION:* If you cannot obtain a reading, report to your supervisor promptly.
16. Record the time and your reading. The reading is written as a fraction, with systolic over

diastolic. For example, BP 124/72 (or 124/80/72).
17. Remove the cuff. Expel any remaining air by squeezing the cuff. Use alcohol to clean the stethoscope earpieces and diaphragm/bell. Replace all equipment.
18. Check patient for safety and comfort before leaving.
19. Wash hands.
20. Record all required information on the patient's chart or agency form, for example, date, time, B. P. 126/74, your signature and title. Report any abnormal readings immediately to your supervisor.

PRACTICE Go to the workbook and use the evaluation sheet for 13:7, Measuring and Recording Blood Pressure, to practice this procedure. When you feel you have mastered this skill, sign the sheet and give it to your instructor for further action.

✔ *Final Checkpoint* Using the criteria listed on the evaluation sheet, your instructor will grade you on your performance.

UNIT 13 SUMMARY

Vital signs are important indicators of health states of the body. The four main vital signs are temperature, pulse, respirations, and blood pressure.

Temperature is a measurement of the balance between heat lost and heat produced by the body. It can be measured orally, rectally, aurally (by way of the ear), and between folds of skin. An abnormal body temperature can indicate disease.

Pulse is the pressure of the blood felt against the wall of an artery as the heart contracts or beats. Pulse can be measured at various body sites, but the most common site is the radial pulse, which is at the wrist. The rate, rhythm, and volume (strength) should be noted each time a pulse is taken. An apical pulse is taken with a stethoscope and at the apex of the heart. The stethoscope is used to listen to the heart beat. Apical pulse is frequently taken on infants and small children with rapid pulse rates.

Respiration refers to the breathing process. Each respiration consists of an inspiration (breathing in) and an expiration (breathing out). The rate, rhythm, and character, or type, of respirations should always be noted.

Blood pressure is the force exerted by the heart against the arterial walls when the heart contracts or relaxes. Two measurements are noted: systolic and diastolic. An abnormal blood pressure can indicate disease.

Vital signs are major indications of body function. The health care worker must use precise methods to measure vital signs so results are as accurate as possible. A thorough understanding of vital signs and what they indicate will allow the health care worker to be alert to any abnormalities so they can be immediately reported to the correct individual.

UNIT 13 SUGGESTED REFERENCES

American Heart Association. *Office Evaluation of Hypertension.* Dallas, TX: American Heart Association, 1992.

American Heart Association. *Recommendations for Human Blood Pressure Determination by Sphygmomanometers.* Dallas, TX: American Heart Association, 1992.

Cooper, Marian G., and David E. Cooper. *The Medical Assistant.* 6th ed. New York, NY: McGraw-Hill, 1993.

Hegner, Barbara, and Esther Caldwell. *Nursing Assistant: A Nursing Process Approach.* 7th ed. Albany, NY: Delmar Publishers, 1995.

Huber, Helen, and Audree Spatz. *Homemaker-Home Health Aide.* 4th ed. Albany, NY: Delmar Publishers, 1994.

Keir, Lucille, Connie Krebs, and Barbara A. Wise. *Medical Assisting: Clinical and Administrative Competencies.* 3rd ed. Albany, NY: Delmar Publishers, 1993.

Long, Barbara C., and Wilma J. Phipps. *Medical Surgical Nursing.* 3rd ed. St. Louis, MO: C. V. Mosby, 1993.

Memmler, Ruth Lundeen, and D. L. Wood. *The Human Body in Health and Disease.* 7th ed. Philadelphia, PA: J. B. Lippincott, 1992.

Zakus, Sharron. *Procedures for Medical Assistants.* 3rd ed. St. Louis, MO: C. V. Mosby, 1994.

UNIT 14

First Aid

UNIT OBJECTIVES

After completing this unit of study, you should be able to:

- ◆ Demonstrate cardiopulmonary resuscitation for one-person rescue, two-person rescue, infants, children, and obstructed-airway victims
- ◆ Describe first aid for
  — bleeding and wounds
  — shock
  — poisoning
  — burns
  — heat exposure
  — cold exposure
  — bone and joint injuries, including fractures
  — specific injuries to the eyes, head, nose, ears, chest, abdomen, and genital organs
  — sudden illness including heart attack, stroke, fainting, convulsions, and diabetic reactions
- ◆ Apply dressings and bandages, observing all safety precautions and using the circular, spiral, figure-eight, and recurrent, or finger, wrap
- ◆ Define, pronounce, and spell all of the key terms

KEY TERMS

abrasion
   (ah"-bray´-shun)
amputation
avulsion
   (ay"-vul´-shun)
bandages
burn
cardiopulmonary resuscitation
   (car´-dee-oh-pull´-meh-nah-
   ree ree"-suh-sih-tay´-shun)
cerebrovascular accident
   (seh-ree´-bro-vass"-ku-lehr
   ax´-ih-dent)

convulsion
diabetic coma
diaphoresis
   (dy"-ah-feh-ree´-sis)
dislocation
dressing
fainting
first aid
fracture
frostbite
heart attack
heat cramps
heat exhaustion

heat stroke
hemorrhage
hypothermia
incision
infection
insulin shock
laceration
poisoning
puncture
shock
sprain
strain
wound

INFORMATION

14:1 *Providing First Aid*

In every health care career you may have experiences that require a knowledge of first aid. This section provides basic guidelines for all of the first aid topics discussed in the remaining sections of this unit. All students are strongly encouraged to take the First Aid Certification Course through their local Red Cross divisions to become proficient in providing first aid.

First aid is not full and complete treatment. Rather, **first aid** is best defined as "immediate care that is given to the victim of an injury or illness to minimize the effect of the injury or illness until experts can take over." Application of correct first aid can often mean the difference between life and death or recovery versus permanent disability. In addition, by knowing the proper first aid measures, you can help yourself and others in a time of emergency.

C In any situation where first aid treatment is necessary, it is essential that you remain calm. Avoid panic. Evaluate the situation thoroughly. Always have a reason for anything you do. The treatment you provide will vary depending on the type of injury or illness, the environment, others present, equipment or supplies on hand, and the availability of medical help. Therefore, it is important for you to think about all of these factors and determine what action is necessary.

The first step of first aid is to recognize that an emergency exists. Many senses can alert you to an emergency. Listen for unusual sounds such as screams, calls for help, breaking glass, screeching tires, or changes in machinery or equipment noises. Look for unusual sights such as an empty medicine container, damaged electrical wires, a stalled car, smoke or fire, a person lying motionless, blood, or spilled chemicals. Note any unusual, unfamiliar, or strange odors such as those of chemicals, natural gas, or pungent fumes. Watch for unusual appearances or behaviors in others such as difficulty in breathing, clutching of the chest or throat, abnormal skin colors, slurred or confused speech, unexplained confusion or drowsiness, excessive perspiration, signs of pain, and any symptoms of distress. Sometimes, signs of an emergency are clearly evident. An example is an automobile accident with victims in cars or on the street. Other times, signs are less obvious and require an alert individual to note that something is different or wrong. An empty medicine container and a small child with slurred speech, for example, are less obvious signs.

⚠ After determining that an emergency exists, the next step is to take appropriate action to help the victim or victims. Check the scene and make sure it is safe to approach. A quick glance at the area can provide information on what has occurred, dangers present, number of people involved, and other important factors. If live electrical wires are lying on the ground around an accident victim, for example, a rescuer could be electrocuted while trying to assist the victim. An infant thrown from a car during an automobile accident may be overlooked. A rescuer who pauses briefly to assess the situation will avoid such dangerous pitfalls and provide more efficient care. If the scene is not safe, call for medical help. Do not endanger your own life or the lives of other bystanders. Allow professionals to handle fires, dangerous chemicals, damaged electrical wires, and other life-threatening situations. If the scene appears safe, approach the victim. Determine whether the victim is conscious (see figure 14-1). If the victim shows no sign of consciousness, tap him gently and call to him. If the victim shows signs of consciousness, try to find out what happened and what is wrong. Never move an injured victim unless the victim is in a dangerous area such as an area filled

Figure 14-2 Call for emergency medical services (EMS) as soon as possible.

with fire and/or smoke, flood waters, or carbon monoxide or poisonous fumes, or one with dangerous traffic, where vehicles cannot be stopped. If it is necessary to move the victim, do so as quickly and carefully as possible. Victims have been injured more severely by improper movement at the scenes of accidents, so avoid any unnecessary movement.

Ⓒ In an emergency, it is essential to call the emergency medical services (EMS) as soon as possible (see figure 14-2). Use a telephone or CB radio to contact the police, ambulance or rescue squad, fire department, utility company, or other resources. In many areas of the country, the emergency number 911 can be used to contact any of the emergency medical services. Sometimes, it may be necessary to instruct others to contact authorities while you are giving first aid. Make sure that complete, accurate information is given to the correct authority. Describe the situation, actions taken, exact location and telephone number from which you are calling, assistance required, number of people involved, and other similar information. Do not hang up the receiver or end the CB radio call until the other party has all of the necessary information. If you are alone and providing urgent emergency care such as controlling severe bleeding or providing cardiopulmonary resuscitation (CPR), shout for

Figure 14-1 Determine whether the victim is conscious by gently tapping and by calling to him or her.

help. If no one arrives to call EMS, continue providing care for approximately 1 minute, and then get to the nearest telephone, call for EMS, and return immediately to the victim.

After calling for help, provide care to the victim. If possible, obtain the victim's permission before providing any care. Introduce yourself and ask if you can help. If the victim can respond, he or she should give you permission before you provide care. If the victim is a child or minor, and a parent is present, obtain permission from the parent. If the victim is unconscious, confused, or seriously ill and unable to consent to care, and no other relative is available to give permission, you can assume that you have permission. It is important to remember that every individual has the right to refuse care. If a person refuses to give consent for care, do not proceed. If possible, have someone witness the refusal of care. If a life-threatening emergency exists, call EMS, alert them to the situation, and allow the professionals to take over.

Always attend to life-threatening emergencies first. Examples include no breathing or difficulty in breathing, no pulse, and/or severe bleeding. Proper care for these emergencies is described in the sections that follow. If the victim is conscious, breathing, and able to talk, reassure the victim and try to determine what has happened. Ask the victim about pain or discomfort. Check for signs of poisoning and provide first aid as needed.

Check the victim for other types of injuries. Examples include fractures (broken bones), burns, shock, specific injuries, and other similar conditions. Always have a sound reason for anything you do. Examine the victim thoroughly and note any abnormal signs or symptoms. Check vital signs. Note the temperature, color, and moistness of the skin. Check and compare the pupils of the eyes. Look for fluids or blood draining from the mouth, nose, or ears. Gently examine the body for cuts, bruises, swelling, and painful areas. Report any abnormalities noted to emergency medical services when they arrive at the scene.

Obtain as much information regarding the accident, injury, or illness as possible. This information can then be given to the correct authorities. Information can be obtained from the victim, other persons present, or by examination of items present at the scene. Emergency medical identification contained in a bracelet, necklace, medical card, or Vial-of-Life is an important source of information. Empty medicine containers, bottles of chemicals or solutions, or similar items also can reveal important information. Be alert to all such sources of information. Use this information to determine how you may help the victim.

Some general principles of care should be observed whenever first aid is necessary. Some of these principles are:

a. Obtain qualified assistance as soon as possible. Report all information obtained, observations noted, treatment given, and other important facts to the correct authorities. It may sometimes be necessary to send someone at the scene to obtain help.

b. Avoid any unnecessary movement of the victim. Keep the victim in a position that will allow for providing the best care for the type of injury or illness.

c. Reassure the victim. A confident, calm attitude will help relieve the victim's anxiety.

d. If the victim is unconscious or vomiting, do not give him or her anything to eat or drink. It is best to avoid giving a victim anything to eat or drink while providing first aid treatment, unless the specific treatment requires that fluids or food be given.

e. Protect the victim from cold or chilling, but avoid overheating the victim.

f. Work quickly, but in an organized and efficient manner.

g. Do not make a diagnosis or discuss the victim's condition with observers at the scene. It is essential to maintain confidentiality and protect the victim's right to privacy while providing treatment.

h. Make every attempt to avoid further injury.

 CAUTION: Provide only the treatment that you are qualified to provide.

STUDENT *Go to the workbook and complete the assignment sheet for 14:1, Providing First Aid.*

INFORMATION

14:2 *Performing Cardiopulmonary Resuscitation*

Figure 14-3 Open the airway by using the head-tilt/chin-lift method.

At some time in your life, you may find an unconscious victim who is not breathing. This is an emergency situation. Correct action can save a life. Certification courses in cardiopulmonary resuscitation (CPR) are offered by the Red Cross and American Heart Association. This section provides the basic facts about cardiopulmonary resuscitation.

The word parts of cardiopulmonary resuscitation provide a fairly clear description of the procedure: cardio (the heart) plus pulmonary (the lungs) plus resuscitation (to remove from apparent death or unconsciousness). When you administer CPR, you breathe for the person *and* circulate the blood. The purpose is to keep oxygenated blood flowing to the brain and other vital body organs until the heart and lungs start working again, or until medical help is available.

Clinical death occurs when the heart stops beating and the victim stops breathing. Biological death refers to the death of the body cells. Biological death occurs 4 to 6 minutes after clinical death and can result in permanent brain damage as well as damage to other vital organs. If CPR can be started immediately after clinical death occurs, the victim may be revived.

Cardiopulmonary resuscitation is as simple as ABC. In fact, the *ABC*s serve as guides to lifesaving techniques for persons who have stopped breathing and have no pulse.

a. *A* stands for airway. To open the victim's airway, use the head-tilt/chin-lift method (see figure 14-3). Put one hand on the victim's forehead and put the fingertips of the other hand under the bony part of the jaw, near the chin. Tilt the head back without closing the victim's mouth. This action prevents the tongue from falling back and blocking the air passage. If the victim has a suspected neck or upper spinal cord injury, try to open the airway by lifting the chin without tilting the head back. If it is difficult to keep the jaw lifted with one hand, use a modified jaw-thrust maneuver to open the airway. Grasp the angles of the victim's lower jaw by positioning one hand on each side. Lift with both hands to move the lower jaw forward, making every attempt to avoid excessive backward tilting or side-to-side movement of the head.

b. *B* stands for breathing. Breathing means that you breathe into the victim's mouth or nose to supply needed oxygen or provide ventilations. To avoid loss of air when providing mouth-to-mouth breathing, it is important to pinch the victim's nose shut and make a tight seal around the victim's mouth with your mouth.

c. *C* stands for circulation. By applying pressure to a certain area of the breastbone (sternum), the heart is compressed between the sternum and vertebral column. Blood is squeezed out of the heart and into the blood vessels. In this way, oxygen is supplied to blood cells.

Care must be taken to evaluate the victim's condition before CPR is started. First, determine whether the victim is conscious. Tap the victim gently and ask, "Are you okay?" If you know the victim, call the victim by name and speak loudly. If there is no response and the victim is unconscious, call out for help. Immediately check for breathing. Try not to move the victim while you check breathing. If the victim is breathing, leave the victim in the same position and proceed with other needed care. If the victim is not breathing, or you are unable to determine whether the victim is breathing, position the victim on his or her back. If you must turn the victim, support the victim's head and neck and keep the victim's body in as straight a line as possible while turning. Then, open the airway by tilting the victim's head back. This step will sometimes start the victim breathing. To check for breathing, use a three-point evaluation for approximately 5 seconds. Look for chest movement. Listen for breathing through the nose or mouth. Feel for movement of air from the nose or mouth. If the victim is not breathing, give two slow, full breaths, each breath lasting approximately 1½ seconds. Then, check the carotid pulse in the neck to determine whether cardiac compression is needed. Take at least 5 to 10 seconds to determine whether the pulse is absent before starting compressions.

! *CAUTION:* Cardiac compressions are not given if the pulse can be felt. If a person has stopped breathing but still has a pulse, it may be necessary to give only pulmonary respiration.

Correct hand placement is essential before performing chest compressions. For adults and children over 1 year of age, the hand is placed on the lower half of the sternum. While kneeling alongside the victim, find the correct position by using the middle finger of your hand that is closest to the victim's feet to follow the ribs up to where the ribs meet the sternum, at the substernal notch. Keep the middle finger on the notch and position the index finger above it so two fingers are on the sternum. Then place the heel of your opposite hand (the hand closest to the victim's head) on the sternum, next to the index finger. Measuring in this manner minimizes the danger of applying pressure to the tip of the sternum, called the xiphoid process.

! *CAUTION:* The xiphoid process can be broken off quite easily and therefore should not be pressed.

Cardiopulmonary resuscitation can be performed on adults, children, and infants. In addition, it can be done by one person or two persons. Rates of ventilations and compressions vary according to the number of persons giving CPR and the age of the victim.

a. One-person rescue: For adults, the person performing the rescue should provide fifteen compressions followed by two ventilations, for a cycle ratio of 15:2. If fifteen compressions are given at the *rate* of approximately 80 to 100 per minute, this will allow time for the rescuer to stop for two ventilations and still complete a 15:2 cycle in approximately 15 seconds. Four 15:2 cycles should be completed every minute. The hands should be positioned correctly on the sternum. The two hands should be interlaced and only the heel of the palm should rest on the sternum. Pressure should be applied straight down to compress the sternum approximately 1½ to 2 inches, or 3.8 to 5.0 centimeters.

b. Two-person rescue: For adults, two people performing a rescue can provide more frequent ventilations, because one breath is given after every five compressions. One rescuer applies the compressions at the rate of 80 to 100 per minute. After every fifth compression, the rescuer applying compressions pauses, and the second rescuer provides one ventilation. Thus, there is a 5:1 ratio.

c. Infants: Cardiopulmonary resuscitation for an infant is different than that for an adult because of the infant's size. Ventilations are given by covering both the infant's nose and mouth; a seal is made by the mouth of the rescuer. Breaths are given slowly until the infant's chest rises gently. The brachial pulse site in the arm is used to check pulse. Compressions are given by placing two fingers on the sternum one finger's width below an imaginary line drawn between the nipples. The sternum should be compressed ½ to 1 inch (approximately 1.4 to 2.5 centimeters). Compressions are given at a rate of approximately 100 per minute. Even with a one-person rescue, one respiration is given after every five compressions, for a 5:1 ratio. The infant's back must be supported at all times when giving compressions. In addition, the infant's head should not be tilted as far back as an adult's because this can obstruct the infant's airway.

d. Children: Cardiopulmonary resuscitation for children depends on the size of the child. The CPR method for an adult is usually used if the child is relatively large or is older than 8. The initial steps of CPR for a child are the same steps used in adult CPR, except that the head is not tilted as far back when the airway is opened. The main differences relate to compressions. The heel of one hand is placed on the sternum above the substernal-notch, that is, in the same position used for adult compressions. The sternum is compressed 1 to 1½ inches (approximately 2.5 to 3.8 centimeters). Compressions are given at a rate of 80 to 100 per minute. After each five compressions, one slow breath is given until the chest rises gently. This provides a 5:1 ratio. Each cycle of five compressions and one ventilation should take approximately 5 seconds, and ten to twelve cycles should be completed every minute.

OBRA There are times when a victim has an obstructed airway (an object blocking the airway). Special measures must be taken to clear this obstruction.

a. If the victim is conscious, coughing, and able to breathe, the airway is not completely obstructed. Remain calm and encourage the victim to remain calm. Encourage the victim to cough hard. Coughing is the most effective method of expelling the object from the airway.

b. If the victim is conscious but not able to talk, breathe, or cough, the airway is completely obstructed. The victim usually grasps his or her throat and appears cyanotic. Immediate action must be taken to clear the airway. Abdominal thrusts, as described in Procedure 14:2E, are given to provide a force of air to push the object out of the airway.

c. If the victim is unconscious and has an obstructed airway, a sequence of steps is performed to remove the obstruction. The sequence includes giving five abdominal thrusts, performing a mouth sweep, opening the airway, and attempting to ventilate (give

breaths). The sequence, described in detail in Procedure 14:2F, is repeated until the object is expelled, ventilations are successful, or other qualified medical help arrives.

d. If an infant (birth to 1 year old) has an obstructed airway, a different sequence of steps is used to remove the obstruction. The sequence includes five back blows; five chest thrusts; a check of the mouth and a finger sweep, if the object is seen; and an attempt to ventilate. The sequence, described in detail in Procedure 14:2F, is repeated until the object is expelled, ventilations are successful, or other qualified medical help arrives.

e. If a child aged 1 to 8 has an obstructed airway, the same sequence of steps used for an adult is followed. However, a finger sweep of the mouth is *not* performed unless the object can be seen in the mouth.

f. Until the airway is cleared, chest compressions have no value. Compressions circulate oxygen to the body cells. Unless the airway is cleared and oxygen is supplied to the lungs, however, there is no oxygen to circulate.

Once CPR is started, it must be continued unless one of the following situations occur:

a. The victim recovers and starts to breathe.

b. Other qualified help arrives and takes over.

c. A doctor or other legally qualified person orders you to discontinue the attempt.

d. The rescuer is so physically exhausted, CPR can no longer be continued.

e. The scene suddenly becomes unsafe.

Even though CPR must be started immediately, it is also essential to obtain medical help for the victim as soon as possible. If another person is available, tell him or her to call for help. If you are alone, call aloud for help and start CPR. If no help has arrived in 1 minute, it may be necessary for you to stop CPR for a brief period to either call emergency medical services (EMS) or find another person who can call. Make every attempt to resume CPR as quickly as possible.

STUDENT Go to the workbook and complete the assignment sheet for 14:2, Performing Cardiopulmonary Resuscitation. Then return and continue with the procedures.

PROCEDURE

Performing CPR— One-Person Rescue *14:2A*

EQUIPMENT AND SUPPLIES

CPR manikin, alcohol or disinfecting solution, gauze sponges

Figure 14-4 Use only training manikins while practicing CPR.

PROCEDURE

! *CAUTION:* Only a CPR training manikin (see figure 14-4) should be used to practice this procedure. *Never* practice CPR on another person.

1. Assemble equipment. Position the manikin on a firm surface, usually the floor.
2. Check for consciousness. Shake the "victim" by tapping the shoulder. Ask, "Are you OK?"
3. Open the airway. Use the head-tilt/chin-lift method. Place one hand on the victim's forehead. Place the fingertips of the other hand under the bony part of the victim's jaw, near the chin. Tilt the head without closing the victim's mouth.

   NOTE: This action moves the tongue away from the back of the throat and prevents the tongue from blocking the airway.

   ! *CAUTION:* If the victim has a suspected neck or upper spinal cord injury, use a modified jaw-thrust maneuver to open the airway. Grasp the angles of the victim's lower jaw by positioning one hand on each side. Lift with both hands to move the lower jaw forward, making every attempt to avoid excessive backward tilting or side-to-side movement of the head.

4. Check for breathing. Put your ear close to the victim's nose and mouth while looking at the chest. Look, listen, and feel for respirations for about 5 seconds.
5. *If the victim is breathing,* keep the airway open and obtain medical help. *If the victim is not breathing,* administer mouth-to-mouth resuscitation as follows:
   a. Keep the airway open.

   b. Resting your hand on the victim's forehead, use your thumb and forefinger to pinch the victim's nose shut.
   c. Seal the victim's mouth with your mouth.
   d. Give two full, slow breaths, each lasting approximately 1 to 1½ seconds (see figure 14-5A).
   e. Watch the chest for movement to be sure the air is entering the victim's lungs.

      NOTE: Obtain medical help for a nonbreathing victim as quickly as possible. Tell someone else to call for help if at all possible.

6. Palpate the carotid pulse: kneeling at the victim's side, place the fingertips of your hand on the victim's voice box. Then slide the fingers toward you and into the groove at the side of the victim's neck, where you should find the carotid pulse. Take at least 5 seconds but not more than 10 seconds to feel for the pulse (see figure 14-5B).

   NOTE: The pulse may be weak, so check carefully.

7. *If the victim has a pulse,* continue providing mouth-to-mouth resuscitation. Give one breath every 5 seconds. Count, "One, one thousand; two, one thousand; three, one thousand; four, one thousand; and breathe," to obtain the correct timing. After 1 minute of rescue breathing (approximately twelve breaths), recheck the pulse to make sure the heart is still beating.

Figure 14-5A If the victim is not breathing, give two slow, full breaths.

Figure 14-5B Palpate the carotid pulse for at least 5 seconds to determine whether the heart is beating.

Figure 14-5C Use smooth, even motions to compress the chest straight down while giving fifteen compressions.

8. *If the victim does not have a pulse,* administer chest compressions as follows:
   a. Locate the correct place on the sternum: while kneeling alongside the victim, use the middle finger of your hand that is closest to the victim's feet to follow the ribs up to where the ribs meet the sternum, at the substernal notch. Keep the middle finger on the notch and position the index finger above it so two fingers are on the sternum. Then, place the heel of the opposite hand (the one closest to the victim's head) on the sternum, next to the index finger.

   ⚠ *CAUTION:* The heel of your hand should be approximately 1 to 1½ inches above the end of the sternum.

   b. Place your other hand on top of the hand that is correctly positioned. Keep your fingers off the victim's chest; it may help to interlock your fingers.
   c. Raise up on your knees so that your shoulders are directly over the victim's sternum. Lock your elbows and keep your arms straight.

   NOTE: This position will allow you to push straight down on the sternum and compress the heart, which lies between the sternum and vertebral column.

   d. Push straight down to compress the chest approximately 1½ to 2 inches, or 3.8 to 5.0 centimeters (see figure 14-5C). Use a smooth, even motion.
   e. Administer fifteen compressions at the rate of 80 to 100 per minute. Count, "One and, two and, three and," etc., to obtain the correct rate.
   f. Allow the chest to relax completely after each compression. Keep your hands on the sternum during the upstroke (chest relaxation period).
   g. The fifteen compressions should be completed in approximately 10 seconds.

9. After administering fifteen compressions, give the victim two ventilations, or respirations. Avoid excessive body movement while giving the ventilations. Keep your knees

in the same position and swing your body upward to give the respirations. Respirations should be completed in approximately 5 seconds.

10. Repeat the cycle of fifteen compressions followed by two ventilations. After four cycles of a 15:2 ratio, take 5 seconds to check the victim for breathing and the presence of a carotid pulse. If no pulse is felt, give two breaths and then continue providing fifteen compressions followed by two respirations.
    NOTE: Remember, cardiac compressions are applied only if the victim has no pulse.

11. After you begin CPR, do not stop unless
    a. The victim recovers.
    b. Help arrives to take over and give CPR.
    c. A physician or other legally qualified person orders you to discontinue the attempt.
    d. You are so physically exhausted, you cannot continue.
    e. The scene suddenly becomes unsafe.

12. Make every effort to obtain medical help for the victim as soon as possible. Shout for help, send someone to telephone for help, or, as a last resort, stop CPR long enough to telephone for help or to locate someone else who can telephone for help.

13. After the practice session, use a gauze pad saturated with 70-percent alcohol or a 10-percent bleach disinfecting solution to clean the manikin. Wipe the face and clean inside the mouth thoroughly. Saturate a clean gauze pad with the solution and lay it on the mouth area for at least 30 seconds. Use another gauze pad to wipe the area dry. Follow manufacturer's instructions for any additional cleaning required.
    NOTE: A 10-percent bleach solution is more effective than alcohol. Some manikins have disposable mouthpieces that are discarded after use. If the mouthpiece is discarded, the remainder of the face should still be disinfected.

14. Replace all equipment used. Wash hands.

PRACTICE   *Go to the workbook and use the evaluation sheet for 14:2A, Performing CPR—One-Person Rescue, to practice this procedure. When you feel you have mastered this skill, sign the sheet and give it to your instructor for further action.*

✔ *Final Checkpoint*   Using the criteria listed on the evaluation sheet, your instructor will grade you on your performance and knowledge.

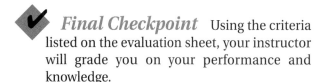

PROCEDURE

Performing CPR— Two-Person Rescue
14:2B

EQUIPMENT AND SUPPLIES

CPR manikin, alcohol or disinfecting solution, gauze sponges

PROCEDURE

⚠ *CAUTION:* Only a CPR training manikin should be used to practice this procedure. *Never* practice CPR on another person.

1. Assemble equipment. Position the manikin on a firm surface, usually the floor.

2. One rescuer begins CPR on the victim. The second rescuer contacts emergency medical services.

3. Shake the victim to check for consciousness. Ask, "Are you OK?"

4. Use the head-tilt/chin-lift method to open the victim's airway. Place one hand on the victim's forehead. Place the fingertips of the other hand under the bony part of the victim's jaw, near the chin. Tilt the victim's head back without closing the victim's mouth.

5. Check for breathing. Look, listen, and feel for breathing for 5 seconds.

6. *If the victim is not breathing,* give two slow, full breaths, each lasting approximately 1 to 1½ seconds. Watch the chest for movement to be sure air is entering the victim's lungs.
   NOTE: You may use a gauze sponge over the victim's mouth for pulmonary resuscitation.

7. Feel for the carotid pulse for at least 5 seconds and not more than 10 seconds.

8. *If there is no pulse,* give chest compressions. Locate the correct hand position on the ster-

num. Until the second rescuer returns, provide compressions and respirations as for a one-person rescue. Give fifteen compressions followed by two respirations.

9. When the second rescuer returns after calling for help, the first rescuer should complete the cycle of fifteen compressions and two respirations.

10. The first rescuer should then take 5 seconds to check for breathing and the presence of a carotid pulse. The first rescuer should then state, "No pulse. Continue CPR." The first rescuer then gives one full, slow breath for approximately 1½ seconds.

11. The second rescuer should get into position for compressions and locate the correct hand placement while the first rescuer is checking for pulse and breathing. After the first rescuer gives one full, slow breath, the second rescuer should begin compressions at the rate of 80 to 100 per minute, or five compressions in approximately 4 seconds (see figure 14-6A). The second rescuer should count out loud, "One and, two and, three and, four and, five." After each five compressions, the second rescuer should pause slightly to allow the first rescuer to give one slow, full breath. Rescue then continues with one breath after each five compressions.

12. Continue with the cycle of five compressions and one ventilation. The rescuer giving breaths should recheck pulse and breathing every few minutes by asking the rescuer giving compressions to pause for 5 seconds.

13. If one rescuer gets tired, the rescuers can change positions. The person giving compressions should provide a clear signal to change positions, such as, "Change, and two, and three, and four, and five." The compressor should complete a cycle of five compressions. The ventilator should give one breath at the end of the five compressions. The ventilator should then move to the chest and locate the correct hand placement for compressions (see figure 14-6B). The compressor should move to the head, open the airway, and check the pulse and breathing for 5 seconds. After checking for pulse and breathing, the person should then give one full slow breath and state, "No pulse. Continue CPR." The new compressor should then give five compressions at the rate of 80 to 100 per

Figure 14-6A In a two-person rescue, one breath is given after every five compressions.

Figure 14-6B When the person doing compressions gets tired, the rescuers can change positions.

minute. The rescue should continue with one ventilation after each five compressions.

14. The rescuers should continue CPR until qualified medical help arrives, the victim recovers, a doctor or other legally qualified person orders CPR discontinued, or the scene suddenly becomes unsafe.

15. After the practice session, use a gauze pad saturated with 70-percent alcohol or a 10-percent bleach disinfecting solution to clean the manikin. Wipe the face and clean inside the mouth thoroughly. Saturate a clean gauze pad with the solution and lay it on the mouth

area for at least 30 seconds. Use another gauze pad to wipe the area dry. Follow manufacturer's instructions for any additional cleaning required.

NOTE: A 10-percent bleach solution is more effective than alcohol. Some manikins have disposable mouthpieces that are discarded after use. If the mouthpiece is discarded, the remainder of the face should still be disinfected.

16. Replace all equipment used. Wash hands.

PRACTICE *Go to the workbook and use the evaluation sheet for 14:2B, Performing CPR—Two-Person Rescue, to practice this procedure. When you feel you have mastered this skill, sign the sheet and give it to your instructor for further action.*

✔ *Final Checkpoint* Using the criteria listed on the evaluation sheet, your instructor will grade you on your performance.

PROCEDURE

Performing CPR on Infants and Children 14:2C&D

EQUIPMENT AND SUPPLIES

CPR infant and child manikins, alcohol or disinfecting solution, gauze pads

PROCEDURE

! *CAUTION:* Only CPR training manikins should be used to practice these procedures. *Never* practice CPR on a human infant or child.

1. Assemble equipment.
2. Gently shake the infant or child or tap the infant's foot (for reflex action) to determine consciousness. Call to the infant or child.

Send for medical assistance as soon as possible if there is no response.

3. Use the head-tilt/chin-lift method to open the infant's or child's airway. Tip the head back gently, taking care not to tip it as far back as you would an adult's head.

! *CAUTION:* Tipping the head too far will cause an obstruction of the infant's airway.

NOTE: For CPR techniques, infants are usually considered to be under 1 year old; children are ages 1 to 8 years. Children over 8 years old usually require the same techniques as do adults. Use your judgment for this age group, depending on the size of the child.

4. Look, listen, and feel for breathing. Check for at least 5 seconds.
5. *If there is no breathing,* give two slow, full breaths, each breath lasting approximately 1½ seconds. For an infant, cover the infant's nose and mouth with your mouth (see figure 14-7A). For a child, cover the child's nose and mouth with your mouth, or pinch the child's nose and cover the child's mouth with your mouth. Breathe until the chest rises gently during each ventilation and allow for chest deflation after each breath.
6. Check the pulse. For an infant, check the pulse over the brachial artery: place your fingertips on the inside of the upper arm and halfway between the elbow and shoulder. Put

Figure 14-7A If an infant is not breathing, cover the infant's mouth and nose with your mouth and give two slow, full breaths.

your thumb on the posterior (outside) of the arm. Squeeze your fingers gently toward your thumb. Feel for the pulse for 5 to 10 seconds. For a child, check the pulse at the carotid pulse site. Feel for the pulse for 5 to 10 seconds.

7. *If a pulse is present,* continue providing ventilations by giving the infant or child one ventilation every 3 seconds. After 1 minute (approximately twenty breaths), recheck the pulse and breathing for 5 seconds.

8. *If no pulse is present,* administer cardiac compressions. For an infant, locate the correct position for compressions by drawing an imaginary line between the nipples. Place 2 fingers on the sternum and one finger's width below this imaginary line. Give compressions at the rate of 100 per minute (see figure 14-7B). For a child, place the heel of one hand one finger's width above the substernal notch of the breastbone. Give compressions at the rate of 80 to 100 per minute. Make sure the infant or child is on a firm surface, or use one hand to support the infant's or child's back while administering compressions. Press hard enough to compress the infant's chest ½ to 1 inch, or 1.4 to 2.5 centimeters, or the child's chest 1 to 1½ inches, or 2.5 to 3.8 centimeters. Give 5 compressions in approximately 3 seconds.

9. After every five compressions, give one slow, full breath until the chest rises gently.

10. Continue the cycle of five compressions followed by one ventilation. To establish the correct rate for an infant, count, "One, two, three, four, five, breathe"; for a child, count, "One and two and three and four and five, breathe."

11. After 1 minute, check for breathing and pulse for 5 seconds. Continue CPR if no breathing or pulse is noted. Recheck the pulse and breathing every few minutes for 5 seconds.

12. Obtain medical help as quickly as possible. Send someone else to telephone or obtain help, or call for someone to assist. If no help is available, stop CPR after 1 minute to telephone for medical assistance. Resume CPR as quickly as possible.

13. After the practice session, use a gauze pad saturated with 70-percent alcohol or a 10-percent bleach disinfecting solution to clean the manikin. Wipe the face and clean inside the mouth thoroughly. Saturate a clean gauze pad with the solution and lay it on the mouth area for at least 30 seconds. Use another gauze pad to wipe the area dry. Follow manufacturer's instructions for specific cleaning. *NOTE:* The 10-percent bleach solution is more effective than alcohol. Some manikins have disposable mouthpieces that are discarded after use. If the mouthpiece is discarded, the remainder of the face should still be disinfected.

14. Replace all equipment used. Wash hands.

Figure 14-7B Use two fingers to give an infant cardiac compressions.

PRACTICE *Go to the workbook and use the evaluation sheets for 14:2C, Performing CPR on Infants and 14:2D, Performing CPR on Children, to practice these procedures. When you feel you have mastered these skills, sign the sheets and give them to your instructor for further action.*

✔ *Final Checkpoint* Using the criteria listed on the evaluation sheet, your instructor will grade you on your performance.

PROCEDURE

Performing CPR—Obstructed Airway on Conscious, Adult Victim

OBRA

14:2E

EQUIPMENT AND SUPPLIES

CPR manikin or choking manikin

PROCEDURE

⚠ *CAUTION:* Only a manikin should be used to practice this procedure. Do not practice on another person. Hand placement can be tried on another person, but the actual abdominal thrust should *never* be performed unless the person is choking.

1. Assemble equipment. Position the manikin in an upright position sitting on a chair.
2. Determine whether the victim has an airway obstruction. Ask, "Are you choking?" Check to see whether the victim can cough or speak.

⚠ *CAUTION:* If the victim is coughing, the airway is not completely obstructed. Encourage the victim to remain calm and cough hard. Coughing is usually very effective for removing an obstruction.

3. If the victim cannot cough, talk, or breathe, call for help.
4. Perform abdominal thrusts to try to remove the obstruction. Follow these steps:
    a. Stand behind the victim.
    b. Wrap both arms around the victim's waist.
    c. Make a fist of one hand (see figure 14-8A). Place the thumb side of the victim's fist in the middle of the victim's abdomen, slightly above the navel (umbilicus) but well below the xiphoid process at the end of the sternum.
    d. Grasp the fist with your other hand. (See figure 14-8B).
    e. Use quick, upward thrusts to press into the victim's abdomen (see figure 14-8C).
        NOTE: The thrusts should be delivered hard enough to cause a force of air to push the obstruction out of the airway.

Figure 14-8A Make a fist of one hand.

Figure 14-8B Place the thumb side of the fist above the umbilicus but well below the xiphoid process at the end of the sternum. Grasp the fist with your other hand.

Figure 14-8C Use quick, upward thrusts to press into the victim's abdomen.

CAUTION: Make sure that your forearms do not press against the victim's rib cage while the thrusts are being performed.

f. If you cannot reach around the victim to give abdominal thrusts (the victim is very obese), or if a victim is in the later stages of pregnancy, give chest thrusts. Stand behind the victim. Wrap your arms under the victim's axilla (armpits) and around to the center of the chest. Make a fist with one hand and place the thumb side of the fist against the center of the sternum but well above the xiphoid process. Grab your fist with your other hand and thrust inward.

g. Repeat the thrusts until the object is expelled or until the victim becomes unconscious. If the victim loses consciousness, follow Procedure 14:2F, Performing CPR— Obstructed Airway on Unconscious Victim. Start with a mouth sweep, try to give two breaths, and then give five abdominal thrusts if you are unable to ventilate the victim.

5. Make every effort to obtain medical help for the victim as soon as possible. Send someone to call for help. If no one is present, yell for help. If no one answers your calls, you may have to stop your efforts for a short period of time to telephone for or obtain assistance.

6. After the practice session, replace all equipment used. Wash hands.

PRACTICE *Go to the workbook and use the evaluation sheet for 14:2E, Performing CPR—Obstructed Airway on Conscious, Adult Victim, to practice this procedure. When you feel you have mastered this skill, sign the sheet and give it to your instructor for further action.*

✔ *Final Checkpoint* Using the criteria listed on the evaluation sheet, your instructor will grade you on your performance.

PROCEDURE

Performing CPR— Obstructed Airway on Unconscious Victim

OBRA

14:2F

EQUIPMENT AND SUPPLIES

CPR manikin, alcohol or disinfecting solution, gauze sponges

PROCEDURE

CAUTION: Only a manikin should be used to practice this procedure. Do *not* practice on another person.

1. Assemble equipment. Place the manikin on a firm surface, usually the floor.
2. Shake the victim gently. Ask, "Are you OK?"
3. Use the head-tilt/chin-lift method to open the airway.
4. Look, listen, and feel for breathing for 5 seconds.
5. If the victim is not breathing, call for help. Give two slow, full breaths. If air does not go into the lungs on the first breath, reposition the victim's head and try to breathe again. If the chest still does not rise, the airway is probably obstructed.
   NOTE: You may place an opened gauze sponge over the mouth, if you wish.
6. Yell for help. If someone responds to your calls for help, send him or her to telephone for emergency medical assistance.
7. Perform five abdominal thrusts. Position the victim on his or her back. Place one of your legs on either side of the hips and thighs and "straddle" the victim (see figure 14-9A). Place the heel of one hand on the victim's abdomen, making sure the heel is positioned well below the tip of the xiphoid process, at the end of the sternum, but slightly above the navel (umbilicus). Place your other hand on top of the first hand. Give five quick, upward thrusts into the abdomen.
   NOTE: This action provides a force of air to help free the object obstructing the airway.

Figure 14-9A Straddle the unconscious victim to give five abdominal thrusts.

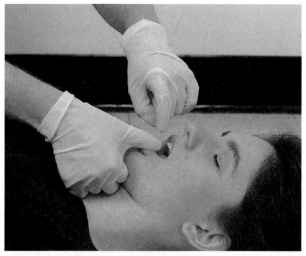

Figure 14-9B Use a C-shaped, or hooking, motion to check the mouth for the object.

NOTE: If the victim is pregnant or very obese, it may be necessary to give chest thrusts instead of abdominal thrusts. Position your hands in the same position used for chest compressions. Push straight down five times.

8. Check the mouth for the object. Open the victim's mouth by grasping the lower jaw between your thumb and fingers and lifting it. This pushes the tongue out of the airway and away from the object that may be lodged there. Use the index finger of your opposite hand to sweep along the inside of the mouth. With a C-shape or hooking motion, bring the finger along one cheek and sweep across the throat from the side and toward the opposite cheek (see figure 14-9B). Remove the object if it is seen.

CAUTION: Take care not to push straight into the throat because this may force the object to lodge deeper in the airway.

9. Open the airway and try to give two slow, full breaths. If the chest rises, check the pulse and continue with ventilations or CPR as needed.

10. *If the chest does not rise,* repeat the sequence. Give five thrusts, check the mouth, and attempt to ventilate. Continue repeating the sequence until you are able to get air into the chest during ventilation.

NOTE: Unless you are able to get oxygen into the lungs of the victim, chest compressions have no value. The purpose of chest compressions is to circulate the oxygen.

NOTE: After a period of time without oxygen, the muscles of the throat will relax and

you may be able to remove the object using the previous methods.

11. To care for an infant who has an obstructed airway, follow these steps:
    a. Gently shake the infant to determine consciousness. Call to the infant. Call for help if there is no response.
    b. Use the head-tilt/chin-lift method to open the airway.
    c. Look, listen, and feel for breathing for 5 seconds.
    d. If there is no breathing, cover the infant's nose and mouth with your mouth and attempt to ventilate. If the breaths do not go in, reposition the infant's head and try to breathe a second time. If the breaths still do not go in, assume that the infant has an obstructed airway.
    e. Give five back blows. Hold the infant face down, with your arm supporting the infant's head and jaw. Position the head lower than the chest (see figure 14-10A). Use the heel of your other hand to give five firm back blows between the infant's shoulder blades.

    CAUTION: When performing CPR on an infant, do not use excessive force.

    f. Give five chest thrusts. Turn the infant face up, holding the head lower than the chest. Position two to three fingers on the sternum one finger's width below an imaginary line drawn between the nipples. Gently press straight down five times (see figure 14-10B), to compress the sternum ½ to 1 inch.

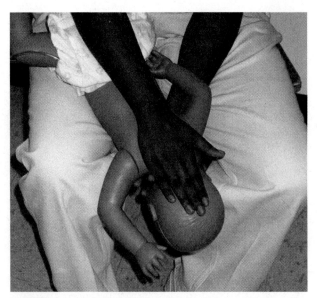

Figure 14-10A To give an infant five back blows, position the infant face down, with the head lower than the chest.

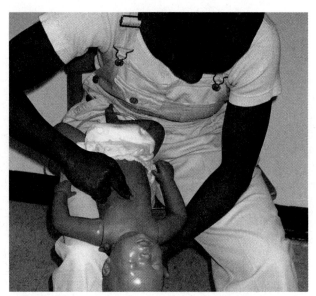

Figure 14-10B Give the infant five chest thrusts, keeping the head lower than the chest.

g. Check the mouth for the object. If you see the object, remove it by using a finger to sweep the mouth.

CAUTION: If you do *not* see the object, do not sweep the mouth with a finger.

h. Attempt to ventilate by giving two slow breaths. If the infant's chest rises, check for pulse and then continue with pulmonary resuscitation or cardiac compressions, as needed. If the chest does not rise, keep repeating the sequence of five back blows, five chest thrusts, checking the mouth, and ventilating until the object can be removed.

12. To care for a child who has an obstructed airway, follow the same procedure used for adult victims *except* look in the mouth during the mouth check. Do *not* perform a finger sweep unless the object can be seen in the mouth. Therefore the sequence of steps is to give five abdominal thrusts, look in the mouth, sweep the mouth if the object is seen, and attempt to ventilate.

13. Make every effort to obtain medical help for the victim as soon as possible. Send someone to telephone for help. If no one is present, yell for help. If no one answers your calls, stop your efforts after 1 minute to telephone for or obtain assistance. Resume CPR as quickly as possible.

14. After the practice session, use a gauze pad saturated with 70-percent alcohol or a 10-percent bleach disinfecting solution to clean the manikin. Wipe the face and clean inside the mouth thoroughly. Saturate a clean gauze pad with the solution and lay it on the mouth area for at least 30 seconds. Use another gauze pad to wipe the area dry. Follow manufacturer's recommendations for specific cleaning or care.

NOTE: A 10-percent bleach solution is more effective than alcohol. Some manikins have disposable mouthpieces that are discarded after use. If the mouthpiece is discarded, the remainder of the face should still be disinfected.

15. Replace all equipment used. Wash hands.

PRACTICE *Go to the workbook and use the evaluation sheet for 14:2F, Performing CPR—Obstructed Airway on Unconscious Victim, to practice this procedure. When you feel you have mastered this skill, sign the sheet and give it to your instructor for further action.*

✔ *Final Checkpoint* Using the criteria listed on the evaluation sheet, your instructor will grade you on your performance.

INFORMATION
14:3 *Providing First Aid for Bleeding and Wounds*

In any health career as well as in your personal life, you may need to provide first aid to control bleeding or care for wounds. This section provides basic information on the principles to observe when providing such first aid.

A **wound** involves injury to the soft tissues. Wounds are usually classified as open or closed. With an open wound, there is a break in the skin or mucous membrane. With a closed wound, there is no break in the skin or mucous membrane but injury occurs to the underlying tissues. Wounds can result in bleeding, infection, and/or tetanus (lockjaw, a serious infection caused by bacteria). First aid care must be directed toward controlling bleeding before the bleeding leads to death, and toward preventing or obtaining treatment for infection.

Open wounds are classified into types according to the injuries that occur. Some main types are abrasions, incisions, lacerations, punctures, avulsions, and amputations.

a. **Abrasion.** With this type of wound the skin is scraped off. Bleeding is usually limited, but infection must be prevented because dirt and contaminants often enter the wound.

b. **Incision.** This is a cut or injury caused by a sharp object such as a knife, scissors, razor blade, or other similar object. If the cut is deep, bleeding can be heavy and can lead to excessive blood loss. In addition, damage to muscles, nerves, and other tissues can occur.

c. **Laceration.** This type of wound involves tearing of the tissues by way of excessive force. The wound often has jagged, irregular edges. Bleeding may be heavy. If the wound is deep, contamination may lead to infection.

d. **Puncture.** This type of wound is caused by a sharp object such as a pin, nail, or pointed instrument. External bleeding is usually limited, but internal bleeding can occur. In addition, the chance for infection is increased and tetanus may develop if the tetanus bacteria enters the wound.

e. **Avulsion.** This type of wound occurs when tissue is torn or separated from the victim's body. It can result in a piece of torn tissue hanging from the ear, nose, hand, or other body part. Bleeding is heavy and usually extensive. It is important to preserve the body part while caring for this type of wound, because a surgeon may be able to reattach it.

f. **Amputation.** This type of injury occurs when a body part is cut off and separated from the body. Loss of a finger, toe, hand, or other body part can occur. Bleeding can be heavy and extensive. Care must be taken to preserve the amputated part because a surgeon may be able to reattach it. The part should be wrapped in a cool, moist dressing (use sterile water or normal saline, if possible), and placed in a plastic bag. The plastic bag should be kept cool or placed in ice water and transported with the victim. The body part should never be placed directly on ice.

Controlling bleeding is the first priority in caring for wounds, because it is possible for a victim to bleed to death in a short period of time. Bleeding can come from arteries, veins, and capillaries. Arterial blood usually spurts from a wound, results in heavy blood loss, and is bright red in color. Arterial bleeding is life-threatening and must be controlled quickly. Venous blood is slower, steadier, and dark red or maroon in color. Venous bleeding is easier to control. Capillary blood "oozes" from the wound slowly, is less red than arterial blood, and clots easily. The four main methods for controlling bleeding are listed in the order in which they should be used: direct pressure, elevation, pressure bandage, and pressure points. *CAUTION:* If possible, use some type of protective barrier, such as gloves or plastic wrap, while controlling bleeding. If this is not possible in an emergency, use thick layers of dressings and try to avoid contact of blood with your skin. Wash your hands thoroughly and as soon as possible after giving first aid to a bleeding victim.

a. Direct pressure: Using your gloved hand over a thick dressing or sterile gauze, apply pressure directly to the wound. If no dressing is available, use a clean cloth or linen-type towel. In an emergency when no materials are available, it may even be necessary to use a bare hand. Continue to apply pressure for 5 to 10 minutes or until the bleeding stops. If blood soaks through the dressing, apply a second dressing over the first and continue to apply direct pressure. Do *not* disturb blood clots once they have formed. Direct pressure will usually stop most bleeding.

b. Elevation: Raise the injured part above the level of the victim's heart to allow gravity to aid in stopping the blood flow from the wound. Continue applying direct pressure while elevating the injured part. *CAUTION:* If fractures (broken bones) are present or suspected, the part should *not* be elevated.

c. Pressure bandage: When the bleeding is under control, apply a pressure bandage. Maintain direct pressure and elevation while applying the pressure bandage. Apply additional dressings over the other dressings on the wound. Use a roller bandage to hold the dressings in place by wrapping the roller bandage around the dressings. Use overlapping turns to cover the dressings and to hold them securely in place. Tie off the ends of the bandage by placing the tie directly over the dressings. Make sure the pressure bandage is secure. Check a pulse site below the pressure bandage to make sure the bandage is not too tight. The pulse should be present and there should be no discoloration of the skin to indicate impaired circulation. If any signs of impaired circulation are present, loosen and replace the pressure bandage.

d. Pressure points: If direct pressure, elevation, and the pressure bandage do not stop severe bleeding, it may be necessary to apply pressure to pressure points. By applying pressure to a main artery and pressing it against an underlying bone, the main blood supply to the injured area can be cut off. However, because this technique also stops circulation to other parts of the limb, it should *not* be used any longer than is absolutely necessary. Direct pressure and elevation should also be continued while pressure is being applied to the pressure point.

The main pressure point for the arm is the brachial artery. It is located on the inside of the arm, approximately halfway between the armpit and the elbow (see figure 14-11A). The main pressure point for the leg is the femoral artery. The pulsation can be felt at the groin (the front middle point of the upper leg, in the crease where the thigh joins the body), see figure 14-11B. When bleeding stops, slowly release pressure on the pressure point. Continue using direct pressure and elevation. If bleeding starts again, be ready to reapply pressure to the correct pressure point.

Figure 14-11A The main pressure point for the arm is the brachial artery. Pressure is applied at the point shown.

Figure 14-11B The main pressure point in the leg is the femoral artery. Pressure is applied with the heel of the hand.

After severe bleeding has been controlled, obtain medical help for the victim. Do not disturb any blood clots or remove the dressings that were used to control the bleeding, because this may result in additional bleeding. Make no attempt to clean the wound, because this too is likely to result in additional bleeding.

In treating minor wounds that do not involve severe bleeding, prevention of infection is the first priority. Wash your hands thoroughly before treating the wound. Put on gloves to avoid contamination from blood or fluid draining from the wound. Use soap and water and sterile gauze, if possible, to wash the wound. Wipe in an outward direction, away from the wound. Discard the wipe after each use. Rinse the wound thoroughly with cool water. Use sterile gauze to gently blot the wound dry. Apply a sterile dressing or bandage. Watch for any signs of infection. Be sure to tell the victim to obtain medical help if any signs of infection appear.

Infection can develop in any wound. It is important to recognize the signs of infection and to seek medical help if they appear. Some signs and symptoms are swelling, heat, redness, pain, fever, pus, and red streaks leading from the wound. Prompt medical care is needed if any of these symptoms occur.

Tetanus bacteria can enter an open wound and lead to serious illness and death. Tetanus infection is most common in puncture wounds and wounds that involve damage to tissue underneath the skin. When this type of wound occurs, it is important to obtain information from the patient regarding his or her last tetanus shot and to get medical advice regarding protection in the form a tetanus shot or booster.

With some wounds, objects can remain in the tissues or become embedded in the wound. Examples of such objects include splinters, small pieces of glass, small stones, and other similar objects. If the object is at the surface of the skin, remove it gently with sterile tweezers or tweezers wiped clean with alcohol. Any objects embedded in the tissues should be left in the skin and removed by a physician.

Closed wounds (those not involving breaks in the skin) can occur anywhere in the body as a result of injury. If the wound is a bruise, cold applications can be applied to reduce swelling. Other closed wounds can be extremely serious and cause internal bleeding that may lead to death. Signs and symptoms may include pain, tenderness, swelling, deformity, cold and clammy skin, rapid and weak pulse, uncontrolled restlessness, excessive thirst, vomited blood, or blood in the urine or feces. Get medical help for the victim as soon as possible. Check breathing, treat for shock, avoid unnecessary movement, and avoid giving any fluids or food to the victim.

While caring for any victim with severe bleeding or wounds, always be alert for the signs of shock. Be prepared to treat shock while providing care to control bleeding and prevent infection in the wound.

C At all times, remain calm while providing first aid. Reassure the victim. Obtain appropriate assistance or medical care as soon as possible in every case requiring additional care.

STUDENT Go to the workbook and complete the assignment sheet for 14:3, Providing First Aid for Bleeding and Wounds. Then return and continue with the procedure.

PROCEDURE

Providing First Aid for Bleeding and Wounds *14:3*

EQUIPMENT AND SUPPLIES

Sterile dressings and bandages, disposable gloves

PROCEDURE

Severe Wounds

1. Follow the steps of priority care, if indicated.
   a. Check the scene. Move the victim only if absolutely necessary.
   b. Check the victim for consciousness and breathing.
   c. Call emergency medical services (EMS).
   d. Provide care to the victim.
2. To control severe bleeding, proceed as follows:
   a. If possible, put on gloves or wrap your hands in plastic wrap to provide a protective barrier while controlling bleeding. If this is not possible in an emergency, use thick layers of dressings and try to avoid contact of blood with your skin.
   b. Using your hand over a thick dressing or sterile gauze, apply pressure directly to the wound.
   c. Continue to apply pressure to the wound for approximately 5 to 10 minutes. Do *not* release the pressure to check whether the bleeding has stopped.
   d. If blood soaks through the first dressing, apply a second dressing and continue to apply direct pressure.
      NOTE: If sterile gauze is *not* available, use clean material or a bare hand.
      CAUTION: Do *not* disturb blood clots once they have formed. This will cause the bleeding to start again.
3. Elevate the injured part above the level of the victim's heart unless a fracture or broken bone is suspected.
   NOTE: This allows gravity to help stop the blood flow to the area.

NOTE: Direct pressure and elevation are used together (see figure 14-12). Do *not* stop direct pressure while elevating the part.

4. When the bleeding is under control, apply a pressure bandage (see figure 14-13). Maintain direct pressure and elevation while applying the pressure bandage. To apply a pressure bandage, proceed as follows:
   a. Apply additional dressings over the dressings already on the wound.
   b. Use a roller bandage to hold the dressings in place by wrapping the roller bandage around the dressings. Use overlapping turns to cover the dressings and to hold them securely in place.
   c. Tie off the ends of the bandage by placing the tie directly over the dressings.
   d. Make sure the pressure bandage is secure. Check a pulse site below the pressure bandage to make sure the bandage is not too tight. A pulse should be present and there should be no discoloration of the skin to indicate impaired circulation. If any signs of impaired circulation are present, loosen and replace the pressure bandage.
5. If the bleeding continues, it may be necessary to apply pressure to the appropriate pressure point. Continue using direct pressure and elevation, and apply pressure to the pressure point as follows:

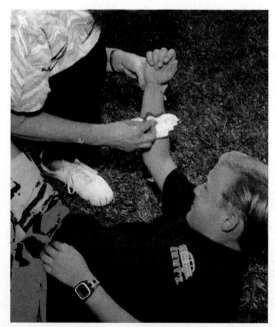

Figure 14-12 By using direct pressure and elevation, most severe bleeding can be controlled.

Figure 14-13 Steps for applying a pressure bandage.

a. If the wound is on the arm or hand, apply pressure to the brachial artery. Place the flat surface of your fingers (not your fingertips) against the inside of the victim's upper arm, approximately halfway between the elbow and axilla area. Position your thumb on the outside of the arm. Press your fingers toward your thumb to compress the brachial artery and decrease the supply of blood to the arm.

b. If the wound is on the leg, place the heel of one hand directly over the femoral artery where it passes over the pelvic bone. The position is on the front, middle part of the upper thigh (groin) where the leg joins the body. Straighten your arm and apply pressure to compress the femoral artery and to decrease the blood supply to the leg.

6. When the bleeding stops, slowly release the pressure on the pressure point while continuing to use direct pressure and elevation. If the bleeding starts again, be ready to reapply pressure to the pressure point.

7. Obtain medical help for the victim as soon as possible. Severe bleeding is a life-threatening emergency.

8. While caring for any victim experiencing severe bleeding, be alert for the signs and symptoms of shock. Treat the victim for shock if any signs or symptons are noted.

9. During treatment, constantly reassure the victim. Encourage the victim to remain calm by remaining calm yourself.

10. After controlling the bleeding, wash your hands as thoroughly and quickly as possible to avoid possible contamination from the blood. Wear gloves and use a disinfectant solution to wipe up any blood spills. Always wash your hands thoroughly after removing gloves.

PROCEDURE

Minor Wounds

1. Wash hands thoroughly with soap and water. Put on gloves.

2. Use sterile gauze, soap, and water to wash the wound. Start at the center and wash in an

outward direction. Discard the gauze after each pass.

3. Rinse the wound thoroughly with cool water to remove all of the soap.

4. Use sterile gauze to dry the wound. Blot it gently.

5. Apply a sterile dressing to the wound.

6. Caution the victim to look for signs of infection. Tell the victim to obtain medical care if any signs of infection appear.

7. If tetanus infection is possible (for example, in cases involving puncture wounds), tell the victim to contact a doctor regarding a tetanus shot.

   ⊗ *CAUTION:* Do *not* use any antiseptic solutions to clean the wound and do *not* apply any substances to the wound unless specifically instructed to do so by your immediate supervisor.

8. Obtain medical help as soon as possible for any victim requiring additional care. Any victim who has particles embedded in a wound, risk of tetanus, severe bleeding, or other complications must be referred for medical care.

9. When care is complete, remove gloves and wash hands thoroughly.

PRACTICE *Go to the workbook and use the evaluation sheet for 14:3, Providing First Aid for Bleeding and Wounds, to practice these procedures. When you feel you have mastered these skills, sign the sheet and give it to your instructor for further action.*

✔ *Final Checkpoint* Using the criteria listed on the evaluation sheet, your instructor will grade you on your performance.

INFORMATION
14:4 *Providing First Aid for Shock*

Shock is a state that can exist with any injury or illness requiring first aid, so it is important that you are able to recognize it and provide treatment. This section provides some basic facts about shock.

Shock can be defined as "a clinical set of signs and symptoms associated with an inadequate supply of blood to body organs, especially the brain and heart." If it is not treated, shock can lead to death, even when a victim's injuries or illness might not themselves be fatal.

Many different things can cause the victim to experience shock: hemorrhage (excessive loss of blood); excessive pain; infection; heart attack; stroke; poisoning by chemicals, drugs, or gases; lack of oxygen; psychological trauma; and dehydration (loss of body fluids) from burns, vomiting, or diarrhea.

The following signs and symptoms can indicate shock:

a. The skin is pale or bluish gray in color. Check the nailbeds and the mucous membrane around the mouth.

b. The skin is cool to the touch.

c. Diaphoresis, or excessive perspiration, may result in a wet, clammy feeling when the skin is touched.

d. The pulse is rapid and weak. A radial pulse is sometimes too weak to be felt. The pulse must be checked at one of the carotid arteries in the neck.

e. Respirations are rapid, shallow, and may be irregular.

f. Blood pressure is very low or below normal, and may not be obtainable.

g. The victim experiences general weakness. As shock progresses, the victim becomes listless and confused. Eventually, the victim loses consciousness.

h. The victim experiences anxiety and extreme restlessness.

i. The victim may complain of excessive thirst.

j. The victim may experience nausea and/or vomiting.

k. The victim may complain of blurred vision. As shock progresses, the victim's eyes may appear sunken and have a vacant or confused expression. The pupils may dilate or become large.

It is essential to get medical help for the victim as soon as possible. Treatment for shock is directed toward (1) eliminating the cause of shock; (2) improving circulation, especially to the brain and heart; (3) providing an adequate oxygen supply; and (4) maintaining body temperature. Some of the basic principles for treatment are as follows:

a. The position for treating shock must be based on the victim's injuries.

> **!** *CAUTION:* If neck or spine injuries are suspected, the victim should not be moved unless it is necessary to remove him or her from danger.

The best position for treating shock is usually to keep the victim lying flat on the back, because this improves circulation. Raising the feet and legs 12 inches can also provide additional blood for the heart and brain. However, if the victim is vomiting or has bleeding and injuries of the jaw or mouth, the victim should be positioned on the side to prevent him or her from choking on blood and/or vomitus. If a victim is experiencing breathing problems, it may be necessary to raise the victim's head and shoulders to make breathing easier. If the victim has a *head* (not neck) injury and has difficulty breathing, the victim should be positioned lying flat or with the head raised slightly. It is important to position the victim based on the injury or illness involved.

b. Cover the patient with blankets or additional clothing to prevent chilling or exposure to the cold. Blankets may also be placed between the ground and the victim. However, it is important to avoid overheating the victim. If the skin is very warm to the touch and perspiration is noted, remove some of the blankets or coverings.

c. Avoid giving the victim anything to eat or drink if medical help will be available in a reasonable period of time. If the victim complains of excessive thirst, a wet cloth can be used to provide some comfort by moistening the lips and mouth. If medical help will not be available for 1 hour or more, the victim's condition is deteriorating, and dehydration is evident, it may be necessary to provide some fluids. A salt/soda solution composed of 1 teaspoon of salt and ½ teaspoon of baking soda per 1 quart of water may be prepared. Give small quantities of the solution every 15 minutes.

> **!** *CAUTION:* If the victim is unconscious, vomiting, or convulsing; has a brain or abdominal injury; or may require surgery, *provide no fluids* and give nothing by mouth to the victim.

Remember that it is important to look for signs of shock while providing first aid for any injury or illness. Provide care that will reduce the effect of shock. Obtain medical help for the victim as soon as possible.

STUDENT *Go to the workbook and complete the assignment sheet for 14:4, Providing First Aid for Shock. Then return and continue with the procedure.*

PROCEDURE
Providing First Aid for Shock 14:4

EQUIPMENT AND SUPPLIES

Blankets, watch with second hand (optional), disposable gloves

PROCEDURE

1. Follow the steps of priority care, if indicated.
   a. Check the scene. Move the victim only if absolutely necessary.
   b. Check the victim for consciousness and breathing.
   c. Call emergency medical services (EMS).
   d. Provide care to the victim.
   e. Control severe bleeding.

◈ *CAUTION:* If possible, wear gloves or use a protective barrier while controlling bleeding.

2. Obtain medical help for the victim as soon as possible. Call or send someone to obtain help.

3. Observe the victim for any signs of shock. Look for a pale or bluish color to the skin. Touch the skin and note if it is cool, moist, or clammy to the touch. Note diaphoresis, or excessive perspiration. Check the pulse to see if it is rapid, weak, or irregular. If you are unable to feel a radial pulse, check the carotid pulse. Check the respirations to see if they are rapid, weak, irregular, shallow, or labored. If equipment is available, check blood pressure to see if it is low. Observe the victim for signs of weakness, apathy, confusion, or consciousness. Note if the victim is nauseated or vomiting, complaining of excessive thirst, restless or anxious, or complaining of blurred vision. Examine the eyes for a sunken, vacant, or confused appearance, and dilated pupils.

4. Try to reduce the effects or eliminate the cause of shock: control bleeding by applying pressure at the site; provide oxygen, if possible; attempt to ease pain through position changes and comfort measures; give emotional support.

5. Position the victim based on the injuries or illness present
   a. If an injury of the neck or spine is present or suspect, do not move the victim.
   b. If the victim has bleeding and injuries to the jaw or mouth, or is vomiting, position the victim's body on either side. This allows fluids, vomitus, and/or blood to drain and prevents the airway from becoming blocked by these fluids.
   c. If the victim is having difficulty breathing, position the victim on the back, but raise the head and shoulders slightly to aid breathing.
   d. If the victim has a head injury, position the victim lying flat or with the head raised slightly.
      NOTE: Never allow the head to be positioned lower than the rest of the body.
   e. If none of these conditions exist, position the victim lying flat on the back. To improve circulation, raise the feet and legs 12 inches (see figure 14-14). If raising the legs causes pain or leads to difficult breathing, however, lower the legs to the flat position.

Figure 14-14 Position a shock victim flat on the back and elevate the feet and legs 12 inches. Do *not* use this position if the victim has a neck, spinal, head, or jaw injury, or if the victim is having difficulty breathing.

❗ *CAUTION:* Do not raise the legs if the victim has head, neck, or back injuries, or if there are possible fractures of the hips or legs.

   f. If in doubt on how to position a victim according to the injuries involved, keep the victim lying down flat or in the position in which you found him or her. Avoid any unnecessary movement.

6. Place enough blankets or coverings on the victim to prevent chilling. Sometimes, a blanket can be placed between the victim and the ground. Avoid overheating the patient, however.

7. If medical help will be available in a reasonable period of time, do not give the patient anything to eat or drink. If the patient complains of excessive thirst, use a moist cloth to wet the lips, tongue, and inside of the mouth. If medical help will be delayed for 1 hour or more, the patient's condition is deteriorating, and dehydration is evident, prepare a 2:1 solution of salt-soda by putting 1 teaspoon of salt and ½ teaspoon of baking soda in 1 quart of water. If the victim is conscious, *not* nauseated or vomiting, *not* convulsing, *not* likely to have surgery for the injuries or illness, and *not* showing signs of a brain or abdominal injury, give small amounts of the salt-soda solution. If any nausea or vomiting develops, stop giving the solution immediately.

8. Observe and provide care to the victim until medical help is obtained.

9. Replace all equipment used. Wash hands.

INFORMATION
14:5 *Providing First Aid for Poisoning*

Poisoning can occur anywhere, anytime—not only in health care settings, but also in your personal life. Thus, you may at some time be required to provide first aid for a poisoning victim. This section provides basic information regarding first aid for poisoning.

Poisoning can happen to any individual, regardless of age. It can be caused by swallowing various substances, inhaling poisonous gases, injecting substances, or contacting the skin with poison. Any substance that causes a harmful reaction when applied or ingested can be called a poison. Immediate action is necessary for any poisoning victim. Treatment varies depending on the type of poison, the injury involved, and the method of contact.

C If a poison has been swallowed, immediate care must be provided before the poison can be absorbed into the body. Call a poison control center (PCC) or a physician immediately. If you cannot contact a PCC, call emergency medical services (EMS). Most areas have poison control centers that provide information on specific antidotes and treatment. Save the label or container of the substance taken so this information can be given to the PCC or physician. It is also helpful to know or estimate how much was taken and the time at which the poisoning occurred. If the victim vomits, save a sample of the vomited material.

If the poisoning victim is unconscious, check for breathing. Provide artificial respiration if the victim is not breathing. Obtain medical help as soon as possible. If the unconscious victim is breathing, position the victim on his or her side so fluids can drain from the mouth. Obtain medical help quickly.

If the poison control center tells you to induce vomiting, get the victim to vomit. When inducing vomiting, place the victim on one side with the head slightly downward. Syrup of ipecac followed by a glass of water can be given to induce vomiting. (Follow dosage recommended on bottle.) Syrup of ipecac is available in most drug stores and can be kept in a first aid kit for poisoning victims. If syrup of ipecac is not available, tickle the back of the victim's throat or administer warm salt water.

! *CAUTION:* Vomiting must *not* be induced in unconscious victims, victims who swallowed an acid or alkali, victims who swallowed petroleum products, victims who are convulsing, or victims who have burns on the lips and mouth.

Because vomiting removes only about one-half of the poison, the PCC may recommend using activated charcoal to counteract the remaining poison. Activated charcoal is available in most drug stores and helps absorb any remaining poison. Follow the directions on the bottle to determine the correct dosage.

If poisoning is due to inhalation of dangerous gases, the victim must be immediately removed from the area before being treated. Carbon monoxide is a gas that causes poisoning when inhaled. It is odorless, colorless, and very difficult to detect. Before entering the danger area, take a deep breath of fresh air and do *not* breathe the gas while you are removing the victim from the area. After rescuing the victim, immediately check for breathing. Provide artificial respiration if needed. Obtain medical help immediately; death may occur very quickly with this type of poisoning.

If poisoning is due to chemicals or poisons coming in contact with the victim's skin, use large amounts of water to wash the skin, thereby diluting the substance and removing it from the skin. Remove any clothing and jewelry that contains the substance. Call a PCC or physician for additional information. Obtain medical help as soon as possible for burns or injuries that may result from contact with the poison.

Contact with a poisonous plant such as poison ivy, oak, or sumac can cause a serious skin reaction (see figure 14-15). If such contact occurs, wash the area thoroughly with soap and water. If a rash or weeping sores develop, lotions such as Calamine or Caladryl, or a paste made from baking soda and water may help relieve the discomfort. If the condition is severe and affects large areas of the body or face, obtain medical help.

If poisoning is due to injection from an insect bite or sting or a snakebite, and an arm or leg is affected, position the affected area below the level of the heart. For an insect bite, remove any embedded stinger and wash the area well with soap and water. Apply a sterile dressing and a cold pack to reduce swelling. For a snakebite, wash the wound and immobilize the injured area, positioning it lower than the heart, if possible. Do not cut the wound or apply a tourniquet. Monitor the breathing of the victim and give artificial respiration if necessary. Obtain medical help for the victim as soon as pos-

Figure 14-15 Contact with a poisonous plant such as poison oak, ivy, or sumac can cause a serious skin reaction. *(Courtesy of Timothy Berger, MD, Associate Clinical Professor, University of California, San Francisco)*

sible. Watch for allergic reaction in all victims. Signs and symptoms of allergic reaction include redness and swelling at the site, itching, hives, pain, swelling of the throat, difficult or labored breathing, dizziness, and a change in the level of consciousness. Maintain respirations and obtain medical help as quickly as possible for the victim who experiences an allergic reaction.

C In all poisoning victims, observe for signs of shock. Treat the victim for shock, if necessary. Try to remain calm and confident while providing first aid for poisoning victims. Reassure the victim as needed. Act quickly and in an organized, efficient manner.

STUDENT Go to the workbook and complete the assignment sheet for 14:5, Providing First Aid for Poisoning. Then return and continue with the procedure.

PROCEDURE

Providing First Aid for Poisoning 14:5

EQUIPMENT AND SUPPLIES

Telephone
disposable gloves

PROCEDURE

1. Follow the steps of priority care, if indicated:
   a. Check the scene. Move the victim only if absolutely necessary.
   b. Check the victim for consciousness and breathing.
   c. Call emergency medical services.
   d. Provide care to the victim.
   e. Control severe bleeding.

♲ *CAUTION:* If possible, wear gloves or use a protective barrier while controlling bleeding.

2. Check the victim for signs of poisoning. Signs may include burns on the lips or mouth, odor, a container of poison, or presence of the poisonous substance on the victim or in the victim's mouth. Information may also be obtained from the victim or from an observer.

3. If the victim is conscious, not convulsing, and has swallowed a poison:
   a. Try to determine the type of poison, how much was taken, and when the poison was taken. Look for the container near the victim.
   b. Call a PCC or physician immediately for specific information on how to treat the poisoning victim. Provide as much information as possible.
   c. Follow the instructions received from the PCC. Obtain medical help if needed.
   d. If the victim vomits, save a sample of the vomited material.

4. If the PCC tells you to get the victim to vomit, induce vomiting. Give the victim syrup of ipecac or warm salt water, or tickle the back of the victim's throat.
   CAUTION: Do *not* induce vomiting if the victim is unconscious or convulsing, has burns on the lips or mouth, or has swallowed an acid, alkali, or petroleum product.

5. If the victim is unconscious:
   a. Check for breathing. If the victim is not breathing, give artificial respiration.
   b. If the victim is breathing, position the victim on his or her side to allow fluids to drain from the mouth.
   c. Call a PCC or physician for specific treatment. Obtain medical help immediately.
   d. If possible, save the poison container and a sample of any vomited material. Check with any observers to find out what was taken, how much was taken, and when the poison was taken.

6. If chemicals or poisons have splashed on the victim's skin, wash the area thoroughly with large amounts of water. Remove any clothing and jewelry containing the substance. If a large area of the body is affected, a shower or tub may be used to rinse the skin. Obtain medical help immediately for burns or injuries caused by the poison.

7. If the victim has come in contact with a poisonous plant such as poison ivy, oak, or sumac, wash the area of contact thoroughly with soap and water. Remove any contaminated clothing. If a rash or weeping sores develop, lotions such as Calamine or Caladryl, or a paste made from baking soda and water, may help relieve the discomfort. If the condition is severe and affects large areas of the body or face, obtain medical help.

8. If the victim has inhaled poisonous gas, do not endanger your life by trying to treat the victim in the area of the gas. Take a deep breath of fresh air before entering the area and hold your breath while you remove the victim from the area. When the victim is in a safe area, check for breathing. Provide artificial respiration, if necessary. Obtain medical help immediately.

9. If poisoning is due to injection from an insect bite or sting or a snakebite, proceed as follows:
   a. If an arm or leg is affected, position the affected area below the level of the heart.
   b. For an insect bite, use a tweezer to remove any embedded stinger. The stinger can also be removed by scraping it off with an object like a credit card. Wash the area well with soap and water. Apply a sterile dressing and a cold pack to reduce swelling.
   c. For a snakebite, wash the wound. Immobilize the injured area, positioning it lower than the heart, if possible. Monitor the breathing of the victim and give artificial respiration if necessary. Obtain medical help for the victim as soon as possible.
   d. Watch for the signs and symptoms of allergic reaction in all victims. Signs and symptoms of allergic reaction include redness and swelling at the site, itching, hives, pain, swelling of the throat, difficult or labored breathing, dizziness, and a change in the level of consciousness. Maintain respirations and obtain medical help as quickly as possible for the victim experiencing an allergic reaction.
   e. Watch for signs of shock in all victims and treat for shock as necessary.

10. Observe for signs of shock while treating any poisoning victim. Treat for shock as necessary.

11. Remain calm while treating the victim. Reassure the victim.

12. Always obtain medical help for any poisoning victim. Some poisons may have delayed reactions. Always keep the telephone numbers of a PCC and other sources of medical assistance in a convenient location so you will be prepared to provide and follow up on first aid for poisoning.

PRACTICE *Go to the workbook and use the evaluation sheet for 14:5, Providing*

First Aid for Poisoning, to practice this procedure. When you feel you have mastered this skill, sign the sheet and give it to your instructor for further action.

✔ *Final Checkpoint* Using the criteria listed on the evaluation sheet, your instructor will grade you on your performance.

INFORMATION
14:6 *Providing First Aid for Burns*

Burns are common injuries. Therefore, you may at some time be required to provide first aid care to a burn victim. This section provides the main facts about burns.

A **burn** is an injury that can be caused by fire, heat, chemical agents, radiation, and/or electricity.

Burns are classified as either first, second, or third degree (see figure 14-16). Characteristics of each type of burn are as follows:

a. First-degree, or superficial, burn: This is the least severe type of burn. It involves only the top layer of skin, the epidermis, and usually heals in 5 to 6 days without permanent scarring. The skin is usually reddened or discolored. There may be some mild swelling, and the victim feels pain. Three common causes are overexposure to the sun (sunburn), brief contact with hot objects or steam, and exposure of the skin to a weak acid or alkali.

b. Second-degree, or partial-thickness, burn: This type of burn involves injury to the top layers of skin, including both the epidermis and dermis. A blister or vesicle forms. The skin is red or has a mottled appearance. Swelling usually occurs, and the surface of the skin frequently appears to be wet. This is a painful burn. Frequent causes include excessive exposure to the sun, a sunlamp, or artificial radiation; contact with hot or boiling liquids; and contact with fire.

c. Third-degree, or full-thickness, burn: This is the most severe type of burn and involves injury to all layers of the skin plus the underlying tissue. The area involved has a white or charred appearance. This type of burn can be either extremely painful or, if nerve endings are destroyed, relatively painless. Frequent causes include exposure to fire or flames, prolonged contact with hot objects, contact with electricity, and immersion in hot or boiling liquids.

First aid treatment for burns is directed toward removing the source of heat, cooling the affected skin area, covering the burn, relieving pain, observing and treating for shock, and preventing infection. Medical treatment is not usually required for first-degree, or superficial, burns. However, medical care should be obtained if more than 15 percent of the surface of an adult's body is burned (10 percent in a child), if the burns affect the face or respiratory tract, if the victim has difficulty breathing, if burns cover more than one body part, or if the burns resulted from chemicals, explosions, or electricity. All victim's suffering from full-thickness, or third-degree, burns should receive medical care.

The main treatment for first-degree and mild second-degree burns is to cool the area by flushing it with large amounts of cool water. Do

Epidermis

Dermis

Subcutaneous
fat, muscle

Skin Red, Dry

First degree, superficial

Blistered, Skin Moist, Pink or Red

Second degree,
partial thickness

Charring, Skin Black, Brown, Red

Third degree, full thickness

Figure 14-16 Types of burns.

not use ice or ice water on burns because doing so causes the body to lose heat. After the pain subsides, use dry, sterile gauze to blot the area dry. Apply a dry, sterile dressing to prevent infection. If nonadhesive dressings are available, it is best to use them because they will not stick to the injured area. If possible, elevate the affected part to reduce swelling caused by inflammation. If necessary, obtain medical help.

⬣! *CAUTION:* Do *not* apply cotton, tissues, ointment, powders, oils, grease, butter, or any other substances to the burned area unless you are instructed to do so by a physician or your immediate supervisor. Do *not* break or open any blisters that form on burns because doing so will just cause an open wound that is prone to infection.

Call for medical help immediately if the victim has third-degree burns. Cover the burned areas with thick, sterile dressings. Elevate the hands or feet if they are burned. If the feet or legs are burned, do *not* allow the victim to walk. If particles of clothing are attached to the burned areas, do *not* attempt to remove these particles. Watch the victim closely for signs of respiratory distress and/or shock. Provide artificial respiration and treatment for shock, as necessary. Watch the victim closely until medical help arrives.

For burns caused by chemicals splashing on the skin, use large amounts of water to flush the affected areas for 15 to 30 minutes or until medical help arrives. Gently remove any clothing or jewelry that contains the chemical to minimize the area injured. Continue flushing the skin with cool water and watch the victim for signs of shock until medical help can be obtained.

If the eyes have been burned by chemicals or irritating gases, flush the eyes with large amounts of water for at least 15 to 30 minutes or until medical help arrives. If only one eye is injured, be sure to tilt the victim's head in the direction of the injury so the injured eye can be properly flushed. Start at the inner corner of the eye and allow the water to run over the surface of the eye and to the outside. Continue flushing the eye with cool water and watch the victim for signs of shock until medical help can be obtained.

⚠ *CAUTION:* Make sure that the water (or remaining chemical) does not enter the *uninjured* eye.

Loss of body fluids (dehydration) can occur very quickly with severe burns, so shock is frequently noted in burn victims. Be alert for any signs of shock and treat the burn victim for shock immediately.

Ⓒ Remain calm while treating the burn victim. Reassure the victim. Obtain medical help as quickly as possible for any burn victim requiring medical assistance.

STUDENT *Go to the workbook and complete the assignment sheet for 14:6, Providing First Aid for Burns. Then return and continue with the procedure.*

PROCEDURE

Providing First Aid for Burns   14:6

EQUIPMENT AND SUPPLIES

Water, sterile dressings, disposable gloves

PROCEDURE

1. Follow the priorities of care, if indicated:
   a. Check the scene. Move the victim only if absolutely necessary.
   b. Check the victim for consciousness and breathing.
   c. Call emergency medical services (EMS) if necessaary.
   d. Provide care to the victim.
   e. Check for bleeding. Control severe bleeding.
   ☣ *CAUTION:* If possible, wear gloves or use a protective barrier while controlling bleeding.
2. Check the burned area carefully to determine the type of burn. A reddened or discolored area is usually a superficial, or first-degree, burn. If the skin is wet, red, swollen, painful, and blistered, the burn is usually a partial-thickness, or second-degree, burn. If the skin is white or charred and there is destruction of tissue, the burn is a full-thickness, or third-degree, burn.
   NOTE: Victims can have more than one type of burn at one time. Treat for the most severe type of burn present.
3. For a first-degree or second-degree burn:
   a. Cool the burn by flushing it with large amounts of cool water. If this is not possible, apply clean or sterile cloths that are cold and wet. Continue applying cold water until the pain subsides.

b. Use sterile gauze to gently blot the injured area dry.

c. Apply dry, sterile dressings to the burned area. If possible, use nonadhesive (non-stick) dressings, because they will not stick to the burn.

d. If blisters are present, do *not* break or open them.

e. If possible, elevate the burned area to reduce swelling caused by inflammation.

f. Obtain medical help for burns to the face, or if burns cover more than 15 percent of the surface of an adult's body or 10 percent of the surface of a child's body. If the victim is having difficulty breathing, or any other distress is noted, obtain medical help.

g. Do *not* apply any cotton, ointment, powders, grease, butter, or similar substances to the burned area.

   NOTE: These substances may increase the possibility of infection.

4. For a third-degree burn:
   a. Call for medical help immediately.
   b. Use thick, sterile dressings to cover the injured areas.
   c. Do *not* attempt to remove any particles of clothing that have stuck to the burned areas.
   d. If the hands and arms or legs and feet are affected, elevate these areas.
   e. If the victim has burns on the face or is experiencing difficulty in breathing, elevate the head.
   f. Watch the victim closely for signs of shock and provide care if necessary.

5. For a burn caused by a chemical splashing on the skin:
   a. Using large amounts of water, immediately flush the area for 15 to 30 minutes or until medical help arrives.
   b. Remove any articles of clothing or jewelry contaminated by the substance.
   c. Continue flushing the area with large amounts of cool water.
   d. Obtain medical help immediately.

6. If the eye has been burned by chemicals or irritating gases:
   a. Tilt the victim's head toward the injured side.
   b. Hold the eyelid of the injured eye open. Pour cool water from the inner part of the eye (the part closest to the nose) toward the outer part (see figure 14-17).

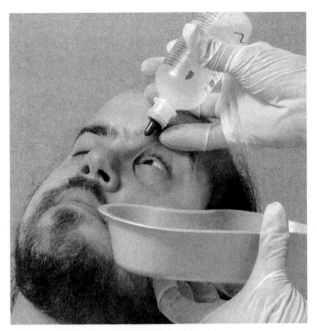

Figure 14-17 To irrigate an eye, hold the eyelid open and irrigate from the inner part of the eye toward the outer part.

c. Use cool water to irrigate the eye for 15 to 30 minutes or until medical help arrives.

   CAUTION: Take care that the water or chemicals do not enter the uninjured eye.

d. Obtain medical help immediately.

7. Observe for the signs of shock in all burn victims. Treat for shock as necessary.

8. Reassure the victim as you are providing treatment. Remain calm and encourage the victim to remain calm.

9. Obtain medical help immediately for any burn victim with extensive burns, third-degree burns, burns to the face, signs of shock, respiratory distress, eye burns, and/or chemical burns to the skin.

PRACTICE *Go to the workbook and use the evaluation sheet for 14:6, Providing First Aid for Burns, to practice this procedure. When you feel you have mastered this skill, sign the sheet and give it to your instructor for further action.*

✔ *Final Checkpoint* Using the criteria listed on the evaluation sheet, your instructor will grade you on your performance.

14:7 INFORMATION
Providing First Aid for Heat Exposure

Excessive exposure to heat or high external temperatures can lead to a life-threatening emergency. This section provides basic facts on conditions that may result from heat exposure and on providing first aid for such conditions.

Overexposure to heat can cause a chemical imbalance in the body. In some instances, such a chemical imbalance can eventually lead to death. Harmful reactions can occur when water or salt are lost through perspiration or when the body cannot eliminate excess heat.

Heat cramps are caused by exposure to heat. They are muscle pains and spasms that result from the loss of salt through perspiration. Firm pressure applied to the cramped muscle will provide relief from the discomfort. The victim should rest and move to a cooler area. In addition, small sips of water can be given to the victim.

Heat exhaustion occurs when a victim is exposed to heat and experiences a loss of fluids through sweating. Signs and symptoms include pale and clammy skin, profuse perspiration (diaphoresis), fatigue or tiredness, weakness, headache, muscle cramps, nausea and/or vomiting, and dizziness and/or fainting. Body temperature is about normal. Treatment methods include moving the victim to a cooler area whenever possible; applying cool, wet cloths; lying the victim down and elevating the victim's feet 12 inches; and giving the victim small sips of cool water, approximately 4 ounces every 15 minutes if the victim is alert and conscious. If the victim vomits, develops shock, or experiences respiratory distress, obtain medical help immediately.

Heat stroke is caused by prolonged exposure to high temperatures. It is a medical emergency. The body is unable to eliminate the excess heat, and internal body temperature rises to 105°F (41°C) or higher. Normal body defenses such as the sweating mechanism no longer function. Signs and symptoms in addition to the high body temperature include red, hot, and dry skin. The pulse is usually rapid, but may remain strong. The victim may lose consciousness. Treatment is geared primarily toward ways of cooling the body quickly, because such high body temperature can cause convulsions and/or death in a very short period of time. The victim can be placed in a tub of cool water, or the skin can be sponged with cool water. Be alert for signs of shock at all times. Obtain medical help immediately.

C After victims have recovered from any condition caused by heat exposure, they must be warned to avoid abnormally warm or hot temperatures for several days. They should also be encouraged to drink sufficient amounts of water and to consume adequate amounts of salt.

STUDENT *Go to the workbook and complete the assignment sheet for 14:7, Providing First Aid for Heat Exposure. Then return and continue with the procedure.*

PROCEDURE
Providing First Aid for Heat Exposure 14:7

EQUIPMENT AND SUPPLIES

Water, salt,
wash cloths or small towels

PROCEDURE

1. Follow the priorities of care, if indicated:
   a. Check the scene. Move the victim only if absolutely necessary.
   b. Check the victim for consciousness and breathing.
   c. Call emergency medical services (EMS) if necessary.

d. Provide care to the victim.

e. Check for bleeding. Control severe bleeding.

◈ *CAUTION:* If possible, wear gloves or use a protective barrier while controlling bleeding.

2. Observe the victim closely for signs and symptoms of heat exposure. Information may also be obtained directly from the victim or from observers. If the victim has been exposed to heat or has been exercising strenuously, and is complaining of muscular pain or spasm, he or she is probably experiencing heat cramps. If the victim has close-to-normal body temperature but has pale and clammy skin, is perspiring excessively, and complains of nausea, headache, weakness, dizziness, or fatigue, he or she is probably experiencing heat exhaustion. If body temperature is high (105°F, or 41°C, or higher); skin is red, dry, and hot; and the victim is weak or unconscious, he or she is experiencing heat stroke.

3. If the victim has heat cramps:

a. Use your hand to apply firm pressure to the cramped muscle(s). This helps relieve the spasms.

b. Encourage relaxation. Allow the victim to lie down in a cool area, if possible.

c. If the victim is alert and conscious and is not nauseated or vomiting, give him or her small sips of water, approximately 4 ounces every 15 minutes.

d. If the heat cramps continue or get worse, obtain medical help.

4. If the victim has heat exhaustion:

a. Move the victim to a cool area, if possible. An air-conditioned room is ideal, but a fan can also help circulate air and cool the victim.

b. Help the victim lie down flat on the back (that is, in the supine position). Elevate the victim's feet and legs 12 inches.

c. Loosen any tight clothing. Remove excessive clothing such as jackets and sweaters.

d. Apply cool, wet cloths to the victim's face.

e. If the victim is conscious and is not nauseated or vomiting, give him or her small sips of water, approximately 4 ounces every 15 minutes.

f. If the victim complains of nausea and/or vomits, discontinue water. Obtain medical help.

5. If the victim has heat stroke:

a. Immediately move the victim to a cool area, if at all possible.

b. Remove excessive clothing.

c. Sponge the bare skin with cool water. The victim can also be placed in a tub of cool water to lower body temperature.

❗ *CAUTION:* Watch that the victim's head is not submerged in water. If the victim is unconscious, you may need assistance to place him or her in the tub.

d. If vomiting occurs, position the victim on his or her side. Watch for signs of difficulty in breathing and provide care as indicated.

e. Obtain medical help immediately. This is a life-threatening emergency.

6. Shock can develop quickly in all victims of heat exposure. Be alert for the signs of shock and treat as necessary.

❗ *CAUTION:* Obtain medical help for heat cramps that do not subside, heat exhaustion with signs of shock or vomiting, and *all* heat stroke victims as soon as possible.

7. Reassure the victim as you are providing treatment. Remain calm.
ⓒ

PRACTICE Go to the workbook and use the evaluation sheet for 14:7, Providing First Aid for Heat Exposure, to practice this procedure. When you feel you have mastered this skill, sign the sheet and give it to your instructor for further action.

✔ *Final Checkpoint* Using the criteria listed on the evaluation sheet, your instructor will grade you on your performance.

INFORMATION
14:8 *Providing First Aid for Cold Exposure*

Prolonged exposure to cold external temperatures can damage body tissues and lead to death. This section provides basic information on conditions caused by cold exposure and on providing first aid for such conditions.

Exposure to cold external temperatures can cause body tissues to freeze and body processes to slow. If treatment is not provided immediately, the victim can die. Factors such as wind velocity, amount of humidity, and length of exposure all affect the degree of injury.

Prolonged exposure to the cold can result in hypothermia. Elderly individuals are more susceptible to hypothermia than are younger individuals (see figure 14-18). Signs and symptoms include shivering, numbness, weakness or drowsiness, low body temperature, confusion, and loss of consciousness. If prolonged exposure continues, body processes will slow down and death can occur. Treatment consists of getting the victim to a warm area, removing wet clothing, slowly warming the victim by wrapping in blankets or putting on dry clothing, and, if the victim is fully conscious, giving warm liquids by mouth.

Frostbite is actual freezing of tissue fluids accompanied by damage to the skin and underlying tissues. It is caused by exposure to the cold. Early signs and symptoms include redness and tingling. As frostbite progresses, signs and symptoms include pale, glossy skin, white or grayish-yellow in color; in some cases, blisters; skin that is cold to the touch; numbness; and, sometimes, pain that gradually subsides until the victim does not feel any pain. If exposure continues, the victim may become confused, lethargic, and incoherent. Shock may develop followed by unconsciousness and death. First aid for frostbite is directed at maintaining respirations, treating for shock, warming the affected parts, and preventing further injury. Frequently, small areas of the body are affected by

Figure 14-18 Elderly individuals are more susceptible to hypothermia than are younger individuals.

frostbite. Common sites include the fingers, toes, ears, nose, and cheeks. Extreme care must be taken to avoid further injury to areas damaged by frostbite. Because the victim usually does not feel pain, the part must be warmed carefully, taking care not to burn the injured tissue. The parts affected may be immersed in warm water at 100°F to 105°F (37.8°C to 40.6°C).

⚠ *CAUTION:* Heat lamps, hot water above 105°F (40.6°C), or heat from a stove or oven should *not* be used. Furthermore, the parts should *not* be rubbed or massaged, because this may cause gangrene (death of the tissue). Avoid opening or breaking any blisters that form, because doing so will create an open wound. Do *not* allow the victim to walk or stand if the feet, legs, or toes are affected. Dry, sterile dressings can be placed between toes or fingers to prevent them from rubbing and causing further injury. Medical help should be obtained as quickly as possible.

Shock is frequently noted in victims exposed to the cold. Be alert for all signs of shock and treat for shock as necessary.

STUDENT Go to the workbook and complete the assignment sheet for 14:8, Providing First Aid for Cold Exposure. Then return and continue with the procedure.

PROCEDURE

Providing First Aid for Cold Exposure

14:8

EQUIPMENT AND SUPPLIES

Blankets, bath water and thermometer, sterile gauze sponges

PROCEDURE

1. Follow the priorities of care, if indicated:
   a. Check the scene. Move the victim only if absolutely necessary.
   b. Check the victim for consciousness and breathing.
   c. Call emergency medical services (EMS) if necessary.
   d. Provide care to the victim.
   e. Check for bleeding. Control severe bleeding.

   CAUTION: If possible, wear gloves or use a protective barrier while controlling bleeding.

2. Observe the victim closely for signs and symptoms of cold exposure. Information may also be obtained directly from the victim or observers. Note shivering, numbness, weakness or drowsiness, confusion, low body temperature, and lethargy. Check the skin, particularly on the toes, fingers, ears, nose, and cheeks. Suspect frostbite if any areas are pale, glossy, white or grayish-yellow, and cold to the touch, and if the victim complains of any part of the body feeling numb or painless.

3. Move the victim to a warm area as soon as possible.

4. Immediately remove any wet or frozen clothing. Loosen any tight clothing that decreases circulation.

5. Slowly warm the victim by wrapping the victim in blankets or dressing the victim in dry, warm clothing. If a body part is affected by frostbite, immerse the part in warm water measuring 100°F to 105°F (37.8°C to 40.6°C).

CAUTION: Warm a victim of hypothermia slowly, because rapid warming can cause heart problems or increase circulation to the surface of the body, which causes additional cooling of vital organs.

CAUTION: Do *not* use heat lamps, hot water above the stated temperatures, or heat from stoves or ovens. Excessive heat can burn the victim.

6. After the body part affected by frostbite has been thawed and the skin becomes flushed, discontinue warming the area because swelling may develop rapidly. Dry the part by blotting gently with a towel or soft cloth. Gently wrap the part in clean or sterile cloths. Use sterile gauze to separate the fingers and/or toes to prevent them from rubbing together.

CAUTION: *Never* rub or massage the frostbitten area, because doing so can cause gangrene.

7. Help the victim lie down. Do not allow the victim to walk or stand if the legs, feet, or toes are injured. Elevate any injured areas.

8. Observe the victim for signs of shock. Treat for shock as necessary.

9. If the victim is conscious and is not nauseated or vomiting, give warm liquids to drink.

CAUTION: Do *not* give beverages containing alcohol or caffeine. Give the victim warm broth, water, or milk.

10. Reassure the victim while providing treatment. Remain calm and encourage the victim to remain calm.

11. Obtain medical help as soon as possible.

> **PRACTICE** *Go to the workbook and use the evaluation sheet for 14:8, Providing First Aid for Cold Exposure, to practice this procedure. When you feel you have mastered this skill, sign the sheet and give it to your instructor for further action.*

✔ *Final Checkpoint* Using the criteria listed on the evaluation sheet, your instructor will grade you on your performance.

INFORMATION
14:9
Providing First Aid for Bone and Joint Injuries

Injuries to bones and joints are common in accidents and falls. This section provides basic information on these types of injuries, including information on providing appropriate first aid.

A variety of injuries can occur to bones and joints. Such injuries sometimes occur together; other times, these injuries occur by themselves. Examples of injuries to bones and joints are fractures, dislocations, sprains, and strains.

A fracture is a break in a bone. A closed, or simple, fracture is a bone break that is not accompanied by an external or open wound on the skin. A compound, or open, fracture is a bone break that is accompanied by an open wound on the skin. Main facts regarding fractures are as follows:

a. Signs and symptoms of fractures can vary. Not all signs and symptoms will be present in every victim. Common signs and symptoms include deformity, limited motion or loss of motion, pain and tenderness at the fracture site, swelling and discoloration, and the protrusion of bone ends through the skin. Additional information obtained from the victim may include hearing a bone break or snap, feeling a grating sensation, and abnormal movements within a part of the body.

b. Treatment for fractures is directed toward maintaining respirations, treating for shock, keeping the broken bone from moving, and preventing further injury. Devices such as splints and slings can be utilized to prevent movement of the injured part. Whenever a fracture is evident or suspected, medical help must be obtained.

A dislocation is when the end of a bone is either displaced from a joint or moves out of its normal position within a joint. This injury is frequently accompanied by a tearing or stretching of ligaments, muscles, and other soft tissue.

a. Signs and symptoms that may occur include deformity, limited or abnormal movement, swelling, discoloration, pain, tenderness, and a shortening or lengthening of the affected arm or leg.

b. First aid for dislocations is basically the same as that for fractures. No attempt should be made to reduce the dislocation (that is, replace the bone in the joint). The affected part must be immobilized in the position in which it was found. Immobilization is accomplished by using splints and/or slings. Movement of the injured part can lead to additional injury to nerves, blood vessels, and other tissue in the area. Obtain medical help immediately.

A sprain is an injury to the tissues surrounding a joint; it usually occurs when the part is forced beyond its normal range of movement. Ligaments, tendons, and other tissues are stretched or torn. Common sites for sprains include the ankles and wrists.

a. Signs and symptoms of a sprain include swelling, pain, discoloration and, sometimes, impaired motion. Frequently, sprains resemble fractures or dislocations. If in doubt, treat the injury as a fracture.

b. First aid for a sprain includes application of cold to decrease swelling and pain, elevation of the affected part, and rest. In addition, an elastic bandage can be used to provide support for the affected area. If swelling is severe or if there is any question of a fracture, medical help should be obtained.

A strain is the overstretching of a muscle; it is caused by overexertion or lifting. A frequent site for strains is the back.

a. Signs and symptoms of a strain include sudden pain, swelling, and/or bruising.

b. Treatment for a strain is directed toward resting the affected muscle while providing support. Bedrest with a backboard under the mattress is recommended for a strained back. Cold applications can be used initially to reduce the swelling. However, warm, wet applications are the main treatment later, because warmth relaxes the muscles. Different types of cold and heat packs are available (see figure 14-19). Medical help should

Figure 14-19 Disposable heat and cold packs contain chemicals that must be activated before using.

Figure 14-20 Splints should be long enough to immobilize the joint above and below the injured area.

Figure 14-21 Some air splints are inflated by blowing into a nozzle. Care must be taken to avoid overinflating this type of splint. *(Photo by Michael Dzaman)*

be obtained for severe strains and all back injuries.

Splints are devices that can be used to immobilize injured parts when fractures, dislocations, and other similar injuries are present or suspected. Many commercial splints are available, including inflatable, or air, splints, padded boards, and traction splints. Splints can also be made from cardboard, newspapers, blankets, pillows, boards, and other similar materials. Some basic principles regarding the use of splints are:

a. Splints should be long enough to immobilize the joint above and below the injured area (see figure 14-20). By preventing movement in these joints, the injured bone or area is held in position and further injury is prevented.

b. Splints should be padded, especially at bony areas and over the site of injury. Cloths, thick dressings, towels, and similar materials can be used as padding.

c. Strips of cloth, roller gauze, triangular bandages folded into bands or strips, and similar materials can be used to tie splints in place.

d. Splints must be applied so that they do not put pressure directly over the site of injury.

e. If an open wound is present, use a sterile dressing to apply pressure and control bleeding.

CAUTION: Wear gloves or use a protective barrier while controlling bleeding to avoid contamination from the blood.

CAUTION: Leave the dressing in place, and apply the splint in such a way that it does *not* put pressure on the wound.

f. *Never* make any attempt to replace broken bones or reduce a fracture or dislocation; and do *not* move the victim. Splint wherever you find the victim.

g. Inflatable, or air, splints are available in various sizes and shapes for different parts of the arms and legs. Care must be taken to avoid any unnecessary movement while the splint is being positioned. Once the splint is positioned, air pressure is used to inflate the splint (see figure 14-21). Some air splints have nozzles; these splints are inflated by blowing into the nozzles. Other air splints require the use of pressurized material in cans, while still others are inflated with cool air from a refrigerant solution.

NOTE: The coldness reduces swelling, while the splint prevents movement.

Care must be taken to avoid overinflating air splints. To test whether the splint is properly inflated, use a thumb to apply slight pressure to the splint; an indentation mark should result.

h. Traction splints are special devices that provide a pulling or traction effect on the injured bone. They are frequently used for fractures of the femur, or thigh bone.

⚖️ *CAUTION:* Only persons specifically trained in the application of traction splints should apply them.

i. After a splint is applied, it is essential to note the circulation and the effects on the nerve endings of the skin below the splint to make sure the splint is not too tight. Check skin temperature (it should be warm to the touch), skin color (pale or blue indicates poor circulation), swelling or edema, numbness or tingling, and pulse, if possible.

🛑 *CAUTION:* If any signs of impaired circulation or impaired neurological status are present, immediately loosen the ties holding the splint.

Slings are available in many different forms. Commercial slings usually have a series of straps that extend around the neck and/or thoracic (chest) region. A common type of sling used for first aid is the triangular bandage. Slings are usually used to support the arm, hand, forearm, and shoulder (see figure 14-22). They may be used when casts are in place. In addition, they are also used to provide immobility if a fracture of the arm or shoulder is suspected.

a. When a sling is applied to an arm, the sling should be positioned in such a way that the hand is higher than the elbow. The purpose of elevating the hand is to promote circulation, prevent swelling (edema), and decrease pain.

b. Circulation in the limb and nerve supply to the limb must be checked frequently. Specifically, check for skin temperature (should be

Figure 14-22 Slings are used to support the arm, hand, forearm, and shoulder.

warm if circulation is good), skin color (blue or very pale indicates poor circulation), swelling (edema), amount of pain, and tingling or numbness. Nailbeds can also be used to check circulation. When the nailbeds are pressed slightly, they blanch (turn white). If circulation is good, the pink color should return to the nailbeds immediately after the pressure is released.

c. If a sling is being applied because of a suspected fracture, or break, to the bone, extreme care must be taken to move the injured limb as little as possible while the sling is being applied. The victim can sometimes help by holding the injured limb in position while the sling is slipped into place.

d. If a triangular bandage is used, care must be taken so that the knot tied at the neck does not press against a bone. The knot should be tied to either side of the spinal column.

e. When shoulder injuries are suspected, it may be necessary to keep the arm next to the body. After a sling has been applied, another bandage can be placed around the thoracic region to hold the arm against the body.

Injuries to the neck or spine are the most dangerous types of injuries to bones and joints.

CAUTION: If a victim who has such injuries is moved, permanent damage resulting in paralysis can occur. If at all possible, avoid any movement of a victim with neck or spinal injuries. Wait until a backboard and adequate help for transfer is available.

Many victims with injuries to bones and/or joints also experience shock. Always be alert for signs of shock and treat as needed.

C Injuries of this type usually involve a great deal of anxiety, pain, and discomfort, so constantly reassure the victim. Encourage the victim to relax, and position the victim as comfortably as possible. Advise the victim that medical help is on the way. First aid measures are directed toward relieving the pain as much as possible.

Obtain medical help for all victims of bone or joint injuries. The only definite diagnosis of a closed fracture is an X ray of the area. Whenever a fracture and/or dislocation is suspected, treat the victim as though one of these injuries has occured.

STUDENT *Go to the workbook and complete the assignment sheet for 14:9, Providing First Aid for Bone and Joint Injuries. Then return and continue with the procedure.*

PROCEDURE

Providing First Aid for Bone and Joint Injuries 14:9

EQUIPMENT AND SUPPLIES

Blankets, splints of various sizes, air or inflatable splints, triangular bandages, strips of cloth or roller gauze, disposable gloves

PROCEDURE

1. Follow the priorities of care, if indicated:
   a. Check the scene. Move the victim only if absolutely necessary. If the victim must be moved from a dangerous area, pull in the direction of the long axis of the body (that is, from the head or feet). If at all possible, tie an injured leg to the other leg or secure an injured arm to the body before movement.
   CAUTION: If neck or spinal injuries are suspected, avoid any movement of the victim unless movement is necessary to save the victim's life.
   b. Check the victim for consciousness and breathing.
   c. Call emergency medical services (EMS) if necessary.
   d. Provide care to the victim.
   e. Control severe bleeding. If an open wound accompanies a fracture, take care not to push broken bone ends into the wound.
   CAUTION: If possible, wear gloves or use a protective barrier while controlling bleeding.

2. Observe for signs and symptoms of a fracture, dislocation, or joint injury. Note deformities (such as a shortening or lengthening of an extremity), limited motion or loss of motion, pain, tenderness, swelling, discoloration, and bone fragments protruding through the skin. Also, the victim may state that he or she heard a bone snap or crack, or may complain of a grating sensation.

3. Immobilze the injured part to prevent movement.
   CAUTION: Do *not* attempt to straighten a deformity, replace broken bone ends, or reduce a dislocation. Avoid any unnecessary movement of the injured part. If a bone injury is suspected, treat the victim as though a fracture or dislocation has occured. Use splints or slings to immobilize the injury.

4. *To apply splints:*
   a. Obtain commercial splints or improvise splints by using blankets, newspapers, boards, cardboard, or similar supportive materials.
   b. Make sure that the splints are long enough to immobilize the joint both above and below the injury.

c. Position the splints, making sure that they do *not* apply pressure directly at the site of injury. Two splints are usually used. However, if a pillow, blanket, or similar item is used, one such item can be rolled around the area to provide support on all sides.

d. Use thick dressings, cloths, towels, or other similar materials to pad the splints. Make sure bony areas are protected. Avoid direct contact between the splint material and the skin.
NOTE: Many commercial splints are already padded. However, additional padding is often needed to protect the bony areas.

e. Use strips of cloth, triangular bandages folded into scarves or strips, roller gauze, or other similar supportive material to tie or anchor the splints in place. The use of elastic bandage is discouraged because the bandages may cut off or interfere with circulation. If splints are long, as are leg splints, three to five ties may be required. Tie the strips above and below the upper joint and above and below the lower joint. An additional tie should be placed in the center region of the splint.

f. Avoid any unnecessary movement of the injured area while splints are being applied. If possible, have another individual support the area while you are applying the splints.

5. *To apply air (inflatable) splints:*
a. Obtain the correct splint for the injured part.
NOTE: Most air splints are available for full arm, lower arm, wrist, full leg, lower leg, and ankle/foot.

b. Some air splints have zippers for easier application, but others must be slipped into position on the victim. If the splint has a zipper, position the open splint on the injured area, taking care to avoid any movement of the affected part. Use your hand to support the injured area. Close the zipper. If the splint must be slipped into position, slide the splint onto your arm first. Then hold the injured leg or arm and slide the splint from your arm to the victim's injured extremity. This technique prevents unnecessary movement.

c. Inflate the splint. Many splints are inflated by blowing into the nozzle. Others require the use of a pressure solution in a can. Follow instructions provided by the manufacturer of the splint.

d. Check to make sure that the splint is not overinflated. Use your thumb to press a section of the splint. Your thumb should leave a slight indentation if the splint is inflated correctly.

6. *To apply a sling,* follow the manufacturer's instructions for commercial slings. To use a triangular bandage for a sling (see figure 14-23), proceed as follows:
a. If possible, obtain the help of another individual to support the injured arm while the sling is being applied. Sometimes, the victim can hold the injured arm in place.

b. Place the long straight edge of the triangular bandage on the uninjured side. Allow one end to extend over the shoulder of the uninjured arm. The other end should hang down in front of the victim's chest. The short edge of the triangle should extend back and under the elbow of the injured arm.

CAUTION: Avoid excessive movement of the injured limb while positioning the sling.

c. Bring the long end of the bandage up and over the injured arm. Then bring it up and over the shoulder of the injured arm.

d. Use a square knot to tie the two ends together near the neck. Make sure the knot is not over a bone. Tie it to either side of the spinal column. Make sure the hand is kept slightly elevated.

e. The point of the bandage is now near the elbow. Bring the point forward, fold it, and pin it to the front of the sling. If no pin is available, coil the end and tie it in a knot.

CAUTION: If you use a pin, put your hand between the pin and the victim's skin while inserting the pin.

f. Check the position of the sling. The fingers of the injured hand should extend beyond the edge of the triangular bandage. In addition, the hand should be slightly elevated to prevent swelling (edema).

7. After splints and/or slings have been applied, check for signs of impaired circulation. Skin color should be pink. A pale or bluish color is a sign of poor circulation. The skin should be warm to the touch. Swelling can indicate poor circulation. If the victim complains of

Figure 14-23 Steps for applying a triangular bandage as a sling.

pain or pressure from the splints and/or slings, or of numbness or tingling in the area below the splints/sling, circulation may be impaired. Slightly press the nailbeds on the foot or hand so they temporarily turn white. If circulation is good, the pink color will return to the nailbeds immediately after pressure is released. If you note any signs of impaired circulation, loosen the splints and/or sling immediately.

8. Watch for signs of shock in any victim with a bone and/or joint injury. Remember, inade-

quate blood flow is the main cause of shock; so watch for signs of impaired circulation, such as a bluish tinge around the lips or nailbeds. Treat for shock, as necessary.

9. If medical help is delayed, cold applications such as cold compresses or an ice bag can be used on the injured area to decrease swelling. *CAUTION:* To prevent injury to the skin, make sure that the ice bag is covered with a towel or other material.

10. Place the victim in a comfortable position, but avoid any unnecessary movement. *CAUTION:* Avoid *any* movement if a neck or spinal injury is suspected.

11. Reassure the victim while providing first aid. Try to relieve the pain by carefully positioning the injured part, avoiding unnecessary movement, and applying cold.

12. Obtain medical help as quickly as possible.

PRACTICE *Go to the workbook and use the evaluation sheet for 14:9, Providing First Aid for Bone and Joint Injuries, to practice this procedure. When you feel you have mastered this skill, sign the sheet and give it to your instructor for further action.*

 Final Checkpoint Using the criteria listed on the evaluation sheet, your instructor will grade you on your performance.

INFORMATION
14:10 Providing First Aid for Specific Injuries

Previous sections discussed first aid for various *types* of injuries. This section provides information on treating injuries to specific *areas* of the body.

Although treatment for burns, bleeding, wounds, poisoning, and fractures is basically the same for all regions of the body, injuries to

specific body parts require special care. Examples of these parts are the eyes, ears, nose, brain, chest, abdomen, and genital organs.

Any *eye* injury always involves the danger of vision loss, especially if treated incorrectly. In most cases involving serious injury to the eyes, it is best *not* to provide major treatment. Obtaining medical help, preferably from an eye specialist, is a top priority of first aid care.

a. Foreign objects such as dust, dirt, and similar small particles frequently enter the eye. These objects cause irritation and can scratch the eye or become embedded in the eye tissue. Signs and symptoms include redness, a burning sensation, pain, watering or tearing of the eye, and/or the presence of visible objects in the eye. If the foreign body is floating freely, prevent the victim from rubbing the eye, wash your hands thoroughly, and gently draw the upper lid down over the lower lid. This stimulates the formation of tears. The proximity of the lids also creates a wiping action, which may remove the particle. If this does not remove the foreign body, use your thumb and forefinger to grasp the eyelashes and gently raise the upper eyelid. Tell the victim to look down and tilt his or her head toward the injured side. Use water to gently flush the eye or use the corner of a piece of sterile gauze to gently remove the object.

🛑 *CAUTION:* If this does not remove the object or if the object is embedded, make *no* attempt to remove it.

Apply a dry, sterile dressing and obtain medical help for the victim. Serious injury can occur if any attempt is made to remove an object embedded in the eye tissue.

b. Blows to the eye from a fist, accident, or explosion may cause contusions or black eyes as a result of internal bleeding and torn tissues inside the eye. Because this can lead to loss of vision, the victim should be examined as soon as possible by an eye specialist. Apply sterile dressings or an eye shield, keep the victim lying flat, and obtain medical help. It is sometimes best to cover both eyes to prevent involuntary movement of the injured eye.

c. Penetrating injuries that cut the eye tissue are extremely dangerous.

🛑 *CAUTION:* If an object is protruding from the eye, make *no* attempt to remove the object. Rather, support it by *loosely* applying dressings.

Apply dressings to both eyes to prevent involuntary movement of the injured eye. Avoid applying pressure to the eye while applying the dressings. Keep the victim lying flat on his or her back to prevent fluids from draining out of the eye. Obtain medical help immediately.

Injuries to the *ear* can result in rupture or perforation of the eardrum. These injuries also require medical care. Treatment for specific types of ear injuries is as follows:

a. Wounds of the ear frequently result in torn or detached tissue. Apply sterile dressings with light pressure to control bleeding.

☣ *CAUTION:* If possible, wear gloves or use a protective barrier while controlling bleeding.

Save any torn tissue and use sterile water or sterile normal saline solution to keep it cool and moist. Send the torn tissue to the medical facility along with the victim.

NOTE: If sterile water is not available, use cool, clean water.

Keep the victim lying flat, but raise his or her head (if no other conditions prohibit raising the head).

b. If the eardrum is ruptured or perforated, place sterile gauze loosely in the outer ear canal. Do *not* allow the victim to hit the side of the head in an attempt to restore hearing and do *not* put any liquids into the ear. Obtain medical help for the victim.

c. Clear or blood-tinged fluid draining from the ear can be a sign of skull or brain injury. Allow the fluid to flow from the ear. Keep the victim lying down. If possible, turn the victim on his or her injured side and slightly elevate the head and shoulders to allow the fluid to drain. Obtain medical help immediately and report the presence and description of the fluid.

☣ *CAUTION:* Wear gloves or use a protective barrier to avoid skin contact with fluid draining from the ear.

Wounds or blows to the *head or skull* can result in injury to the brain. Again, it is important to obtain medical help as quickly as possible for the victim.

a. Signs and symptoms of brain injury include clear or blood-tinged cerebrospinal fluid draining from the nose or ears, loss of consciousness, headache, visual disturbances, pupils unequal in size, muscle paralysis, speech disturbances, convulsions, and nausea and vomiting.

b. Keep the victim lying flat and treat for shock. If there is no evidence of neck or spinal injury, raise the victim's head slightly by supporting the head and shoulders on a small pillow or a rolled blanket or coat.

c. Watch closely for signs of respiratory distress and provide artificial respiration as needed.

d. Make *no* attempt to stop the flow of fluid. Loose dressings can be positioned to absorb the flow.

☣ *CAUTION:* Wear gloves or use a protective barrier to avoid contamination from the cerebrospinal fluid.

e. Do *not* give the victim any liquids. If the victim complains of excessive thirst, use a clean, cool, wet cloth to moisten the lips, tongue, and inside of the mouth.

f. Note how long the victim is unconscious and report this to the ambulance or emergency rescue personnel.

Injuries to the *nose* frequently cause nosebleeds. Nosebleeds are usually more frightening than they are serious. Nosebleeds can also be caused by change in altitude, strenuous activity, high blood pressure, and rupture of small blood vessels after a cold.

a. Keep the victim quiet and remain calm.

b. If possible, place the victim in a sitting position with the head leaning slightly forward.

c. Apply pressure to control bleeding by pressing the bleeding nostril toward the midline. If both nostrils are bleeding, press both nostrils toward the midline.

NOTE: If both nostrils are blocked, tell the victim to breathe through the mouth.

☣ *CAUTION:* Wear gloves or use a protective barrier to avoid contamination from blood.

d. If application of pressure against the midline or septum does not stop the bleeding, insert a small piece of gauze in the nostril and then apply pressure on the outer surface of the nostril.

❗ *CAUTION:* Do not use cotton because the fibers will shed and stick.

Be sure to leave a portion of the gauze extending out of the nostril so that the packing can be removed later.

e. Apply a cold compress to the bridge of the nose. A covered ice pack or a cold, wet cloth can be used.

f. If the bleeding does not stop or a fracture of the nose is suspected, obtain medical assistance. If a person has repeated nosebleeds, a referral for medical attention should be made. Nosebleeds can indicate an underlying condition that requires medical care and treatment, such as high blood pressure.

Injuries to the *chest* are usually medical emergencies because the heart, lungs, and major blood vessels may be involved. Chest injuries include sucking chest wounds, penetrating wounds, and crushing injuries. In all cases, obtain medical help immediately.

a. A sucking chest wound is a deep, open chest wound that allows air to flow directly in and out with breathing. The vacuum that is usually present in the pleura (sacs surrounding the lungs) is destroyed, causing the lung on the injured side to collapse. Immediate medical help must be obtained. An airtight dressing must be placed over the wound to prevent air flow in and out of the wound. Aluminum foil, plastic wrap, or other nonporous material should be used to cover the wound. Tape or a bandage can be used to hold the nonporous material in place. Maintain an open airway (through the nose or mouth) and provide artificial respiration as needed. If possible, position the victim on his or her injured side and elevate the head and chest slightly. This allows the uninjured lung to expand more freely and prevents pressure on the uninjured lung from blood and damaged tissue.

b. Penetrating injuries to the chest can result in sucking chest wounds or damage to the heart and blood vessels. If an object (for example, a knife) is protruding from the chest, do *not* attempt to remove the object. If possible, immobilize the object by placing dressings around it and taping the dressings in position (see figure 14-24). Place the victim in a comfortable position, maintain respirations, and obtain medical help immediately.

c. Crushing chest injuries can be caused in vehicular accidents or when heavy objects strike the chest. Fractured ribs and damage to the lungs and/or heart can occur. Place

Figure 14-24 Immobilize an object protruding from the chest by placing dressings around the object and taping the dressings in place.

the victim in a comfortable position and, if possible, elevate the head and shoulders to aid breathing. If an injury to the neck or spine is suspected, avoid moving the victim. Obtain medical help immediately.

Abdominal injuries can damage internal organs and cause bleeding in major blood vessels. The intestines and other abdominal organs may protrude from an open wound. Medical help must be obtained immediately; bleeding, shock, and organ damage can lead to death in a short period of time.

a. Signs and symptoms include severe abdominal pain or tenderness, protruding organs, open wounds, nausea and vomiting (particularly of blood), abdominal muscle rigidity, and symptoms of shock.

b. Position the victim flat on his or her back. Place a pillow or rolled blanket around the knees. This helps relax the abdominal muscles. Elevate the head and shoulders to aid breathing.

c. Remove clothing from around the wound or protruding organs. Use a large sterile dressing moistened with sterile water or normal saline solution to cover the area. If sterile water or normal saline is not available, use warm tap water to moisten the dressings.

! *CAUTION:* Make no attempt to reposition protruding organs.

d. Avoid giving the victim any fluids or food. If the victim complains of excessive thirst, use a cool, wet cloth to moisten the lips, tongue, and inside of the mouth.

Injuries to *genital organs* can result from falls, blows, or explosions. Zippers catching on genitals and other accidents sometimes bruise the genitals. Because injuries to the genitals may cause severe pain, bleeding, and shock, medical help is required. Basic principles of first aid include the following:

a. Control severe bleeding by using a sterile (or clean) dressing to apply direct pressure to the area.

CAUTION: Wear gloves or use a protective barrier to avoid contamination from blood.

b. Treat the victim for shock.

c. Do not remove any penetrating or inserted objects.

d. Save any torn tissue and use sterile water or sterile normal saline to keep it cool and moist. Send the torn tissue to the medical facility along with the victim.

e. Use a covered ice pack or other cold applications to decrease bleeding and relieve pain.

f. Obtain medical help.

Shock frequently occurs in victims with specific injuries to the eyes, ears, chest, abdomen, or other vital organs. Be alert for the signs of shock and immediately treat all victims.

C Most of the specific injuries discussed in this section result in extreme pain for the victim. It is essential that you reassure the victim constantly and encourage the victim to relax as much as possible. Direct first aid care toward providing as much relief from pain as possible.

STUDENT *Go to the workbook and complete the assignment sheet for 14:10, Providing First Aid for Specific Injuries. Then return and continue with the procedure.*

PROCEDURE

Providing First Aid for Specific Injuries *14:10*

EQUIPMENT AND SUPPLIES

Blankets, pillows, dressings, bandages, tape, aluminum foil or plastic wrap, eye shields or sterile dressings, sterile water, disposable gloves

PROCEDURE

1. Follow the priorities of care, if indicated:
   a. Check the scene. Move the victim only if absolutely necessary.
   b. Check the victim for consciousness and breathing.
   c. Call emergency medical services (EMS), if necessary.
   d. Provide care to the victim.
   e. Check for bleeding. Control severe bleeding.

   CAUTION: If possible, wear gloves or use a protective barrier while controlling bleeding.

2. Observe the victim closely for signs and symptoms of specific injuries. Do a systematic examination of the victim. Always have a reason for everything you do. Explain what you are doing to the victim and/or observers.

3. If the victim has an eye injury, proceed as follows:
   a. If the victim has a free-floating particle or foreign body in the eye, warn the victim *not* to rub the eye. Wash your hands thoroughly to prevent infection. Gently grasp the upper eyelid and draw it down over the lower eyelid. If this does not remove the object, use your thumb and forefinger to grasp the eyelashes and gently raise the upper eyelid. Tell the victim to look down and tilt his or her head slightly to the injured side. Use water to gently flush the eye or use the corner of a piece of sterile gauze to gently remove the object. If this does not remove the object or if the object is embedded, proceed to step b.

   b. If an object is embedded in the eye, make *no* attempt to remove it. Rather, apply a dry, sterile dressing to loosely cover the eye. Obtain medical help.
   c. If an eye injury has caused a contusion, a black eye, internal bleeding, and/or torn tissue in the eye, apply sterile dressings or eye shields to both eyes. Keep the victim lying flat. Obtain medical help.
   NOTE: Both eyes are covered to prevent involuntary movement of the injured eye.
   d. If an object is protruding from the eye, make *no* attempt to remove the object. If possible, support the object in position by loosely placing dressings around it. A paper cup with the bottom removed can also be used to surround and prevent any movement of the object. Apply dressings to the uninjured eye to prevent movement of the injured eye. Keep the victim lying flat. Obtain medical help immediately.

4. If the victim has an ear injury:
   a. Control severe bleeding from an ear wound by using a sterile dressing to apply light pressure.

   CAUTION: Wear gloves or use a protective barrier to prevent contamination from the blood.

   b. If any tissue has been torn from the ear, preserve the tissue by placing it in cool, sterile water or normal saline solution. The tissue may also be put in sterile gauze that has been moistened with sterile water. Send the torn tissue to the medical facility along with the victim.
   NOTE: If sterile water is not available, use cool, clean water.
   c. If a rupture or perforation of the eardrum is suspected or evident, place sterile gauze loosely in the outer ear canal. Caution the victim against hitting the side of the head to restore hearing. Obtain medical help.
   d. If cerebrospinal fluid is draining from the ear, make no attempt to stop the flow of the fluid. If no neck or spinal injury is suspected, turn the victim on his or her injured side and slightly elevate the head and shoulders to allow the fluid to drain. A dressing may be positioned to absorb the flow. Obtain medical help immediately.

⊛ *CAUTION:* Wear gloves or use a protective barrier to prevent contamination from the cerebrospinal fluid.

5. If the victim has a brain injury:

   a. Keep the victim lying flat. Treat for shock. If there is no evidence of a neck or spinal injury, place a small pillow or a rolled blanket or coat under the victim's head and shoulders to elevate the head slightly.

   ⬡ *CAUTION:* Never position the victim's head lower than the rest of the body.

   b. Watch closely for signs of respiratory distress. Provide artificial respiration if needed.

   NOTE: Remove the pillow if artificial respiration is given.

   c. If cerebrospinal fluid is draining from the ears, nose, and/or mouth, make *no* attempt to stop the flow. Position dressings to absorb the flow.

   ⊛ *CAUTION:* Wear gloves or use a protective barrier to prevent contamination from the cerebrospinal fluid.

   d. Avoid giving the victim any fluids by mouth. If the victim complains of excessive thirst, use a cool, wet cloth to moisten the lips, tongue, and inside of the mouth.

   e. If the victim is unconscious, note for how long and report this information to the emergency rescue or ambulance personnel.

   f. Obtain medical help as quickly as possible.

6. If the victim has a nosebleed:

   a. Try to keep the victim calm. Remain calm yourself.

   b. Position the victim in a sitting position, if possible. Lean the head forward slightly. If the victim cannot sit up, slightly elevate the head.

   c. Apply pressure by pressing the nostril(s) toward the midline. Continue applying pressure for at least 5 minutes and longer if necessary to control the bleeding.

   NOTE: If both nostrils are bleeding and must be pressed toward the midline, tell the victim to breathe through the mouth.

   ⊛ *CAUTION:* Wear gloves or use a protective barrier to prevent contamination from the blood.

   d. If application of pressure does not control the bleeding, insert gauze into the bleed-

ing nostril, taking care to allow some of the gauze to hang out. Then apply pressure again by pushing the nostril toward the midline.

   e. Apply cold compresses to the bridge of the nose. Use cold, wet cloths or a covered ice bag.

   f. If the bleeding does not stop, a fracture is suspected, or the victim has repeated nosebleeds, obtain medical help.

   NOTE: Nosebleeds can indicate a serious underlying condition that requires medical attention, such as high blood pressure.

7. If the victim has a chest injury:

   a. If the wound is a sucking chest wound, apply a nonporous dressing. Use plastic wrap or aluminum foil to create an airtight seal. Use tape or a bandage to hold the dressing in place.

   b. Maintain an open airway. Constantly be alert for signs of respiratory distress. Provide artificial respiration as needed.

   c. If there is no evidence of a neck or spinal injury, position the victim with his or her injured side down. Slightly elevate the head and chest by placing small pillows or blankets under the victim.

   d. If an object is protruding from the chest, make *no* attempt to remove it. If possible, immobilize the object with dressings, and tape around it.

   e. Obtain medical help immediately for all chest injuries.

8. If the victim has an abdominal injury:

   a. Position the victim flat on the back. Place a small pillow or a rolled blanket or coat under the victim's knees to slightly flex them. Slightly elevate the head and shoulders to aid breathing. If movement of the legs causes pain, leave the victim lying flat.

   b. If abdominal organs are protruding from the wound, make *no* attempt to reposition the organs. Remove clothing from around the wound or protruding organs. Use a sterile dressing that has been moistened with sterile water or normal saline solution to cover the area. If sterile water or normal saline is not available, use warm tap water to moisten the dressings.

   c. Avoid giving the victim any fluids or food. If the victim complains of excessive thirst, use a cool, wet cloth to moisten the lips, tongue, and inside of the mouth.

d. Obtain medical help immediately.

9. If the victim has an injury to the genital organs:

a. Control severe bleeding by using a sterile dressing to apply direct pressure.

☣ *CAUTION:* Wear gloves or use a protective barrier to prevent contamination from the blood.

b. Position the victim flat on the back. Separate the legs to prevent pressure on the genital area.

c. If any tissue is torn from the area, preserve the tissue by placing it in cool, sterile water or normal saline solution or in gauze moistened with sterile water. Put the tissue on ice and send it to the medical facility along with the victim.

d. Apply cold compresses such as covered ice bags to the area to relieve pain and reduce swelling.

e. Obtain medical help for the victim.

10. Be alert for the signs of shock in all victims. Treat for shock immediately.

11. Constantly reassure all victims while providing care. Remain calm. Encourage the victim to relax as much as possible.

Ⓒ

12. Always obtain medical help as quickly as possible. Shock, pain, and injuries to vital organs can cause death in a very short period of time.

> **PRACTICE** *Go to the workbook and use the evaluation sheet for 14:10, Providing First Aid for Specific Injuries, to practice this procedure. When you feel you have mastered this skill, sign the sheet and give it to your instructor for further action.*

✔ *Final Checkpoint* Using the criteria listed on the evaluation sheet, your instructor will grade you on your performance.

INFORMATION
14:11 *Providing First Aid for Sudden Illness*

The victim of a sudden illness requires first aid until medical help can be obtained. This section provides basic information about sudden illnesses, including heart attack, stroke, fainting, convulsions, and diabetic reactions.

Sudden illness can occur in any individual. At times, it is difficult to determine the exact illness being experienced by the victim. However, by knowing the signs and symptoms of some major disorders, you should be able to provide appropriate first aid care. Information regarding a specific condition or illness may also be obtained from the victim, medical alert bracelets or necklaces, or medical information cards. Be alert to all of these factors while caring for the victim of a sudden illness.

A sudden heart attack is also called a coronary thrombosis, coronary occlusion, or myocardial infarction. It may occur when one of the coronary arteries supplying blood to the heart is blocked. If the attack is severe, the victim may die. If the heart stops beating, cardiopulmonary resuscitation (CPR) must be started. Main facts regarding heart attacks are as follows:

a. Signs and symptoms of a heart attack may vary depending on the amount of heart damage. Severe, painful pressure under the breastbone (sternum) with pain radiating to the shoulders, arms, neck, and jaw is a common symptom (see figure 14-25). The victim usually experiences intense shortness of breath. The skin, especially near the lips and nailbeds, becomes pale or bluish in color. The victim feels very weak but is also anxious and apprehensive. Nausea, vomiting, diaphoresis (excessive perspiration), and loss of consciousness may occur.

b. First aid for a heart attack is directed toward encouraging the victim to relax, placing the victim in a comfortable position to relieve pain and assist breathing, and obtaining medical help. Shock frequently occurs, so provide treatment for shock. Prevent any

Figure 14-25 Severe pressure under the sternum with pain radiating to the shoulders, arms, neck, and jaw is a common symptom of a heart attack.

unnecessary stress and avoid excessive movement because any activity places additional strain on the heart. Reassure the victim constantly, and obtain appropriate medical assistance as soon as possible.

A stroke is also called a **cerebrovascular accident** (CVA), apoplexy, or cerebral thrombosis. It is caused by either the formation of a clot in a cerebral artery that provides blood to the brain or hemorrhage from a blood vessel in the brain.

a. Signs and symptoms of a stroke vary depending on the part of the brain affected. Some common signs and symptoms are numbness, paralysis, eye pupils unequal in size, mental confusion, slurred speech, nausea, vomiting, difficult breathing and swallowing, and loss of consciousness.

b. First aid for a stroke victim is directed toward maintaining respirations, lying the victim flat on the back with the head slightly elevated or on the side to allow secretions to drain from the mouth, avoiding any fluids

by mouth, and obtaining medical assistance. Reassure the victim, prevent any unnecessary stress, and avoid any unnecessary movement.

NOTE: Always remember that although the victim may be unable to speak or may appear to be unconscious, he or she may be able to hear and understand what is going on.

Fainting occurs when there is a temporary reduction in the supply of blood to the brain. It may result in partial or complete loss of consciousness. The victim usually regains consciousness after being in a supine position (that is, lying flat on the back).

a. Early signs of fainting include dizziness, extreme pallor, diaphoresis, coldness of the skin, nausea, and a numbness and tingling of the hands and feet.

b. If early symptoms are noted, help the victim to lie down or to sit in a chair and position his or her head at the level of the knees.

c. If the victim loses consciousness, try to prevent injury. Provide first aid by keeping the victim in a supine position. Loosen any tight clothing and maintain an open airway. Use cool water to gently bathe the victim's face. Check for any injuries that may have been caused by the fall. Permit the victim to remain flat and quiet until color improves and the victim has recovered. Then allow the victim to gradually get up. If recovery is not prompt, if other injuries occur or are suspected, or if fainting occurs again, obtain medical help. Fainting can be a sign of a serious illness or condition that requires medical attention.

A **convulsion,** which is a type of seizure, is a violent, involuntary contraction of muscles. Convulsions may occur in conjunction with high body temperatures, head injuries, brain disease, and brain disorders such as epilepsy.

a. Convulsions cause a rigidity of body muscles followed by jerking movements. During a convulsion, a person may stop breathing, bite the tongue, lose bladder and bowel control, and injure body parts. The face and lips may develop a bluish color. The victim loses consciousness. After regaining consciousness at the end of the convulsion, the victim may be confused and disoriented, and complain of a headache.

b. First aid is directed toward preventing self-injury. Removing dangerous objects from the area, providing a pillow or cushion under the victim's head, and providing artificial respiration, as necessary, are all ways to assist the victim.

c. Do *not* try to place anything between the victim's teeth. This can cause severe injury to your fingers, and/or damage to the victim's teeth or gums.

d. Do *not* use force to restrain or stop the muscle movements; this only causes the contractions to become more severe.

e. When the convulsion is over, watch the victim closely. Allow the victim to sleep or rest. Obtain medical help if the seizure lasts more than a few minutes, if the victim has repeated seizures, if other severe injuries are apparent, if the victim does not have a history of seizures, or if the victim does not regain consciousness.

Diabetes is a metabolic disorder caused by a lack or insufficient production of insulin (a hormone produced by the pancreas). Insulin helps the body break down glucose, a form of sugar. When there is a lack of insulin, sugar builds up in the bloodstream. Insulin injections can reduce and control the level of sugar in the blood. Individuals with diabetes are in danger of developing two conditions that require first aid: diabetic coma and insulin shock.

a. **Diabetic coma** is caused by an increase in the level of glucose in the bloodstream. The condition may result from an excess intake of sugar, failure to take insulin, or insufficient production of insulin. Signs and symptoms include confusion; weakness or dizziness; nausea and/or vomiting; rapid, deep respirations; dry, flushed skin; and a sweet or fruity odor to the breath. The victim will eventually lose consciousness and die unless the condition is treated. Medical assistance must be obtained as quickly as possible.

b. **Insulin shock** is caused by an excess amount of insulin (and a low level of glu-

cose) in the bloodstream. It may result from failure to eat the recommended amounts, vomiting after taking insulin, or taking excessive amounts of insulin. Signs and symptoms include muscle weakness; mental confusion; restlessness or anxiety; diaphoresis; pale, moist skin; hunger pangs; and/or palpitations (rapid, irregular heartbeats). The victim may lapse into a coma and develop convulsions. The onset of insulin shock is sudden, and the victim's condition can deteriorate quickly; therefore, immediate first aid care is required. If the victim is conscious, give him or her a drink containing sugar, such as sweetened orange juice. A cube or teaspoon of granulated sugar can also be placed in the victim's mouth. If the victim is confused, avoid giving hard candy.

NOTE: Unconsciousness could occur, and the victim could choke on the hard candy.

The intake of sugar should quickly control the reaction. If the victim loses consciousness or convulsions start, provide care for the convulsions and obtain medical assistance immediately.

c. By observing symptoms carefully and obtaining as much information as possible from the victim, you can usually determine whether the condition is diabetic coma or insulin shock. Ask the victim, "Have you eaten today?" and "Have you taken your insulin?" If the victim has taken insulin but has not eaten, insulin shock is developing because there is too much insulin in the body. If the victim has eaten but has not taken insulin, diabetic coma is developing. In cases when you know that the victim is diabetic but the victim is unconscious and there are no definite symptoms of either condition, you may not be able to determine whether the condition is diabetic coma or insulin shock. In such cases, the recommendation is to put granulated sugar under the victim's tongue before calling for an ambulance. This is the lesser of two evils. If the patient is in diabetic coma, the blood-sugar level can be lowered as needed when the victim is transported for medical care. If the victim is in insulin shock, however, brain damage can occur if the blood-sugar level is not raised immediately. Medical care cannot correct brain damage.

C In all cases of sudden illness, constantly reassure the victim and make every attempt to encourage the victim to relax and avoid further stress. Be alert for the signs of shock and provide treatment for shock to all victims. The pain, anxiety, and fear associated with sudden illness can contribute to shock.

STUDENT *Go to the workbook and complete the assignment sheet for 14:11, Providing First Aid for Sudden Illness. Then return and continue with the procedure.*

PROCEDURE

Providing First Aid for Sudden Illness

14:11

EQUIPMENT AND SUPPLIES

Blankets, pillows, padded tongue blade, sugar, clean cloth, cool water, disposable gloves

PROCEDURE

1. Follow the priorities of care, if indicated.
   a. Check the scene. Move the victim only if absolutely necessary.
   b. Check the victim for consciousness and breathing.
   c. Call emergency medical services (EMS), if necessary.
   d. Provide care to the victim.
   e. Check for bleeding. Control severe bleeding.
   CAUTION: If possible, wear gloves or use a protective barrier while controlling bleeding.
2. Closely observe the victim for specific signs and symptoms. If the victim is conscious, obtain information about the history of the illness, type and amount of pain, and other pertinent details. If the victim is unconscious, check for a medical bracelet or necklace or a medical information card. Always have a reason for everything you do. Explain your actions to any observers, especially if it is necessary to check the victim's wallet for a medical card.

3. If you suspect the victim is having a heart attack, provide first aid as follows:
   a. Place the victim in the most comfortable position possible but avoid unnecessary movement. Some victims will want to lie flat, but others will want to be in a partial or complete sitting position. If the victim is having difficulty breathing, use pillows or rolled blankets to elevate the head and shoulders.
   b. Obtain medical help for the victim immediately. Advise EMS that oxygen may be necessary.
   c. Encourage the victim to relax. Reassure the victim. Remain calm and encourage others to remain calm.
   d. Watch for signs of shock and treat for shock as necessary. Avoid overheating the victim.
   e. If the victim complains of excessive thirst, use a wet cloth to moisten the lips, tongue, and inside of the mouth. Small sips of water can also be given to the victim, but avoid giving large amounts of fluid.
   CAUTION: Do *not* give the victim ice water or very cold water because the cold can intensify shock.
4. If you suspect that the victim has had a stroke:
   a. Place the victim in a comfortable position. Keep the victim lying flat or slightly elevate the victim's head and shoulders to aid breathing. If the victim has difficulty swallowing, turn the victim on his or her side to allow secretions to drain from the mouth and, thus, prevent choking on the secretions.

b. Reassure the victim. Encourage the victim to relax.

c. Avoid giving the victim any fluids or food by mouth. If the victim complains of excessive thirst, use a cool, wet cloth to moisten the lips, tongue, and inside of the mouth.

d. Obtain medical help for the victim as soon as possible.

5. If the victim has fainted:

a. Keep the victim in a supine position (that is, lying flat on the back).

b. Check for breathing. Provide artificial respiration, if necessary.

c. Loosen any tight clothing.

d. Use cool water to gently bathe the face.

e. Check for any other injuries.

f. Encourage the victim to continue lying down until his or her skin color improves.

g. If no other injuries are suspected, allow the victim to get up slowly. First, elevate the head and shoulders. Then place the victim in a sitting position. Allow the victim to slowly stand. If any signs of dizziness, weakness, or pallor are noted, return the victim to the supine position.

h. If the victim does not recover quickly, or if any other injuries occur, obtain medical care. If fainting has occurred frequently, refer the victim for medical care.
NOTE: Fainting can be a sign of a serious illness or condition.

6. If the victim is having a convulsion:

a. Remove any dangerous objects from the area. If the victim is near heavy furniture or machinery that cannot be moved, move the victim to a safe area.

b. Place soft material such as a blanket, small pillow, rolled jacket, or other similar material under the victim's head to prevent injury.

c. Closely observe respirations at all times. During the convulsion, there will be short periods of apnea (cessation of breathing).
NOTE: If breathing does not resume quickly, artificial respiration may be necessary.

d. Do *not* try to place anything between the victim's teeth. This can cause injury to the teeth and/or gums.

e. Do *not* attempt to restrain the muscle contractions.

f. Note how long the convulsion lasts and what parts of the body are involved. Be sure to report this information to the EMS personnel.

g. After the convulsion ends, closely watch the victim. Encourage the victim to rest.

h. Obtain medical assistance if the seizure lasts more than a few minutes, if the victim has repeated seizures, if other severe injuries are apparent, if the victim does not have a history of seizures, or if the victim does not regain consciousness.

7. If the victim is in diabetic coma:

a. Place the victim in a comfortable position. If the victim is unconscious, position him or her on either side to allow secretions to drain from the mouth.

b. Frequently check respirations. Provide artificial respiration as needed.

c. Obtain medical help immediately so the victim can be transported to a medical facility.

8. If the victim is in insulin shock:

a. If the victim is conscious and can swallow, offer a drink containing sugar.

b. If the victim is unconscious, place a small amount of granulated sugar under the victim's tongue.

c. Place the victim in a comfortable position. Position an unconscious victim on either side to allow secretions to drain from the mouth.

d. If recovery is not prompt, obtain medical help immediately.

9. Observe all victims of sudden illness for signs of shock. Treat for shock as necessary.

10. Constantly reassure any victim of sudden illness. Encourage relaxation to decrease stress.

PRACTICE *Go to the workbook and use the evaluation sheet for 14:11, Providing First Aid for Sudden Illness, to practice this procedure. When you feel you have mastered this skill, sign the sheet and give it to your instructor for further action.*

✔ ***Final Checkpoint*** Using the criteria listed on the evaluation sheet, your instructor will grade you on your performance and knowledge.

14:12 *Applying Dressings and Bandages*

Figure 14-26 Folding a cravat bandage from a triangular bandage.

In many cases requiring first aid, it will be necessary for you to apply dressings and bandages. This section provides basic information on types of bandages and dressings and on application methods.

A *dressing* is a sterile covering placed over a wound or an injured part. It is used to control bleeding, absorb blood and secretions, prevent infection, and ease pain. Materials that may be used as dressings include gauze pads in a variety of sizes and compresses of thick, absorbent material. Fluff cotton should *not* be used as a dressing because the loose cotton fibers may contaminate the wound. In an emergency when no dressings are available, an ironed handkerchief or pillowcase may be used. The dressing is held in place with tape or a bandage.

Bandages are materials used to hold dressings in place, to secure splints, and to support and protect body parts. Bandages should be applied snugly enough to control bleeding and prevent movement of the dressing, but not so tightly that they interfere with circulation. Types of bandages include roller gauze bandages, triangular bandages, and elastic bandages.

a. Roller gauze bandages come in a variety of widths, most commonly 1-, 2-, and 3-inch widths. They can be used to hold dressings in place on almost any part of the body.

b. Triangular bandages can be used to secure dressings on the head/scalp or as slings. A triangular bandage is sometimes used as a covering for a large body part such as a hand, foot, or shoulder. By folding the triangular bandage into a band of cloth called a cravat (see figure 14-26), the bandage can be used to secure splints or dressings on body parts.

c. Elastic bandages are easy to apply because they readily conform, or mold, to the injured part. However, they can be quite hazardous; if they are applied too tightly or are stretched during application, they can cut off or constrict circulation. Elastic bandages are sometimes used to provide support and stimulate circulation.

Several methods are used to wrap bandages. The method used depends on the body part involved. Some common wraps include the spiral wrap, the figure-eight wrap for joints, and the finger, or recurrent, wrap. The wraps are described in Procedure 14:12, immediately following this information section.

After any bandage has been applied, it is important to check the part below the bandage to make sure the bandage is not so tight as to interfere with blood circulation. Signs that indicate poor circulation include swelling, a pale or blue (cyanotic) color to the skin, coldness to the touch, and numbness or tingling. If the bandage has been applied to the hand, arm, leg, or foot, press lightly on the nailbeds to blanch them (that is, make them turn white). The pink color should return to the nailbeds immediately after pressure is released. If the pink color does not return or returns slowly, this is an indication of poor or impaired circulation. If any signs of impaired circulation are noted, loosen the bandages immediately.

STUDENT Go to the workbook and complete the assignment sheet for 14:12, Applying Dressings and Bandages. Then return and continue with the procedure.

PROCEDURE

PROCEDURE

Applying Dressings and Bandages   *14:12*

EQUIPMENT AND SUPPLIES

Sterile gauze pads, triangular bandage, roller gauze bandage, elastic bandage, tape, disposable gloves

PROCEDURE

1. Assemble equipment.
2. Wash hands. Put on gloves if there is any chance of contact with blood or body fluids.
3. Apply a dressing to a wound as follows:
   a. Obtain the correct size dressing. The dressing should be large enough to extend at least 1 inch beyond the edges of the wound.
   b. Open the sterile dressing package, taking care not to touch or handle the sterile dressing with your fingers.
   c. Use a pinching action to pick up the sterile dressing so you handle only one part of the outside of the dressing. (The ideal situation would involve the use of sterile transfer forceps or sterile gloves to handle the dressing. However, these items are usually not available in emergency situations).
   d. Place the dressing on the wound. The untouched (sterile) side of the dressing should be placed on the wound. Do *not* slide the dressing into position. Instead, hold the dressing directly over the wound and then lower the dressing onto the wound.
   e. Secure the dressing in place with tape or with one of the bandage wraps.
   ⚠ *CAUTION:* If tape is used, do not wrap it completely around the part. This can lead to impaired circulation.
4. Apply a triangular bandage to the head or scalp (see figure 14-27):
   a. Fold a 2-inch hem on the base (longest side) of the triangular bandage.

Figure 14-27 Steps for applying a triangular bandage to the head or scalp.

   b. Position and secure a sterile dressing in place over the wound.
   c. Keeping the hem on the outside, position the middle of the base of bandage on the forehead, just above the eyebrows.
   d. Bring the point of the bandage down over the back of the head.
   e. Bring the two ends of the base of the bandage around the head and above the ears. Cross the ends when they meet at the back of head. Bring them around to the forehead.
   f. Use a square knot to tie the ends in the center of the forehead.
   g. Use one hand to support the head. Use the other hand to gently but firmly pull down on the point at the back of the head until the bandage is snug against the head.
   h. Bring the point up and tuck it into the bandage where the bandage crosses at the back of the head.

5. Make a cravat bandage from a triangular bandage (review figure 14-26):
   a. Bring the point of the triangular bandage down to the middle of the base (the long end of the bandage).
   b. Continue folding the bandage lengthwise until the desired width is obtained.
6. Apply a circular bandage with the cravat bandage (see figure 14-28):
   a. Place a sterile dressing on the wound.
   b. Place the center of the cravat bandage over the sterile dressing.
   c. Bring the ends of the cravat around the part and cross them when they meet.
   d. Bring the ends back to the starting point.
   e. Use a square knot to tie the ends of the cravat over the dressing.

   ⚠ *CAUTION:* Avoid tying or wrapping the bandage too tightly. This could impair circulation.

   NOTE: Roller gauze bandage can also be used.

   CAUTION: This type of wrap is *never* used around the neck because it could strangle the victim.

7. Apply a spiral wrap using roller gauze bandage or elastic bandage:
   a. Place a sterile dressing over the wound.
   b. Hold the roller gauze or elastic bandage so that the loose end is hanging off the bottom of the roll.
   c. Start at the farthest end (the bottom of the limb) and move in an upward direction.
   d. Anchor the bandage by placing it on an angle at the starting point. To do this, encircle the limb once, leaving a corner of the bandage uncovered. Turn down this free corner and then encircle the part again with the bandage (see figure 14-29A).
   e. Continue encircling the limb. Use a spiral type motion to move up the limb. Overlap each new turn approximately one-half the width of the bandage.
   f. Use one or two circular turns to finish the wrap at the end point.
   g. Secure the end by taping, pinning, or tying. To avoid injury when pins are used, place your hand under the double layer of bandage and between the pin and the skin before inserting the pin (see figure 14-29B). The end of the bandage can also

Figure 14-28 Steps for applying a circular bandage with a cravat bandage.

be cut in half and the two halves brought around opposite sides and tied into place.

8. Use roller gauze bandage or elastic bandage to apply a figure-eight ankle wrap:
   a. Position a dressing over the wound.
   b. Anchor the bandage at the instep of the foot.

Figure 14-29A Anchor the bandage by leaving a corner exposed. This corner is then folded down and covered when the bandage is circled around the limb.

Figure 14-29B Place your hand between the bandage and the victim's skin while inserting a pin.

c. Make one or two circular turns around the instep and foot (see figure 14-30A).
d. Bring the bandage up over the foot in a diagonal direction. Bring it around the back of the ankle and then down over the top of the foot. Circle it under the instep. This creates the figure-eight pattern.

Figure 14-30A Bring the bandage over the foot in a diagonal direction for the start of the figure-eight pattern. *(Photo by Michael Dzaman)*

Figure 14-30B Keep repeating the figure-eight pattern by moving downward and backward toward the heel with each turn. *(Photo by Michael Dzaman)*

e. Repeat the figure-eight pattern. With each successive turn, move downward and backward toward the heel (see figure 14-30B). Overlap the previous turn by one-half to two-thirds the width of the bandage.
NOTE: Hold the bandage firmly but do not pull it too tightly. If you are using elastic bandage, avoid stretching the material during the application.
f. Near completion, use one or two final circular wraps to circle the ankle.
g. Secure the bandage in place by taping, pinning, or tying the ends, as described in 7g, preceding.

⚠ *CAUTION:* To avoid injury to the victim when pins are used, place your hand between the bandage and the victim's skin.

9. Use roller gauze bandage to apply a recurrent wrap to the fingers (see figure 14-31).

   a. Place a sterile dressing over the wound.

   b. Hold the roller gauze bandage so that the loose end is hanging off the bottom of the roll.

   c. Place the end of the bandage on the bottom of the finger. Then bring the bandage up to the tip of the finger and down to the bottom of the opposite side of the finger. With overlapping wraps, fold the bandage backward and forward over the finger three or four times.

   d. Start at the bottom of the finger and use a spiral wrap up and down the finger to hold the recurrent wraps in position.

   e. Complete the bandage by using a figure-eight wrap around the wrist. Bring the bandage in a diagonal direction across the back of the hand. Circle the wrist at least two times. Bring the bandage back over the top of the hand and circle the bandaged finger. Repeat this figure-eight motion at least twice.

   f. Secure the bandage by circling the wrist once or twice. Tie the bandage at the wrist.

10. After any bandage has been applied, check the circulation below the bandage at frequent intervals. Note any signs of impaired circulation, including swelling, coldness, numbness or tingling, pallor or cyanosis, and poor return of pink color after nailbeds are blanched by lightly pressing on them. If any signs of poor circulation are noted, loosen the bandages immediately.

11. Obtain medical help for any victim who may need additional care.

12. Remove gloves and wash hands.

PRACTICE *Go to the workbook and use the evaluation sheet for 14:12, Applying Dressings and Bandages, to practice this procedure. When you feel you have mastered this skill, sign the sheet and give it to your instructor for further action.*

Figure 14-31 Recurrent wrap for the finger.

✔ *Final Checkpoint* Using the criteria listed on the evaluation sheet, your instructor will grade you on your performance.

UNIT 14 SUMMARY

First aid is defined as "the immediate care given to the victim of an injury or illness to minimize the effect of the injury or illness until experts can take over." Nearly everyone at some time experiences situations for which a proper knowledge of first aid is essential. It is important to follow correct techniques while administering first aid and to provide only the treatment you are qualified to provide.

The basic principles of first aid were presented in this unit. Methods of cardiopulmonary resuscitation (CPR) for infants, children, adults, and choking victims were described. Proper first aid for bleeding, shock, poisoning, burns, heat and cold exposure, bone and joint injuries, specific injuries, and sudden illness were covered. Instructions were given for the application of common dressings and bandages. By learning and following the suggested methods, the health care worker can provide correct first aid treatment in emergency situations until the help of experts can be obtained.

UNIT 14 SUGGESTED REFERENCES

American Medical Association. *Handbook of First Aid and Emergency Care.* Chicago, IL: American Medical Association, 1995.

American National Red Cross. *Community CPR.* St. Louis, MO: Mosby Lifeline, 1993.

American National Red Cross. *Community First Aid and Safety.* St. Louis, MO: Mosby Lifeline, 1993.

American National Red Cross. *CPR for the Professional Rescuer.* St. Louis, MO: Mosby Lifeline, 1993.

American National Red Cross. *Emergency Response.* St. Louis, MO: Mosby Lifeline, 1993.

American National Red Cross. *Standard First Aid.* St. Louis, MO: Mosby Lifeline, 1993.

Brunner, Lillian Sholtis, and Doris Suddarth. *The Lippincott Manual of Nursing Practice.* 5th ed. Philadelphia, PA: J. B. Lippincott, 1991.

Chernega, Janet Bridger. *Emergency Guide for Dental Auxiliaries.* 2nd ed. Albany, NY: Delmar Publishers, 1994.

Grant, Harvey. *Action Guide for Emergency Service.* 6th ed. Englewood Cliffs, NJ: Brady Communications, 1994.

Heckman, James (Ed.). *Emergency Care and Transportation of the Sick and Injured.* 6th ed. Park Ridge, IL: American Academy of Orthopaedic Surgeons, 1995.

Instructional Materials Laboratory. *Emergency Victim Care.* Columbus, OH: Ohio State University, n.d.

Jardins, Terry R. *Cardiopulmonary Anatomy and Physiology: Essentials for Respiratory Care.* 2nd ed. Albany, NY: Delmar Publishers, 1993.

National Safety Council. *CPR Manual.* Boston, MA: Jones and Bartlett, 1993.

For additional information on first aid and emergency care, write to:

◆ American Red Cross—contact your local chapter for First Aid and CPR courses and certification.

◆ U.S. Department of Transportation
Emergency Medical Services Branch
N-42-13
Washington, D.C. 20540

UNIT 15

Preparing for the World of Work

After completing this unit of study, you should be able to:

◆ Identify at least five job-keeping skills and explain why employers consider them to be essential skills

◆ Write a letter of application containing all required information and using correct form for letters

◆ Prepare a resumé containing all necessary information and meeting standards for neatness and correctness

◆ Complete a job application form that meets standards of neatness and accuracy

◆ Demonstrate how to participate in a job interview, including wearing correct dress and meeting standards established in this unit

◆ Determine gross and net income

◆ Calculate an accurate budget for a 1-month period, accounting for fixed expenses and variable expenses without exceeding net monthly income

◆ Define, pronounce, and spell all of the key terms

KEY TERMS

application forms	gross income	net income
budget	income	resumé
deductions	job interview	*(rez´-ah-may)*
fixed expenses	letter of application	variable expense

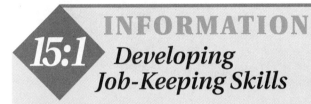

INFORMATION
15:1 *Developing Job-Keeping Skills*

In order to obtain and keep a job, there are certain characteristics that you must develop to be a good employee. This section provides basic information on how to develop good job-keeping skills.

A recent survey of employers asked for information on the deficiencies of high school graduates. The most frequent complaints included poor written grammar, spelling, speech, and math skills. Other complaints included lack of respect for work, lack of self-initiative, poor personal appearance, not accepting responsibility, excessive tardiness and poor attendance, and inability to accept criticism. Any of these defects would be detrimental in a health care worker.

In order to be successful in a health care career, it is essential that you develop good job-keeping skills. Being aware of and striving to achieve the qualities needed for employment are as important as acquiring the knowledge and skills required in your chosen health care profession.

C Correct grammar is a must. This includes both the written and spoken word. Patients often judge ability on how well a person speaks or writes information. Use of words like *ain't* indicates a lack of education and does not create a favorable or professional impression. You must constantly strive to use correct grammar. Listen to how other health care professionals speak and review basic concepts of correct grammar. It may even be necessary to take a communications course to learn to speak cor-

rectly. Because you will be completing legal written records for health care, the use of correct spelling, punctuation, and sentence structure is also essential. Use a dictionary to check spelling, or use the spell check on a computer system. Refer to standard English books or secretarial manuals for information on sentence structure and punctuation. Constantly strive to improve both oral and written communication skills.

Reporting to work on time and when scheduled is also a habit you must develop. Because many health care facilities provide care seven days a week, and often 24-hours per day, an employee who is frequently absent can cause a major disruption in schedule and contribute to an insufficiency of personnel to provide patient care. Most health care facilities have strict rules regarding absenteeism, and a series of absences can result in job loss.

When you arrive at work, be prepared to work. An employer does not pay workers to socialize, make personal telephone calls, consult others about personal or family problems, or work in a sloppy and inefficient manner. Develop a good work ethic. Observe all legal and ethical responsibilities. Follow the policies and procedures of your health care facility. Recognize your limitations and seek help when you need it. Be willing to learn new procedures and techniques. Watch efficient and knowledgeable staff members and learn by their examples. Constantly strive to do the best job possible. A worker who has self-initiative, who sees a job that needs to be done and does it, is a valuable employee who is likely to be recognized and rewarded.

Because health care typically involves a team of different professionals working together to provide patient care, it is also important to have a positive attitude and to be willing to work with others. If you are willing to help others when they need help, they will likely be willing to help you. Two or three people working together can lift a heavy patient much more readily than can one. By being positive, you create a good impression and encourage the same attitude in others. Too often, employees concentrate only on the negative aspects of their jobs. Every job has some bad points; and it is easy to criticize these points as it is easy to criticize the bad points in others with whom you work. However, this leads to a negative attitude and helps create poor morale in everyone. By concentrating on the good aspects of a job and the rewards it can provide, work will seem much more pleasant, and employees will obtain more satisfaction from their efforts.

Most individuals are more than willing to take credit for the good things they have done. In the same manner, it is essential to take responsibility for mistakes. If you make a mistake, report it to your supervisor and make every effort to correct the error. Every human being will do something wrong at some time. Recognizing an error, taking responsibility for it, and making every effort to correct it or prevent it from happening again is a sign of a competent worker. Honesty is essential in health care. Not accepting responsibility for your actions is dishonest. It is often a reason for dismissal and can prevent you from obtaining another position.

A final point essential for obtaining and keeping a job is willingness to learn. Health care changes constantly because of advances in technology and research. Every health care worker must be willing to learn new things. Participating in staff development programs (see figure 15-1), taking courses at technical schools or colleges, attending special seminars or meetings, reading professional journals, and asking questions of other qualified individuals are all

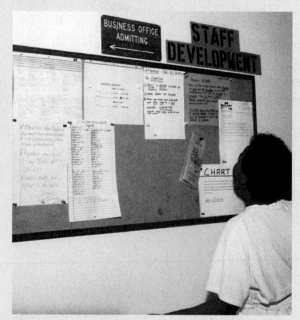

Figure 15-1 Participating in staff development programs is one way to improve your own knowledge and skills.

ways to improve your knowledge and skills. Employers recognize these efforts. Ambition is often rewarded with a higher salary and/or job advancement.

Without good job-keeping skills, no amount of knowledge will help you keep a job. Therefore, it is essential for you to strive to develop the qualities that employers need in workers. Be courteous, responsible, enthusiastic, cooperative, reliable, punctual, and efficient. Strive hard to be the best you can be. If you do this, you will not only be likely to retain your job, but you will probably be rewarded with job advancement, increased salary, and personal satisfaction.

STUDENT *Go to the workbook and complete the assignment sheet for 15:1, Developing Job-Keeping Skills.*

INFORMATION

15:2 Writing a Letter of Application and Preparing a Resumé

In your search for a job, you will often respond in writing to advertisements or sources. This usually involves sending a resume, which should be accompanied by a letter of application, or cover letter. This section provides basic information about this type of letter and the resume.

The purpose of a **letter of application** is to obtain an interview. You must create a good impression in the letter so that the employer will be interested in possibly obtaining you as an employee. In most cases, you will be responding to a job advertised either in the newspaper or through other sources. However, at times a resumé is sent to potential employers even though they have not advertised a job opportunity. A cover letter should accompany all resumés.

The letter should be typewritten on good quality paper. It must be neat, complete, and done according to correct form for letters. Care must be taken to ensure that spelling and punctuation are correct. Remember, this letter is the employer's first impression of you.

If possible, the letter should be addressed to the correct individual. If you know the name of the agency or company, call to obtain this information. Be sure you obtain the correct spelling of the person's name as well as the person's correct title. If you are responding to a box number, follow the instructions in the advertisement. Another possibility is to address the letter to the personnel director or the head of a particular department.

The letter usually contains three to four paragraphs. The contents of each paragraph are described as follows:

a. Paragraph one should state your purpose for writing and should express interest in the position for which you are applying. If you are responding to an advertisement, state the name and date of the publication. If you were referred by another individual, give this person's name and title.

b. The second paragraph should state why you feel you are qualified for the position. It may also state why you want to work for this particular employer. Information should be brief because most of the information will be included on your resumé.

c. Paragraph three should state that a resumé is included. You may also want to draw the employer's attention to one or two important features on your resumé. If you are not including a resumé, state that one is available on request. Whenever possible, it is best to enclose a resumé.

d. The final paragraph closes the letter. Be sure you clearly state how the employer can contact you for additional information. Include a telephone number and the times you will be available to respond to a telephone call. Finally, include a thank you to the potential employer for considering your application.

Figure 15-2 is a sample letter of application to serve as a guide to writing a good letter. However, remember this is only one guide. Letters must be varied to suit each circumstance.

A **resumé** is a record of information about an individual. It is a thorough yet concise summary of an individual's education, experience, and abilities. It is used to provide an employer with basic information that makes you appear qualified as an employee.

A resumé should be typed and attractive in appearance. Like a letter of application, a resumé creates an impression on the employer. Information should be presented in an organized fashion. At the same time, the resumé should be concise and pertinent. Good-quality paper; correct spelling and punctuation; straight, even margins; and an attractive style are essential. If you are sending out a series of resumés, professional copies are permitted. However, be sure the copies are clear, on good-quality paper, and appealing in appearance.

Resumé format can vary. Review sample sources and find a style that you feel best presents your information. For a recent high school graduate with minimum experience, a one-page resumé is usually sufficient.

Parts of a resumé can also vary. Some of the most important parts that should be included

18 Hireme Lane
Job City, Ohio 44444
June 3, 19--

Mr. Prospective Employer
Personnel Director
Health Care Facility
12 Nursing Lane
Dental City, Ohio 44833

Dear Mr. Employer:

In response to your advertisement in the _____
on _____, 19 _____, I would like to apply for
the position of _____.

I recently graduated from _____. I majored in
_____ and feel I am well qualified for this
position. I enjoy working with people and have a sincere
interest in additional training in _____.

My resume is enclosed. I have also enclosed a specific list of
skills which I mastered during my school experience. I feel
that previous positions noted on the resume have provided me
with a good basis for meeting your job requirements.

Thank you for considering my application. If you desire
additional information, or would like to interview me, please
contact me at the above address or by telephone at 589-1111
after 2:00 P.M.

Sincerely,

Iamjob Hunting

Figure 15-2 A sample letter of application.

are shown in figures 15-3A and 15-3B and are described as follows:

a. Personal identification: This includes your name, address, and telephone number. Be sure to include the area code.

b. Employment objective, job desired, or career goal: Briefly state the title of the position for which you are applying.

c. Educational background: List the name and address of your high school. Be sure to in-

FLORENCE NURSE
22 SOUTH MAIN STREET
NURSING, OHIO 33303
(419) 589-1111

EMPLOYMENT OBJECTIVE: NURSING ASSISTANT

SKILLS

RECORDING VITAL SIGNS	MOVING/TRANSFERRING PATIENTS
OBSERVING INFECTION CONTROL	PROVIDING PERSONAL HYGIENE
ADMINISTERING CPR AND FIRST AID	MAKING BEDS
UNDERSTANDING MEDICAL TERMINOLOGY	APPLYING HEAT/COLD APPLICATIONS
ASSISTING WITH ADMISSIONS/DISCHARGES	COLLECTING SPECIMENS

EDUCATION

CAREER HIGH SCHOOL	GRADUATION: JUNE 5, 1993
5 DIAMOND STREET	MAJOR: HEALTH OCCUPATIONS
NURSING, OHIO 33302	GRADE AVERAGE: A'S AND B'S

WORK EXPERIENCE

SUMMER 1992 TO PRESENT	COUNTRY KING FRIED CHICKEN
	5 SOUTHERN LANE
	MANSFIELD, OHIO 33302
FAST FOOD WORKER	DUTIES: OPERATE REGISTER,
	RECORD ORDERS, PROMOTE SALES
SUMMER OF 1991 AND 1992	MADISON RAM HOSPITAL
	602 ESLEY LANE
	MANSFIELD, OHIO 33301
CANDY STRIPER	VOLUNTEER DUTIES: DELIVER MAIL
	AND FLOWERS, ASSISTED NURSES

EXTRACURRICULAR ACTIVITIES

SCHOOL MARCHING BAND	THREE YEARS
VOCATIONAL INDUSTRIAL CLUBS OF AMERICA (VICA)	CLASS TREASURER - TWO YEARS
RED CROSS CLUB MEMBER	THREE YEARS
RED CROSS BLOOD MOBILE	VOLUNTEER WORKER - TWO YEARS
MARCH OF DIMES WALKATHON	WALKER FOR FIVE YEARS
CHURCH YOUTH GROUP	MEMBER FOR SEVEN YEARS

REFERENCES

JANE SMARTO, R.N.	55 EDUCATION LANE
TEACHER	NURSING, OHIO 33303
CAREER HIGH SCHOOL	(419) 589-2134
JEAN SMITH, L.P.N.	432 GERIATRIC PATH
GERIATRIC NURSE	OLDVILLE, OHIO 33300
HAPPY FOLKS HOME	(419) 529-9865
JERRY BROWN	556 EXECUTIVE ROAD
PERSONNEL DIRECTOR	MANSFIELD, OHIO 33300
MADISON HEALTH CARE PROVIDERS	(419) 747-2993

Figure 15-3A A sample resumé with information centered.

clude special courses or majors if they relate to the job position. If you have taken additional courses or special training, list them also. If you have completed college or technical school, this information should be placed first.

THOMAS J. TOOTH

340 DENTAL LANE   FLOSS, OHIO 44598   (524) 333-2435

CAREER GOAL: POSITION AS A DENTAL ASSISTANT IN GENERAL PRACTICE WITH A GOAL OF BECOMING A CERTIFIED DENTAL ASSISTANT

EDUCATION: OHIO JOINT VOCATIONAL SCHOOL, OPPORTUNITY, OHIO 44597
GRADUATED IN JUNE 1992
MAJORED IN DENTAL ASSISTANT PROGRAM FOR TWO YEARS

SKILLS: IDENTIFICATION OF TEETH, CHARTING CONDITIONS OF THE TEETH, MIXING DENTAL CEMENTS AND BASES, POURING MODELS AND CUSTOM TRAYS, PREPARING ANESTHETIC SYRINGE, SETTING UP BASIC DENTAL TRAYS, STERILIZING OF INSTRUMENTS, DEVELOPING AND MOUNTING X RAYS, TYPING BUSINESS LETTERS, COMPLETING INSURANCE FORMS

WORK EXPERIENCE: DENTAL LABORATORY PRODUCTS, 55 MODEL STREET, FLOSS, OHIO 44598
EMPLOYED SEPTEMBER 1991 TO PRESENT AS DENTAL LAB ASSISTANT
PROFICIENT IN MODELS, CUSTOM TRAYS, PROSTHETIC DEVICES

DRUGGIST STORES, 890 PHARMACY LANE, OPPORTUNITY, OHIO 44597
EMPLOYED JUNE 1990 TO AUGUST 1991 AS SALESPERSON
EXPERIENCE IN CUSTOMER RELATIONS, INVENTORY, REGISTER, AND SALES PROMOTION

ACTIVITIES: HEALTH OCCUPATIONS STUDENTS OF AMERICA (HOSA) TREASURER
FIRST PLACE REGIONAL AWARD IN HOSA DENTAL ASSISTANT CONTEST
VOLUNTEER WORKER DURING DENTAL HEALTH WEEK
MEMBER OF SCHOOL PEP CLUB
HOBBIES INCLUDE FOOTBALL, SWIMMING, BASKETBALL, READING

PERSONAL TRAITS: DEPENDABLE, CONSIDERATE OF OTHERS, WILLING TO LEARN, ADAPTABLE TO NEW SITUATIONS, RESPECTFUL AND HONEST, ADEPT AT DENTAL TERMINOLOGY, ABLE TO PERFORM A VARIETY OF DENTAL SKILLS

REFERENCES: REFERENCES WIL BE FURNISHED ON REQUEST

Figure 15-3B A sample resumé with left margin highlights.

d. Work or employment experience: This includes previous positions of employment. Always start with the most recent position and work backward. Each entry should include the name and address of the employer, dates employed, your job title, and a brief description of duties. Avoid use of the word *I*. For example, instead of stating, "I sterilized supplies," state, "sterilized supplies," using action verbs to describe duties.

e. Skills: List special knowledge or work skills you have that can be used in the job you are seeking. The list of skills should be specific and indicate your qualifications and ability to perform the job duties. When work experience is limited, a list of skills is important to show an employer that you are qualified for the position.

f. Other activities: These can include organizations of which you are a member, offices held, special awards received, volunteer work, hobbies, special interests, and other similar facts. Keep this information brief, but do not hesitate to include facts that indicate school, church, and community involvement. This section can show an employer that you are a well-rounded person who participates in activities, assumes leadership roles, strives to achieve, and practices good citizenship. Write out the full names of organizations rather than the identifying letters. For example, write *Vocational Industrial Clubs of America* rather than *V.I.C.A.* and *Health Occupations Students of America* rather than *H.O.S.A.*

g. References: Most sources recommend stating that "references will be furnished on request." For a high school student with limited experience, however, references can provide valuable additional information. Always be sure you have an individual's permission before using that person as a reference. List the full name, title, address, and telephone number of the reference. It is best not to use relatives or high school friends as references. Select professionals in your field, clergy, teachers, or other individuals with responsible positions.

Honesty is always the best policy, and this is particularly true regarding resumes. Never give information that you think will look good but is exaggerated or only partly true. Inaccurate or false information can cost you a job. If you have an A to B average in school, include this information. If your average is lower than an A to B, do *not* state that it is.

Before preparing your resumé, it is important to list all of the information you wish to include. Then select the format that best presents this information. The two sample resumés shown in figures 15-3A and 15-3B are meant to serve as guidelines only. Do not hesitate to evaluate other formats and present your information in the best possible way.

The envelope should be the correct size for your letter of application and resumé. Do *not* fold the letter into small sections and put it in an undersized envelope. This creates a sloppy impression. When possible, it is best to buy standard business envelopes that match your paper. Be sure the envelope is addressed correctly and neatly. It should also be typewritten.

STUDENT *Go to the workbook and complete the assignment sheet for 15:2, Writing a Letter of Application and Resumé. Then return and continue with the procedure.*

PROCEDURE

Writing a Letter of Application and Preparing a Resumé

C

15:2

EQUIPMENT AND SUPPLIES

Good-quality paper, inventory sheet for resumés (see workbook), typewriter with good ribbon (or computer with word processing software and a printer)

PROCEDURE

1. Assemble equipment. Check the typewriter or computer printer to be sure the ribbon is of good quality and is not worn.
2. Re-read the preceding information section on letters of application and resumés.
3. Review the sample letters of application and resumés.
4. Go to the workbook and complete the inventory sheet for resumés. Check dates for accuracy. Be sure that names are spelled correctly. Use the telephone book or other sources to check addresses and zip codes.

5. Carefully evaluate all of your information. Determine the best method of presenting your information. Try different ways of writing your material. Do not hesitate to show several different versions to your instructor or others and get their opinions on which way seems most effective.

6. Type a rough draft of a letter of application. Follow the correct form for letters. Use correct spacing and margins. Check for correct spelling and punctuation.

7. Type a final letter of application. Be sure it contains the required information. Proofread the letter for spelling errors and other mistakes.

8. Type a rough draft of your resumé. Position the information in an attractive manner. Be sure that spacing is standard throughout the resumé and margins are even margins on all sides.

9. Review your sample resumé. Reword any information, if necessary. Be sure all information is pertinent and concise. Ask your instructor or others for opinions regarding suggested changes.

10. Type your final resumé. Take care to avoid errors. If you are not a good typist, it might be wise to have someone else complete the final draft. Proofread the final copy, checking carefully for errors.

    NOTE: Resumés can be copies of the original; but be sure the copies are of good quality. Letters of application must be originals; they are individually tailored for each potential job, and, therefore, are not copied.

11. Replace all equipment.

PRACTICE *Go to the workbook and use the evaluation sheet for 15:2, Writing a Letter of Application and Resumé, to practice this procedure. When you feel you have mastered this skill, sign the sheet and give it to your instructor for further action. Also give your instructor your letter of application and resumé along with the evaluation sheet.*

✔ *Final Checkpoint* Using the criteria listed on the evaluation sheet, your instructor will grade your letter of application and resumé.

INFORMATION
15:3 *Completing Job Application Forms*

Even though you provide each potential employer with a resumé, most employers still require you to complete an application form. Basic information regarding these forms is provided in this section.

Application forms are used by employers to collect specific information. Forms vary from employer to employer, but most request similar information.

Before completing any application form, it is essential that you first read the entire form. Note areas where certain information is to be placed. Read instructions that state how the form is to be completed. Some forms request that the applicant type or print all answers. Others request that the form be completed in the person's handwriting.

Be sure you have all of the required information with you when you go for a job interview. Many employers will ask you to complete the application form at that time. Others will allow you to take the form home. Still others will even send the form to you prior to the interview. The latter two options allow you more time to obtain complete information and print or type the form (unless otherwise requested).

C Fill out each item neatly and completely. Do *not* leave any areas blank. Put "none" or "NA" (meaning "not applicable") when the item requested does not apply to you. Be sure addresses include zip codes and all other required information. Watch spelling and punctuation. Errors will not impress the potential employer. If the application does not state otherwise, it is best to type or to print neatly (see figure 15-4). Use a pen if printing. Be sure you take your time and that all information is legible. Take care *not* to write in spaces that state "office use only" or "do not write below this line." Employers often judge how well you follow directions by your reaction to these sections.

Be sure all information is correct and truthful. Remember, material can be checked and verifed. A simple half-truth can cost you a job.

Always proofread your completed application. Check for completeness, spelling, proper answers to questions, and any errors.

If references are requested, be sure to include all information requested. Before using anyone's name as a reference, it is best to obtain that person's permission. Be prepared to provide reference information when you go for a job interview.

Even though questions vary on different forms, some basic information is usually requested on all of them. In order to be sure you have this information, it is useful to take a "wallet card" with you. A sample card is included in the workbook (as Assignment 1). Employers will not be impressed if you have to ask for a telephone book in order to find requested information; you may appear to be unprepared. Of course, if you are allowed to take the application home or if it is mailed to you, looking for information would not be a problem.

Remember that employers use application forms as a screening method. In order to avoid

Figure 15-4 To complete a job application form, type the information or use blue or black ink.

being eliminated from consideration for a position of employment, be sure your application creates a favorable impression.

STUDENT *Go to the workbook and complete the assignment sheet for 15:3, Completing Job Application Forms. Then return and continue with the procedure.*

PROCEDURE

Completing Job Application Forms
C
15:3

EQUIPMENT AND SUPPLIES

Typewriter or pen
wallet card
    (sample in workbook,
    as Assignment 1)
sample application forms
    (sample in workbook,
    as Assignment 2)

PROCEDURE

1. Assemble equipment. If a typewriter is used, be sure the ribbon is of good quality.
2. Complete all information on the wallet card. A sample is included in the workbook (as Assignment 1). Check dates and be sure information is accurate. List full addresses, zip codes, and names.
3. Review the preceding information section on completing job application forms. Read additional references, as needed.
4. Read the entire sample application form (Assignment 2) in the workbook. Be sure you understand the information requested for each part. Read all directions completely.

5. Unless otherwise directed, type all information requested. If a typewriter is not available, use a blue or black ink pen to print all information.
6. Complete all areas of the form. Use "none" or "NA" as a reply to items that do not apply to you.
7. Take care not to write in spaces labeled "office use only" or "do not write below this line." Leave these areas blank.
8. In the space labeled *"signature,"* sign your name. Note any statement that may be printed by the signature line. Be sure you are aware of what you are signing and the permission you may be giving. Most employers request permission to contact previous employers and/or references, and a verification that information is accurate in this type of signature statement.

9. Recheck the entire application. Be sure information is correct and complete. Note and correct any spelling errors. Be sure you have answered all of the questions.
10. Replace all equipment.

PRACTICE *Go to the workbook and use the evaluation sheet for 15:3, Completing Job Application Forms, to practice this procedure. Obtain sample job application forms from your instructor or other sources. When you feel you have mastered this skill, sign the sheet and give it to your instructor for further action.*

✔ *Final Checkpoint* Using the criteria listed on the evaluation sheet, your instructor will grade your job application form.

INFORMATION
15:4 *Participating in a Job Interview*

A job interview is what you are seeking when you send a letter of application and a resumé. You must prepare for an interview just as hard as you did when composing your resumé. A poor interview can mean a lost job. Some basic facts about the job interview are discussed in this section.

A job interview is usually the last step before getting or being denied a particular position of employment. Usually, you have been screened by the potential employer and have been selected for an interview as a result of your resumé and application form. To the employer, the interview serves at least two main purposes: (1) it provides the opportunity to evaluate you in person, obtain additional information, and ascertain whether you meet the job qualifications; and (2) it allows the employer to tell you about the position in more detail.

Careful preparation is needed before going to an interview. Be sure you have all required information. Your "wallet card," resumé, and completed application form (if you have done one) must be ready. If possible, find out about the position and the agency offering the job. In this way, you will be more aware of the agency's needs.

Be sure of the scheduled date and time of the interview. Know the name of the individual you must contact and the exact place of the interview. Write this information down and take it with you.

Dress carefully. It is best to dress conservatively. Coats and ties are still best for men. Athough pantsuits are sometimes acceptable for women, employers still generally prefer dresses or skirts. Even though it shouldn't be the case, first impressions can affect the employer. All clothes should fit well and be clean and pressed, if needed. Avoid bright, flashy colors and very faddish styles.

Check your entire appearance. Hair should be neat, clean, and styled attractively. Nails should be clean. Women should avoid wearing bright nail polish, too much makeup, and perfume. Men should be clean shaven. Be sure that your teeth are clean and your breath is fresh. Jewelry should not be excessive. And last but not least, use a good antiperspirant! When you are nervous, you perspire.

Leave and arrive early for your interview. It is best to arrive 5 to 10 minutes early. Late arrival could mean a lost job. Allow for traffic, trains blocking the road, and other complications that might interfere with your arriving on time.

During the interview, observe all of the following points:

a. Greet the interviewer by name when you are introduced. Introduce yourself. Shake hands firmly and smile (see figure 15-5).

b. Use correct grammar. Avoid using slang words.

c. Speak slowly and clearly. Don't mumble.

d. Be polite. Practice good manners.

e. **C** Maintain eye contact. Avoid looking at the floor, ceiling, or away from the interviewer. Looking at the middle of the interviewer's forehead or at the tip of the interviewer's nose can sometimes help when you are nervous and experiencing difficulty with direct eye contact.

f. Answer all questions thoroughly, but don't go into long, drawn-out explanations.

g. Do *not* smoke, chew gum, or eat candy during the interview.

h. Be aware of your posture and sit straight.

i. Smile but avoid excessive laughter or giggling.

j. Be yourself. Do not try to assume a different personality or different mannerisms; doing so will only increase your nervousness.

k. Listen closely to the interviewer. Do not interrupt in the middle of a sentence. Allow the interviewer to take the lead.

l. Avoid awkward habits such as swinging your legs, jingling change in your pocket, waving your hands or arms, or patting at your hair.

m. Never discuss personal problems, finances, or other situations in an effort to get the job. This usually has a negative effect on the interviewer.

n. Do not criticize former employers or degrade them in any way.

o. Answer all questions truthfully to the best of your ability.

p. Think before you respond. Try to organize the information you present.

q. Be proud of yourself, to a degree. You have skills and are trained. Make sure the interviewer is aware of this. However, be sure to show a willingness to learn and to gain additional knowledge.

Figure 15-5 Shake hands firmly and smile when you greet an interviewer.

r. Do not immediately question the employer about salary, fringe benefits, insurance, and other similar items. This information is usually mentioned before the end of the interview. If the employer asks whether you have any questions, ask about the job description or responsibilities, type of uniform required, potential for career growth, continuing education or in-service programs, and job orientation. These types of questions indicate a sincere interest in the job rather than a "What's in it for me?" attitude.

s. Do not expect a definite answer at the end of the interview. The interviewer will usually tell you that he or she will contact you.

t. Thank the interviewer for the interview as you leave. If the interviewer extends a hand, shake hands firmly. Smile, be polite, and exit with confidence.

u. Never try to extend the interview if the interviewer indicates that he or she is ready to end it.

After the interview, it is best to send a follow-up note to thank the employer for the interview (see figure 15-6). You may indicate that you are still interested in the position. You may also state that you are available for further questioning. When an employer is evaluating several applicants, a thank-you note is some-times the deciding factor in who gets the job.

C Because you may be asked many different questions during an interview, it is impossible to prepare all answers ahead of time. However, it is wise to think about some potential questions and your responses to them. The following is a suggested list of questions to review. Additional questions may be found in any book on job interviews.

◆ *Tell me a little about yourself.* (Note: Stick to job-related information.)
◆ *What are your strong points/weak points?*
◆ *Why do you feel you are qualified for this position?*
◆ *What jobs have you held in the past? Why did you leave these jobs?* (Note: Avoid criticizing former employers.)
◆ *What school activities are you involved in?*
◆ *What kind of work interests you?*
◆ *Why do you want to work here?*
◆ *What skills do you have that would be of value?*
◆ *What is your attitude toward work?*
◆ *What do you want to know about this job opening?*
◆ *What were your favorite subjects in school and why?*
◆ *What does success mean to you?*
◆ *What are the three most important things to you in a job?*
◆ *Do you prefer to work alone or with others? Why?*
◆ *How many days of school did you miss last year?*
◆ *What do you do in your spare time?*
◆ *Do you have any plans for further education?*

⚖ Any questions that may reflect discrimination or bias do *not* have to be answered during a job interview. Federal law prohibits discrimination with regard to age, cultural or ethnic background, marital status, parenthood, religion, race, and gender. Employers are aware that it is illegal to ask questions of this nature, and the large majority will not ask such questions. If an employer does ask a question of this nature, however, you have the right to refuse to answer. An example of this type of question might be, "I see you married

Figure 15-6 After a job interview, send a thank-you note to the employer.

recently. Do you plan to start having children in the next year or two?" Be polite but firm in your refusal. A statement such as "I prefer not to answer that question" or "Can I ask you how this would affect the job we are discussing?" is usually sufficient.

⚖ At the end of the interview, you may be asked to provide proof of your eligibility to work. Under the Bureau of Immigration Reform Act of 1986, employers are now required by federal law to ask you to complete an Employment Eligibility Verification Form I-9. This form helps the employer verify that you are legally entitled to work in the United States. To complete this form, you must provide documents that indicate your identity. A birth certificate, passport, and/or immigration card can be used for this purpose. You must also have a photo identification, such as a driver's license, and a social security card. The employer must make copies of these documents and include them in your file. Having these forms readily available shows that you are prepared for a job.

STUDENT *Go to the workbook and complete the assignment sheet for 15:4, Participating in a Job Interview. Then return and continue with the procedure.*

PROCEDURE

Participating in a Job Interview

C

15:4

EQUIPMENT AND SUPPLIES

Desk, two chairs, evaluation sheets, lists of questions

PROCEDURE

1. Assemble equipment. Role play a mock interview with four persons. Arrange for two people to evaluate the interview, one person to be the interviewer, and you to be the interviewee.
2. Position the two evaluators in such a way that they can observe both the interviewer and you, the person being interviewed. Make sure they will not interfere with the interview.
3. The interviewer should be seated at the desk and have a list of possible questions to ask during the interview.
4. Play the role of the person being interviewed. Prepare for this role by doing the following:

   ◆ Be sure you have all necessary information. Prepare your wallet card, resumé, and job application form.
   ◆ Dress appropriately for the interview (as outlined in the preceding information section).
   ◆ Arrive at least 5 to 10 minutes early for the interview.

5. When you are called for the interview, introduce yourself. Be sure to refer to the interviewer by name.
6. Sit in the chair indicated. Be aware of your posture, making sure to sit straight.
7. Listen closely to the employer. Answer all questions thoroughly and completely. Think before you speak. Organize your information.
8. Maintain eye contact. Avoid distracting mannerisms.
9. Use correct grammar. Avoid slang expressions. Speak in complete sentences. Practice good manners.
10. When you are asked whether you have any questions, ask questions pertaining to the job responsibilities. Avoid a series of questions on salary, fringe benefits, vacations, time off, etc.
11. At the end of the interview, thank the interviewer for his or her time. Shake hands as you leave.
12. Check your performance by looking at the evaluation sheets completed by the two observers. Study suggested changes.
13. Replace all equipment.

PRACTICE *Go to the workbook and use the evaluation sheet for 15:4, Participating in a Job Interview, to practice this procedure. When you feel you have mastered this skill, sign the sheet and give it to your instructor for further action.*

✔ *Final Checkpoint* Using the criteria listed on the evaluation sheet, your instructor will grade you on your performance.

INFORMATION

15:5 Determining Net Income

1/2 Obtaining a job means, in part, that you will be earning your own money. This often means that you will be, responsible for your own living expenses. To avoid debt and financial crisis, it is important that you learn about managing your money effectively, including understanding how to determine net income. Basic information on this topic is presented in this section.

The term **income** usually means money that you earn or that is available to you. However, the amount you actually earn and the amount you receive to spend may vary. The following two terms explain the difference.

a. **Gross Income:** This is the total amount of money you earn for hours worked. It is the amount determined before any deductions have been taken out of your pay.

b. **Net Income:** This is commonly referred to as "take home pay." It is the amount of money available to you after all payroll **deductions** have been taken out of your salary. Some common deductions are Social Security tax, federal and state taxes, and city taxes. Other deductions may include payroll deductions such as those for United Appeal, medical or life insurance, union dues, and other similar items.

To determine gross income, simply multiply your wage per hour times the number of hours worked. For example, if you earn $4.00 per hour and work a 40 hour week, 4 × 40 = $160.00. In this example, then, $160.00 would be your gross income.

1/2 To determine net income, you must first determine the amounts of the various deductions that will be taken out of your gross pay. Deduction percentages usually vary depending on your income level. You can usually determine approximate deduction percentages and, therefore, your approximate net income by referring to tax charts. Never hesitate to ask about deduction percentages. It is your responsibility to check your own paycheck for accuracy. Starting with the example of gross pay of $160.00, the following shows how net pay may be determined.

Gross Pay $160.00

a. Deduction for federal tax in this income range is usually approximately 15 percent. Check tax tables for accuracy.

15%, or .15, × 160 = $24.00 — 24.00
136.00

b. Deduction for state tax is approximately 2 percent.

2%, or .02, × 160 = $3.20 — 3.20
132.80

c. Deduction for city tax is approximately 1 percent.

1%, or .01, × 160 = 1.60 — 1.60
131.20

d. Deduction for F.I.C.A., or Social Security tax, includes 6.2 percent of the first $60,600 in income and a Medicare deduction of 1.45 percent of the total net in income, for a total deduction of 7.65 percent.

7.65%, or .0765, × 160 = 12.24 — 12.24
118.96

e. Net income after taxes, then, would be $118.96. Therefore, before you even receive your paycheck, $41.04 will be deducted from it. Additional deductions for insurance, union dues, contributions to charity, and other items may also be taken out of your gross pay.

In order to manage your money effectively, it is essential that you be able to calculate your net income. Because this is the amount of money you will have to spend, it will to some extent determine your lifestyle.

STUDENT *Read and complete Procedure 15:5, Determining Net Income.*

PROCEDURE

Determining Net Income

15:5

EQUIPMENT AND SUPPLIES

Assignment sheet for 15:5, Determining Net Income; pen or pencil

PROCEDURE

1. Assemble equipment. If a calculator is available, you may use it to complete this assignment.
2. Read the instructions on the assignment sheet in the workbook for 15:5, Determining Net Income. Use the assignment sheet with this procedure.
3. Determine your wage per hour by using your salary in a current job or an amount assigned by your instructor. Multiply this amount by the number of hours you work per week. This is your gross weekly pay.
4. If your instructor has tax tables, read the tax tables to determine the percentage, or amount of money, that will be withheld for federal tax. If tax tables are not available, check with your employer for this information.
   NOTE: The average withholding tax for an initial income bracket is usually approximately 15 percent. If you cannot find the exact amount or percentage, use this amount (0.15) for an approximate determination.
5. Multiply the percentage for federal tax times your gross weekly pay to determine the amount deducted for federal tax.
6. Determine the deduction for state tax by reading your state tax tables or by consulting your employer.
   NOTE: An average state tax is 2 percent. If you cannot find the exact amount or percentage, use this amount (0.02) for an approximate determination.
7. Multiply the percentage for state tax by your gross weekly pay to determine the amount deducted for state tax.
8. Determine the deduction for any city or corporation tax by reading the city/corporation tax tables or consulting your employer.
   NOTE: An average city/corporation tax is 1 percent. If you cannot find the exact amount or percentage, use this amount (0.01) for an approximate determination.
9. Multiply the percentage for city/corporation tax by your gross weekly pay to determine the amount deducted for city/corporation tax.
10. Check the current deduction for F.I.C.A., or Social Security and Medicare, by checking the tax tables or asking your employer for this information. Determine the deduction for F.I.C.A. by multiplying your gross weekly pay by this percentage.
    NOTE: In 1995, the F.I.C.A. rate was 6.2 percent of the first $60,600 in income and 1.45 percent of total net income for Medicare. Use this total of 7.65 percent, or 0.0765, if you cannot obtain another percentage.
11. List the amounts for any other deductions. Examples include insurance, charitable donations, union dues, and similar items.
12. Add the amounts determined for federal tax, state tax, city/corporation tax, social security, and other deductions together.
13. Subtract the total amount for deductions from your gross weekly pay. The amount left is your net, or take home, pay.
14. Recheck any figures, as needed.
15. Replace all equipment.

PRACTICE *Go to the workbook and use the evaluation sheet for 15:5, Determining Net Income. Practice determining net income according to the criteria listed on the evaluation sheet. When you feel you have mastered this skill, sign the sheet and give it to your instructor for further action.*

✔ *Final Checkpoint* Using the criteria listed on the evaluation sheet, your instructor will grade you on your performance.

INFORMATION

15:6 Calculating a Budget

1/2 In order to use your net income wisely, it is best to prepare a budget. This section provides basic information on this topic.

A budget is an itemized list of living expenses. It must be realistic to be effective.

A budget usually consists of two main types of expenses: fixed expenses and variable expenses. Fixed expenses include items such as rent or house payments, utilities, food, car payments, and insurance payments. Variable expenses include items such as entertainment, clothing purchases, and donations.

The easiest way to prepare a budget is to simply list all anticipated expenses for a 1-month period. Then, determine your net monthly pay. Allow a fair percentage of the net monthly pay for each of the budget items listed.

Savings should be incorporated into every budget. If saving money is regarded as an obligation, it is easier to set aside money for this purpose. When an emergency occurs, money is then available to cover the unexpected expenditure.

Some payments are due once or twice a year. An example is insurance payments. To be realistic, a monthly amount should be budgeted for this purpose. To determine a monthly amount, divide the total yearly cost for the insurance by twelve. Then, budget this amount each month. In this way, when insurance payments are due, the money is available for payment, and one month's budget will not have to bear the full amount of the insurance payment.

It is important that budgeted expenses do *not* exceed net monthly income. It may sometimes be necessary to limit expenses that are not fixed. Entertainment, clothing purchases, and similar items are examples of expenses that can be limited.

The final step is to live by your budget and avoid any spending over the allotted amounts. This is one way to prevent financial problems and excessive debt. If your fixed expenses or net income increases, you will have to revise your budget. Remember, creating a budget leads to careful management of hard-earned money.

STUDENT *Read Procedure 15:6, Calculating a Budget. Then go to the workbook and complete the corresponding assignment sheet.*

PROCEDURE

Calculating a Budget **1/2** 15:6

EQUIPMENT AND SUPPLIES

Assignment sheet for 15:6, Calculating a Budget; pen or pencil

INTRODUCTION

1. Assemble equipment. If a calculator is available, you may use it to complete this procedure.
2. Go to the workbook and read the instructions on the assignment sheet for 15:6, Calculating a Budget.

3. Determine your fixed expenses for a 1-month period. This includes amounts you must pay for rent, utilities, loans, charge accounts, insurance, and similar items. List these expenses.
4. Determine your variable expenses for a 1-month period. This includes amounts for clothing purchases, personal items, donations, entertainment, and similar items. List these expenses.
5. List any other items that must be included in your monthly budget. Be sure to list a reasonable amount for each item.
6. Determine a reasonable amount for savings. Many people prefer to set aside a certain percentage of their net monthly pay as savings.
7. Determine your net monthly pay. Double-check all figures for accuracy.
8. Add all of your monthly budget expenses together. The sum represents your total expenditures per month.

9. Compare your expense total to your net monthly income. If your expense total is higher than your net income, you will have to revise your budget and reduce any expenses that are not fixed. If your expense total is lower than your net income, you may increase the dollar amounts of your budget items. If the other figures in your budget are realistic, it may be wise to increase the dollar amount of savings.

10. When the expense total in your budget equals your monthly net income, you have a balanced budget. Live by this budget and avoid any expenditures not listed on the budget.

11. Replace all equipment.

PRACTICE *Go to the workbook and use the evaluation sheet for 15:6, Calculating a Budget, to practice this procedure. When you feel you have mastered this skill, sign the sheet and give it to your instructor for further action.*

✔ *Final Checkpoint* Using the criteria listed on the evaluation sheet, your instructor will grade you on your performance.

UNIT 15 SUMMARY

Even if an individual is proficient in many skills, it does not necessarily follow that the individual will obtain the "ideal" job. Just as it is important to learn the skills needed in your chosen health care career, it is important to learn the skills necessary to obtain a job.

Job-keeping skills important to an employer include using correct grammar in both oral and written communications, reporting to work on time and when scheduled, being prepared to work, following correct policies and procedures, having a positive attitude, working well with others, taking responsibility for your actions, and being willing to learn. Without good job-keeping skills, no amount of knowledge will help you keep a job.

One of the first aspects of obtaining a job involves preparing a letter of application and a resume. These are the "press releases" that tell a potential employer about your skills and abilities. A properly prepared resumé will help you obtain an interview.

It is important to prepare for an interview. Careful consideration should be given to dress and appearance. Answers should be prepared for common interview questions. The applicant should also try to learn as much as possible about the potential employer; this way, the applicant will be able to match his or her skills and abilities to the needs of the employer. Finally, practice completing job application forms. A neat, correct, and thorough application form will also help you get a job.

Certain other skills become essential when a person has a job. Everyone should be able to calculate gross and net income. In addition, everyone should be able to develop a budget based on needs and income. Having and following a budget makes it more likely that money earned will be spent wisely and minimizes the chance of debt. Learn the job-seeking and job-keeping skills well. They will benefit you throughout your life as you seek new positions of employment and advance in your chosen health career.

UNIT 15 SUGGESTED REFERENCES

Bailey, Larry J. *Working: Skills for a New Age.* Albany, NY: Delmar Publishers, 1990.

Davis, Rene V., Rosemary T. Fruehling, and Nield B. Oldham. *Psychology: Human Relations and Work Adjustments.* 7th ed. New York, NY: McGraw-Hill, 1989.

Hing-McGowan, Joyce. *Writing for Employment.* Cincinnati, OH: Southwestern, 1993.

Krantman, Stan. *The Resumé Writer's Workbook.* Albany, NY: Delmar Publishers, 1995.

Kushner, John. *How to Find and Apply for a Job.* 6th ed. Cincinnati, OH: Southwestern, 1996.

Masters, L. Ann. *Applying and Interviewing for a Job.* Cincinnati, OH: Southwestern, 1993.

Perrin, Carl, and Peter Dublin. *Successful Resumés and Interviews.* Albany, NY: Delmar Publishers, 1994.

Ransbottom, LuEllen. *Budgeting Your Time and Money.* Cincinnati, OH: Southwestern, 1993.

Simmers, Louise. *Practical Problems in Mathematics for Health Occupations.* Albany, NY: Delmar Publishers, 1996.

APPENDIX A
Vocational Student Organizations

Vocational student organizations provide both secondary (high school) and postsecondary (after high school) vocational students with the opportunity to associate with other students enrolled in the same programs or career areas. Some purposes of these organizations are to develop student leadership, improve the quality and relevance of education, develop citizenship responsibilities, and overcome sexual and racial discrimination and stereotyping.

The United States Department of Education recognizes and supports the following nine vocational student organizations:

◆ American Industrial Arts Student Association (AIASA)
◆ Distributive Education Clubs of America (DECA)
◆ Future Business Leaders of America (FBLA)
◆ Future Farmers of America (FFA)
◆ Future Homemakers of America (FHA)
◆ Health Occupations Students of America (HOSA)
◆ National Post-Secondary Agriculture Student Organization (NPSASO)
◆ Office Education Association (OEA)
◆ Vocational Industrial Clubs of America (VICA)

Two organizations that supplement Health Occupations education are discussed: Health Occupations Students of America (HOSA) and Vocational Industrial Clubs of America (VICA).

HEALTH OCCUPATIONS STUDENTS OF AMERICA

Health Occupations Students of America (HOSA, pronounced *Ho'sa*) is the national organization for students enrolled in Health Occupations programs.

Membership begins at the local level, where students who are enrolled in a Health Occupations education program join together under the supervision of their classroom instructor, who serves as the HOSA local chapter advisor. Local chapters associate with the HOSA state association and the HOSA national organization.

Members of HOSA are involved in community-oriented, career-related, and leadership-development activities. All HOSA activities relate to the classroom instructional program and the health care delivery system. Furthermore, HOSA is an integral part of the Health Occupations education program, meaning that HOSA activities motivate students and enhance what the students learn in the classroom and on the job.

The mission of HOSA is "to enhance the delivery of quality health care to all Americans." The HOSA motto is "The hands of HOSA mold the health of tomorrow." Goals that HOSA believes are vital for each member are:

◆ To promote physical, mental, and social well being.
◆ To develop effective leadership qualities and skills.
◆ To develop the ability to communicate effectively with people.
◆ To develop character.
◆ To develop responsible citizenship traits.
◆ To understand the importance of pleasing oneself as well as being of service to others.
◆ To build self-confidence and pride in one's work.
◆ To make realistic career choices and seek successful employment in the health care field.
◆ To develop an understanding of the importance of interacting and cooperating with other students and organizations.
◆ To encourage individual and group achievement.
◆ To develop an understanding of current health care issues, environmental concerns, and sur-

vival needs of the community, the nation, and the world.

◆ To encourage involvement in local, state, and national health care and education projects.

In addition to providing activities that allow members to develop occupational skills, leadership qualities, and fellowship through social and recreational activities, HOSA also encourages skill development and a healthy competitive spirit through participation in the National Competitive Events Program. Competition is held at the local, district/regional, state, and national levels. Some of the competitive events include contests in prepared and extemporaneous speaking, job-seeking skills, standard first aid/CPR, dental assisting, clerical and clinical medical assisting, medical laboratory assisting, nursing assisting, practical nursing, dental spelling and terminology, medical spelling and terminology, extemporaneous health display, community awareness project (of health-related issues), parliamentary procedure, and the HOSA Bowl.

HOSA has an official emblem, shown in figure A-1. The circle represents the continuity of health care; the triangle represents the three aspects of human well-being: social, physical, and mental; and the hands signify the caring of each HOSA member. The colors of HOSA—maroon, medical white, and navy blue—are represented in the emblem. The background of the outer circle is ma-

roon. Medical white is used for the letters in the outer circle; the area around the triangle; and the hands, figure, and "HOSA" inside the triangle. The triangle and the "Founded 1976" are navy blue.

The HOSA handbook provides detailed information about the structure, purposes, competitive events, and activities of HOSA. Students interested in further details should refer to this handbook.

VOCATIONAL INDUSTRIAL CLUBS OF AMERICA

Some states do not have HOSA organizations. Students in Health Occupations education programs in these states can participate in VICA. Vocational Industrial Clubs of America (VICA, pronounced *Vik'a*) is a national organization for students enrolled in trade, industrial, technical, and Health Occupations courses that are vocationally and occupationally oriented. Examples of these courses include auto mechanics, auto body, cosmetology, drafting, machine trades, welding, and Health Occupations. Membership begins with local clubs that affiliate with a state association and then the national organization.

The Vocational Industrial Clubs of America bring students together to exchange ideas, discuss problems, and share common purposes. The clubs provide opportunities for leadership and skill development, offer chances to excel through an achievement and recognition program, and promote high standards and values.

The VICA mission statement states, "VICA is an active partnership among people who are involved in the education, training, and employment of vocational-technical students to influence the quality and relevance of vocational education." The VICA motto is "Preparing for leadership in the world of work." Some of VICA's purposes include:

◆ To unite in a common bond all students enrolled in trade, industrial, technical, and health education.

◆ To develop leadership abilities through participation in educational, vocational, civic, recreational, and social activities.

◆ To foster a deep respect for the dignity of work.

◆ To assist students in establishing realistic vocational goals.

Figure A-1 The HOSA emblem. *(With permission of Health Occupations Students of America)*

◆ To help students attain purposeful lives.

◆ To create enthusiasm for learning.

◆ To promote high standards in trade ethics, workmanship, scholarship, and safety.

◆ To develop the ability of students to plan together, organize, and carry out worthy activities and projects through the use of the democratic process.

◆ To develop patriotism through a knowledge of our nation's heritage and the practice of democracy.

In addition to individual- and club-achievement programs, VICA offers skill competition in both leadership and job areas. Competition is held at the local, district/regional, state, and national levels. Examples of leadership contests include prepared and extemporaneous speech, VICA ceremonies, club business procedure, job interview, and safety promotion. Examples of job-centered contests for Health Occupations students include medical assisting, dental assisting, nurse assisting, practical nurse, basic health care skills, and, in some states, first aid and CPR.

The official emblem of VICA is shown in figure A-2. The shield represents patriotism, or a belief in democracy, liberty, and the American way of life. The torch represents knowledge. The orbital circles represent technology and the training needed to master new technical frontiers along with the need for continuous education. The gear represents the industrial society and the cooperation of the individual working with labor and management for the betterment of humankind. The hands represent youth and the search for knowledge along with the desire to acquire a skill.

The VICA Leadership Handbook and other VICA publications provide more information on the various activities and programs. Students interested in further details should refer to these sources of information.

Figure A-2 The VICA emblem. *(With permission of Vocational Industrial Clubs of America, Inc.)*

OTHER SOURCES OF INFORMATION

◆ Health Occupations Students of America
4108 Amon Carter Boulevard, Suite 202
Fort Worth, Texas 76155

◆ Vocational Industrial Clubs of America
P.O. Box 3000
Leesburg, Virginia 22075

—SUGGESTED REFERENCES—

Health Occupations Students of America. *HOSA Handbook: Sections A, B, C.* Fort Worth, Texas: HOSA.

Vocational Industrial Clubs of America. *VICA Leadership Handbook.* Falls Church, Virginia: VICA.

Metric Conversion Charts

The metric system is gradually replacing other systems of measurement. The following information and charts will assist you in converting measurements.

1. Temperature measurements:
   ◆ To convert Fahrenheit (F) temperatures to Celsius (C) temperatures, subtract 32 from the Fahrenheit temperature and then multiply the result by 5/9, or 0.5556.
   ◆ To convert Celsius (C) temperatures to Fahrenheit (F) temperatures, multiply the Celsius temperature by 9/5, or 1.8, and then add 32 to the total.
   ◆ The following chart provides some major temperature equivalents

2. Linear measurements:
   ◆ To convert inches to centimeters, multiply the number of inches by 2.54 (1 inch = 2.54 centimeters).
   ◆ To convert feet to centimeters, multiply the number of feet by 30.48 centimeters (1 foot = 30.48 centimeters).
   ◆ To convert centimeters to inches, divide the number of centimeters by 2.54.
   ◆ To convert centimeters to feet, divide the number of centimeters by 30.48.

3. Weight measurements:
   ◆ To convert pounds to kilograms, divide the number of pounds by 2.2 (1 kilogram = 2.2 pounds).
   ◆ To convert kilograms to pounds, multiply the number of kilograms by 2.2.

4. Liquid measurements:
   ◆ Note that 1 cubic centimeter (cc) is equal to 1 milliliter (mL)
   ◆ To convert household measurements (e. g., cups, ounces, quarts, or pints) to metric measurements, multiply the the household measurement by the equivalent number of cubic centimeters or milliliters. For example, 1 teaspoon equals 5 cubic centimeters. Therefore, 3 teaspoons converted to metric would be 3 × 5, or 15 cubic centimeters or milliliters.
   ◆ To convert metric measurements to household measurements, divide the metric measurement by the number of metric units in one of the household units. For example, there are 30 cubic centimeters or milliliters in 1 ounce. Therefore, 180 cubic centimeters or milliliters converted to ounces would be 180 ÷ 30, or 6 ounces.

Fahrenheit-Centigrade Equivalents

F	C	F	C	F	C
32	0	102	38.9	116	46.7
70	21.1	103	39.4	117	47.2
75	23.9	104	40	118	47.8
80	26.7	105	40.6	119	48.3
85	29.4	106	41.1	120	48.9
90	32.2	107	41.7	125	51.7
95	35	108	42.2	130	54.4
96	35.6	109	42.8	135	57.2
97	36.1	110	43.3	140	60
98	36.7	111	43.9	150	65.6
98.6	37	112	44.4	212	100
99	37.2	113	45		
100	37.8	114	45.6		
101	38.3	115	46.1		

Linear English—Metric Equivalents

1 inch (in) = 0.0254 meters (m)
12 inches = 1 foot (ft) = 0.3048 meters (m)
3 feet = 1 yard (yd) = 0.914 meters (m)
5,280 feet = 1 mile = 1601.6 meters (m)
39.372 inches = 3.281 feet = 1 meter (m)
1.094 yards = 1 meter (m)
0.621 miles = 1 kilometer (km)

Liquid English—Metric Equivalents

1 drop (gtt) = 0.0667 milliliters (ml)
15 drops (gtts) = 1.0 milliliters (ml)
1 teaspoon (tsp) = 5.0 milliliters (ml)
3 teaspoons = 1 tablespoon (tbsp) = 15.0 milliliters (ml)
1 ounce (oz) = 30.0 milliliters (ml)
8 ounces (oz) = 1 cup (cp) = 240.0 milliliters (ml)
2 cups (cp) = 1 pint (pt) = 500.0 milliliters (ml)
2 pints (pt) = 1 quart (qt) = 1,000.0 milliliters (ml)

24-Hour Clock (Military Time) Conversion Chart

Time	24-Hour Time	Time	24-Hour Time
12:01 AM	0001	12:01 PM	1201
12:05 AM	0005	12:05 PM	1205
12:30 AM	0030	12:30 PM	1230
12:45 AM	0045	12:45 PM	1245
1:00 AM	0100	1:00 PM	1300
2:00 AM	0200	2:00 PM	1400
3:00 AM	0300	3:00 PM	1500
4:00 AM	0400	4:00 PM	1600
5:00 AM	0500	5:00 PM	1700
6:00 AM	0600	6:00 PM	1800
7:00 AM	0700	7:00 PM	1900
8:00 AM	0800	8:00 PM	2000
9:00 AM	0900	9:00 PM	2100
10:00 AM	1000	10:00 PM	2200
11:00 AM	1100	11:00 PM	2300

A

abbreviation—A shortened form of a word, usually just letters.

abdominal—Pertaining to the cavity or area in front of body and containing the stomach, the small intestine, part of the large intestine, the liver, the gallbladder, the pancreas, and the spleen.

abduction—Movement away from the midline.

abrasion—Injury caused by rubbing or scraping the skin.

absorption—Act or process of sucking up or in; taking in of nutrients.

abuse—Any care that results in physical harm or pain, or mental anguish.

accelerator—A chemical substance that increases the rate of a chemical reaction.

acceptance—The process of receiving or taking; approval; belief.

Acetest—Reagent tablet containing chemicals that react with ketones; used to check for presence of ketones in urine.

acidosis—A pathological condition resulting from a disturbance in the acid-base balance in the blood and body tissues.

activities of daily living (ADL)—Daily activities necessary to meet basic human needs, e.g., feeding, dressing, and elimination.

acute—Lasting a short period of time but relatively severe (e.g., an acute illness).

addiction—State of being controlled by a habit, as can happen with alcohol and drugs.

adduction—Movement toward the midline.

adenitis—Inflammation of a gland or lymph node.

adipose—Fatty tissue; fat.

adolescence—Period of development from 12 to 20 years of age; teenage years.

adrenal—One of two endocrine glands located one above each kidney.

advanced directive—A legal document designed to indicate a person's wishes regarding care in case of a terminal illness or during the dying process.

aerobic—Requiring oxygen in order to live and grow.

afebrile—Without a fever.

affection—A warm or tender feeling toward another; fondness.

agar plate—Special laboratory dish containing agar, a gelatinous colloidal extract of a red alga, which is used to provide nourishment for growth of organisms.

agent—Someone who has the power or authority to act as the representative of another.

agglutination—Clumping together, as in the clumping together of red blood cells.

air compressor—Machine that provides air under pressure; used in dental areas to provide air pressure to operate handpieces and air syringe.

alginate—Irreversible, hydrocolloid, dental-impression material.

alignment—Positioning and supporting the body so that all body parts are in correct anatomical position.

alimentary canal—The digestive tract from the esophagus to the rectum.

alveoli—Microscopic air sacs in the lungs.

Alzheimer's disease—Progressive, irreversible disease involving memory loss, disorientation, deterioration of intellectual function, and speech and gait disturbances.

amalgam—Alloy (mixture) of various metals and mercury; restoration or filling material used primarily on posterior teeth.

ambulate—To walk.

amino acid—The basic component of proteins.

amputation—The cutting off or separation of a body part from the body.

anaerobic—Not requiring oxygen in order to live and grow; able to thrive in the absence of oxygen.

analgesia—The state of inability to feel pain yet still being conscious.

anatomy—The study of the structure of an organism.

anemia—Disease caused by lack of blood or an insufficient number of red blood cells.

anesthesia—The state of inability to feel sensation, especially the sensation of pain.

anger—Feeling of displeasure or hostility; mad.

anorexia—Loss of appetite.

anorexia nervosa—Psychological disorder involving loss of appetite and excessive weight loss not caused by a physical disease.

anoxia—Without oxygen; synonymous with suffocation.

antecubital—The space located on the inner part of the arm and near the elbow.

anterior—Before or in front of.

anterior teeth—Teeth located toward the front of the mouth; includes incisor and cuspids.

antibody—Substance, usually a protein, formed by the body to produce an immunity to an antigen or pathogen.

antibody screen—Test that checks for antibodies in the blood prior to a transfusion.

anticoagulant—Substance that prevents clotting of the blood.

antigen—Substance that causes the body to produce antibodies; may be introduced into the body or formed within the body.

antisepsis—Aseptic control that inhibits, retards growth of, or kills pathogenic organisms; not effective against spores and viruses.

anuria—Without urine; producing no urine.

anus—External opening of the anal canal, or rectum.

aorta—Largest artery in the body; carries blood away from the heart.

aortic valve—Flap or cusp located between the left ventricle of the heart and the aorta.

apathy—Indifference; lack of emotion.

apex—The pointed extremity of a conelike structure; the rounded, lower end of the heart, below the ventricles.

aphasia—Language impairment; loss of ability to comprehend or speak normally.

apical foramen— The opening in the apex of a tooth; allows nerves and blood vessels to enter tooth.

apical pulse—Pulse taken with a stethoscope and near the apex of the heart.

apnea—Absence of respirations; temporary cessation of respirations.

apoplexy—A stroke; *see* **cerebral vascular accident**.

appendicular skeleton—The bones that form the limbs or extremities of the body.

application form—A form or record completed when applying for a job.

appointment—A schedule to do something on a particular day and time.

aquamatic pad—Temperature-controlled unit that circulates warm liquid through a pad to provide dry heat.

aqueous humor—Watery liquid that circulates in the anterior chamber of the eye.

arterial—Pertaining to an artery.

arteriole—Smallest branch of an artery; vessel that connects arteries to capillaries.

arteriosclerosis—Hardening and/ or narrowing of the walls of arteries.

artery—Blood vessel that carries blood away from the heart.

arthritis—Inflammation of a joint.

asepsis—Being free from infection.

aspirate—To remove by suction.

aspirating syringe—Special dental anesthetic syringe designed to hold carpules.

assault—Physical or verbal attack on another person; treatment or care given to a person without obtaining proper consent.

assistant—Level of occupational proficiency where an individual can work in an occupation after a period of education or on-the-job training.

associate's degree—Degree awarded by a vocational-technical school or community college after successful completion of a 2-year course of study or its equivalent.

astigmatism—Defect or blurring of vision due to irregularity of the cornea of the eye.

atherosclerosis—Form of arteriosclerosis characterized by accumulation of fats or mineral deposits on the inner walls of the arteries.

atrium—Also called an *auricle*; an upper chamber of the heart.

atrophy—Wasting away of tissue; decrease in size.

audiologist—Individual specializing in diagnosis and treatment of hearing disorders.

audiometer—Instrument used to test hearing and determine hearing defects.

aural temperature—Measurement of body temperature at the tympanic membrane in the ear.

auricle—Also called the *pinna;* external part of the ear.

auscultation—Process of listening for sounds in the body.

autoclave—Piece of equipment used to sterilize articles by way of steam under pressure and/or dry heat.

autonomic nervous system—That division of the nervous system concerned with reflex, or involuntary, activities of the body.

avulsion—A wound that occurs when tissue is separated from the body.

axial skeleton—The bones of the skull, rib cage, and spinal column; the bones that form the trunk of the body.

axilla—Armpit; that area of the body under the arm.

ayer blade—Wooden or plastic blade used to scrape cells from the cervix of the uterus; used for Pap tests.

bachelor's degree—Degree awarded by a college or university after a person has completed a 4-year course of study or its equivalent.

bacteria—One-celled microorganisms, some of which are beneficial and some of which cause disease.

bandage—Material used to hold dressings in place, secure splints, and support and protect body parts.

bandage scissors—Special scissors with a blunt lower end used to remove dressings and bandages.

bargaining—Process of negotiating an agreement, sale, or exchange.

Bartholin's glands—Two small mucous glands near the vaginal opening.

basal metabolism—The amount of energy needed to maintain life when the subject is at complete rest.

base—Protective (dental) material placed over the pulpal area of a tooth to reduce irritation and thermal shock.

base of support—Standing with feet 6 to 8 inches apart to provide better balance.

battery—Unlawfully touching another person without that person's consent.

bed cradle—A device placed on a bed to keep the top bed linens from contacting the legs and feet.

benign—Not malignant or cancerous.

bicuspids—Also called *premolars;* the teeth that pulverize or grind food and are located between cuspids and molars.

bifurcated—Having two roots (as in teeth).

bile—Liver secretion that is concentrated and stored in the gallbladder and that aids in the emulsification of fats during digestion.

binders—Devices applied to hold dressings in place, provide support, apply pressure, or limit motion.

biohazardous—Contaminated with blood or body fluid and having the potential to transmit disease.

biopsy—Excision of a small piece of tissue for microscopic examination.

bitewing—Also called a *cavity-detecting X ray;* a dental X ray that shows only the crowns of the teeth.

bladder—Membranous sac or storage area for a secretion (gallbladder); also, the vesicle that acts as the reservoir for urine.

bland diet—Diet containing only mild-flavored foods with soft textures.

block style—Written-letter format in which all parts of the letter start at the left margin.

blood—Fluid that circulates through the vessels in the body to carry substances to all body parts.

blood pressure—Measurement of the force exerted by the heart against the arterial walls when the heart contracts (beats) and relaxes.

blood smear—A drop of blood spread thinly on a slide for microscopic examination.

body—Main content, or message part, of a letter.

body mechanics—The way in which the body moves and maintains balance; proper body mechanics involves the most efficient use of all body parts.

boiling water—Method of aseptic control that disinfects but does not sterilize, or kill spores and viruses.

bolus—Food that has been chewed and mixed with saliva.

bowel—The intestines.

Bowman's capsule—Part of the renal corpuscle in the kidney; picks up substances filtered from the blood by the glomerulus.

brachial—Pertaining to the brachial artery in the arm, which is used to measure blood pressure.

bradycardia—Slow heart rate, usually below sixty beats per minute.

brain—Soft mass of nerve tissue inside the cranium.

brand name—Company or product name given to a medication or product.

breast—Mammary, or milk, gland located on the upper part of the front surface of the body.

bronchi—Two main branches of the trachea; air tubes to and from the lungs.

bronchioles—Small branches of the bronchi; carry air in the lungs.

budget—An itemized list of income and expected expenditures for a period of time.

buccal surface—Outside surface of the posterior teeth; surface facing the cheek; facial surface of bicuspids and molars.

buffer period—Period of time kept open on an appointment schedule to allow for emergencies, telephone calls, and other unplanned situations.

bulimarexia—Psychological condition in which person eats excessively and then uses laxatives or vomits to get rid of the food.

bulimia—Psychological condition in which person alternately eats excessively and then fasts or refuses to eat.

burn—Injury to body tissue caused by heat, caustics, radiation, and/or electricity.

burs—Small, rotating instruments of various types; used in dental handpieces to prepare cavities for filling.

calcaneous—Large tarsal bone that forms the heel.

calculus—Also called *tartar,* hard, calcium-like deposit that forms on the teeth; a stone that forms in various parts of the body from a variety of different substances.

calorie—Unit of measurement of the fuel value of food.

cane—A rod used as an aid in walking.

capillary—Blood vessel that connects arterioles and venules and allows for exchange of nutrients and gases between the blood and the body cells.

carbohydrate-controlled diet—Diet in which the number and types of carbohydrates are restricted or limited.

carbohydrates—Group of chemical substances including sugars, cellulose, and starches; nutrient that provide the greatest amount of energy in the average diet.

cardiac—Pertaining to the heart.

cardiopulmonary—Pertaining to the heart and lungs.

cardiopulmonary resuscitation (CPR)—Procedure of providing oxygen and chest compressions to a victim whose heart has stopped beating.

cardiovascular—Pertaining to the heart and blood vessels.

caries—Tooth decay, an infectious disease that destroys tooth tissue.

carious lesion—An occurrence of tooth decay.

carpal—Bone of the wrist.

carpule—A glass cartridge that contains a premeasured amount of anesthetic solution; used for dental anesthesia.

cataract—Condition of the eye where the lens becomes cloudy or opaque, leading to blindness.

catheter—A rubber, metal, or other type of tube that is passed into a body cavity and used for injecting or removing fluids.

caudal—Pertaining to any tail or tail-like structure.

cavitation—The cleaning process employed in an ultrasonic unit; bubbles explode to drive cleaning solution onto article being cleaned.

cavity—A hollow space, such as a body cavity (which contains organs) or a hole in a tooth.

cell—Mass of protoplasm; the basic unit of structure of all animals and plants.

cell membrane—Outer, protective, semipermeable covering of a cell.

cellulose—Fibrous form of carbohydrate.

cement—Dental material used to seal inlays, crowns, bridges, and orthodontic appliances in place.

cementum—Hard, bonelike tissue that covers the outside of the root of a tooth.

central nervous system—The division of the nervous system consisting of the brain and spinal cord.

central processing unit (CPU)—Unit that controls all of the work of a computer; frequently called the "brains" of the computer.

centrifuge—A machine that uses centrifugal (driving away from the center) force to separate heavier materials from lighter ones.

centrosome—That area of cell cytoplasm that contains two centrioles; important in reproduction of the cell.

cerebellum—The section of the brain that is dorsal to the pons and medulla oblongata; maintains balance and equilibrium.

cerebral vascular accident—Also called a *stroke* or *apoplexy*; an interrupted supply of blood to the brain, caused by formation of a clot, blockage of an artery, or rupture of a blood vessel.

cerebrospinal fluid—Watery, clear fluid that surrounds the brain and spinal cord.

cerebrum—Largest section of brain; involved in sensory interpretation and voluntary muscle activity.

certification—The issuing of a statement or certificate by a professional organization to a person who has met the requirements of education and/or experience and who meets the standards set by the organization.

cervical—Pertaining to the neck portion of the spinal column or to the lower part of the uterus.

cervix—Anatomical part of a tooth where the crown joins with the root; entrance or lower part of the uterus.

chain of infection—Factors that lead to the transmission or spread of disease.

character—The quality of respirations (e.g., deep, shallow, or labored).

charge slip—A record on which charges or costs for services are listed.

check—A written order for payment of money through a bank.

chemical—The method of aseptic control in which substances or solutions are used to disinfect articles; does not kill spores and viruses.

chemical abuse—Use of chemical substances without regard for accepted practice; dependence on alcohol or drugs.

chemotherapy—Treatment of a disease by way of chemical agents.

Cheyne-Stokes respirations—Periods of difficult breathing (dyspnea) followed by periods of no respirations (apnea).

chiropractic—System of treatment based on manipulation of the spinal column and other body structures.

cholelithiasis—Condition of stones in the gallbladder.

choroid—Middle or vascular layer of the eye, between the sclera and retina.

chromatin network—That structure in the nucleus of a cell that contains chromosomes with genes, which carry inherited characteristics.

chronic—Lasting a long period of time; reoccurring.

cilia—Hairlike projections.

citizenship—Status of being a citizen (including associated duties, rights, and privileges).

clavicle—Collarbone.

clean—Free from organisms causing disease.

clear-liquid diet—Diet containing only water-based liquids; nutritionally inadequate.

clinic—Institution that provides care for outpatients; a group of specialists working in cooperation.

Clinitest—Reagent tablet containing chemicals that react with glucose; used to detect glucose (sugar) in the urine.

closed bed—Bed that is made following the discharge of a patient.

coccyx—The tailbone; lowest bones of the vertebral column.

cochlea—Snail-shaped section of the inner ear; contains the organ of Corti, for hearing.

cold-mist inhalation—Treatment providing cool, moist air to relieve respiratory congestion and inflammation.

collection—To receive; a letter requesting payment on an account.

colon—The large intestine.

colostomy—An artificial opening into the colon; allows for the evacuation of feces.

communicable disease—Disease that is transmitted from one individual to another.

communication—Process of transmission; exchange of thoughts or information.

compensation—Something given or received as an equivalent for a loss, service, or debt; defense mechanism involving substitution of one goal for another goal to achieve success.

competent—Able, capable.

complete bed bath—A bath in which all parts of a patient's body are bathed while the patient is confined to bed.

complimentary close—Courtesy closing of a letter (e.g., *Sincerely*).

composite—The dental restoration or filling material used most frequently on anterior teeth.

compress—A folded wet or dry cloth applied firmly to a body part.

computer-assisted instruction (CAI)—Teaching method in which a computer and computer programs are used to control the learning process and deliver the instructional material to the learner.

computerized tomography (CT)—A scanning and detection system that uses a minicomputer and display screen to visualize an internal portion of the human body; formerly known as *CAT (computerized axial tomography)*.

concave—Curved inward; depressed.

confidential—Not to be shared or told; to be held in confidence, or kept to oneself.

congenital—Present at birth (as in a congenital defect).

conjunctiva—Mucous membrane that lines the eyelids and covers the anterior part of the sclera of the eye.

connective tissue—Body tissue that connects, supports, or binds body organs.

constipation—Difficulty in emptying the bowel; infrequent bowel movements.

constrict—To contract or narrow; to make smaller.

consultation—Process of seeking information or advice from another person.

contamination—Containing infection or infectious organisms or germs.

contra angle—Attachment used on dental handpieces to cut and polish.

contract—To shorten, decrease in size, or draw together; an agreement between two or more persons.

contracture—Tightening or shortening of a muscle.

conventional-speed handpiece—Low-speed handpiece in dental units; used to remove caries and for fine-finishing work.

convex—Curved outward; projected.

convulsion—Also called a *seizure;* a violent, involuntary contraction of muscles.

cornea—The transparent section of the sclera; allows light rays to enter the eye.

cortex—The outer layer of an organ or structure.

cost containment—Procedures used to control costs or expenses.

Cowper's glands—The pair of small mucous glands near the male urethra.

cranial—Pertaining to the skull or cranium.

cranium—Part of the skull; the eight bones of the head that enclose the brain.

criticism—Judgment regarding worth; censure, disapproval; evaluation.

cross index/reference—A paper or card used in filing systems to prevent misplacment or loss of records.

cross-match—A blood test that checks the compatibility of the donor's blood and the recipient's blood before a transfusion.

crown—The anatomical portion of a tooth that is exposed in the oral cavity, above the gingiva, or gums.

crust—A scab; outer covering or coat.

crutches—Artificial supports that assist a patient in walking.

culture—Values, beliefs, ideas, customs, and characteristics passed from one generation to the next.

culture specimen—A sample of microorganisms or tissue cells taken from an area of the body for examination.

cuspid—Also called a *canine* or *eyetooth*; the type of tooth located at angle the side of lips and used to tear food.

custom tray—Dental impression tray specially made to fit a particular patient's mouth.

cyanosis—Bluish color of the skin, nailbeds, and/or lips due to an insufficient amount of oxygen in the blood.

cystitis—Inflammation of the urinary bladder.

cystoscope—Instrument for examining the inside of the urinary bladder.

cytoplasm—The fluid inside a cell; contains water, proteins, lipids, carbohydrates, minerals, and salts.

dangling—Positioning the patient in a sitting position with his or her feet and legs over the side of the bed prior to ambulation.

day sheet—A daily record listing all financial transactions and/or patients seen.

daydreaming—Defense mechanism of escape; dreamlike musing while awake.

deciduous teeth—Also called *primary teeth*; the first set of twenty teeth.

decubitus ulcer—A pressure sore; a bedsore.

deduction—Something subtracted or taken out (e.g., monies taken out of a paycheck for various purposes).

defamation—Slander or libel; a false statement that causes ridicule or damage to a reputation.

defecation—Evacuation of fecal material from the bowel; a bowel movement.

defense mechanism—Physical or psychological reaction of an organism used in self defense or to protect self-image.

dehydration—Insufficient amounts of fluid in the tissues.

dementia—Loss of mental ability characterized by decrease in intellectual ability, loss of memory, impaired judgment, and disorientation.

denial—Declaring untrue; refusing to believe.

dental chair—Special chair designed to position a patient comfortably while providing easy access to the patient's oral cavity.

dental hygienist—A licensed individual who works with a dentist to provide care and treatment for the teeth and gums.

dental light—Light used in dental units to illuminate the oral cavity.

dentin—Tissue that makes up the main bulk of a tooth.

dentist—A doctor who specializes in diagnosis, prevention, and treatment of diseases of the teeth and gums.

dentition—The number, type, and arrangement of teeth in the mouth.

denture—An entire set of teeth; usually refers to artificial teeth designed to replace natural teeth.

dependable—Capable of being relied on; trustworthy.

deposit slip—A bank record listing all cash and checks that are to be placed in an account, either checking or savings.

depression—Psychological condition of sadness, melancholy, gloom, or despair.

dermis—The skin.

diabetes mellitus—Metabolic disease caused by an insufficient secretion or utilization of insulin and leading to an increased amount of glucose (sugar) in the blood and urine.

diabetic coma—An unconscious condition caused by an increased level of glucose (sugar) and ketones in the bloodstream of a person with diabetes mellitus.

diagnosis—Determination of the nature of a person's disease.

dialysis—Removal of urine substances from the blood by way of passing solutes through a membrane.

diaphoresis—Profuse or excessive perspiration, or sweating.

diaphysis—The shaft, or middle section, of a long bone.

diarrhea—Frequent bowel movements with watery stool.

diastole—Period of relaxation of the heart.

diastolic pressure—Measurement of blood pressure taken when the heart is at rest; measurement of the constant pressure in arteries.

diencephalon—The section of the brain between the cerebrum and midbrain; contains the thalamus and hypothalamus.

dietitian—An individual who specializes in the science of diet and nutrition.

differential count—Blood test that determines the percentage of each kind of leukocyte (white blood cell).

digestion—Physical and chemical breakdown of food by the body in preparation for absorption.

digital—Pertaining to fingers or toes; examination with the fingers.

dilate—Enlarge or expand; to make bigger.

direct smear—A culture specimen placed on a slide for microscopic examination.

disability—A physical or mental handicap that interferes with normal function; incapacitated, incapable.

disease—Any condition that interferes with the normal function of the body.

disinfection—Aseptic-control method that destroys pathogens but does not usually kill spores and viruses.

dislocation—Displacement of a bone at a joint.

disorientation—Confusion with regard to the identity of time, place, or person.

displacement—Defense mechanism in which feelings about one person are transferred to someone else.

distal—Most distant or farthest from the trunk; center or midline.

distal surface—Side surface of teeth that is toward the back of the mouth, or away from the midline of the mouth.

diuretics—Drugs that increase urinary output; "water pills."

doctorate—Degree awarded by a college or university after completion of a prescribed course of study beyond a bachelor's or master's degree.

dorsal—Pertaining to the back; in back of.

dorsal recumbent position—The patient lies on the back with the knees flexed and separated; used for vaginal and pelvic examinations.

douche—*See* **vaginal irrigation.**

dressing—Covering placed over a wound or injured part.

dry cold—Application that provides cold temperature but is dry against the skin.

dry heat—Application that provides warm temperature but is dry against the skin.

duodenum—First part of the small intestine; connects the pylorus of the stomach and the jejunum.

dyspepsia—Difficulty in digesting food; indigestion.

dysphagia—Difficulty in swallowing.

dyspnea—Difficult or labored breathing.

dystrophy—Progressive weakening (atrophy) of a body part, such as a muscle.

dysuria—Difficult or painful urination.

early adulthood—Period of development from 20 to 40 years of age.

early childhood—Period of development from 1 to 6 years of age.

echocardiography—A diagnostic test that uses ultra-high-frequency sound waves to evaluate the structure and function of the heart.

edema—Swelling; excess amount of fluid in the tissues.

ejaculation—Expulsion of seminal fluid from the male urethra.

ejaculatory duct—In the male, duct or tube from the seminal vesicle to the urethra.

electrocardiogram (EKG or ECG)—Graphic tracing of the electrical activity of the heart.

electroencephalogram (EEG)—Graphic recording of the brain waves or electrical activity in the brain.

emblem—A symbol; identifying badge, design, or device.

embolus—A blood clot or mass of material circulating in the blood vessels.

embryo—Unborn infant during the first 3 months of development.

emesis—Vomiting; expulsion of the contents of the stomach and/or intestine through the mouth and/or nose.

emotional—Pertaining to feelings or psychological states.

empathy—Identifying with another's feelings but being unable to change or solve the situation.

enamel—Hardest tissue in the body; covers the outside of the crown of a tooth.

endocardium—Serous membrane lining of the heart.

endocrine—Ductless gland that produces an internal secretion discharged into the blood or lymph.

endodontics—Branch of dentistry involving treatment of the pulp chamber and root canals of the teeth; root canal treatment.

endometrium—Mucous membrane lining of the inner surface of the uterus.

endoplasmic reticulm—Fine network of tubular structures in the cytoplasm of a cell; allows for the transport of materials in and out of the nucleus and aids in the synthesis and storage of protein.

endorsement—A written signature on the back of a check; required in order to receive payment.

endoscope—An instrument used to examine the inside of the body.

endosteum—Membrane lining the medullary canal of a bone.

enema—An injection of fluid into the large intestine through the rectum.

enthusiasm—Intense interest or excitement.

entrepreneur—Individual who organizes, manages, and assumes the risk of a business.

enunciate—To speak clearly, using correct pronunciation.

enzyme—A chemical substance that causes or increases the rate of a chemical reaction.

epidermis—The outer layer of the skin.

epididymus—Tightly coiled tube in the scrotal sac; connects the testes with the vas or ductus deferens.

epigastric—Pertaining to the area of the abdomen above the stomach.

epiglottis—Leaf-shaped structure that closes over the larynx during swallowing.

epilepsy—A chronic disease of the nervous system characterized by motor and sensory dysfunction, sometimes accompanied by convulsions and unconsciousness.

epiphysis—The end or head at the extremity of a long bone.

epistaxis—Nosebleed.

epithelial tissue—Tissue that forms the skin and parts of the secreting glands, and that lines the body cavities.

erythema—Redness of the skin.

erythrocyte—Red blood cell (RBC).

erythrocyte count—Blood test that counts the number of red blood cells (normally 4 to 6 million per cubic millimeter of blood).

erythrocyte sedimentation rate (ESR)—Blood test that determines the rate at which red blood cells settle out of the blood.

esophagus—Tube that extends from the pharynx to the stomach.

essential nutrients—Those elements in food required by the body for proper function.

esteem—Place a high value on; respect.

ethics—Principles of right or good conduct.

etiology—The study of the cause of a disease.

eustachian tube—Tube that connects the middle ear and the pharynx, or throat.

eversion—Turning a body part outward.

exocrine—Gland with a duct that produces a secretion.

expectorate—To spit; to expel mucus, phlegm, or sputum from the throat or respiratory passages.

expiration—The expulsion of air from the lungs; breathing out air.

extension—Increasing the angle between two parts; straightening a limb.

external auditory canal—Passageway or tube extending from the auricle of the ear to the tympanic membrane.

facial surface—The tooth surface nearest the lips or cheek; includes the labial and buccal surfaces.

fainting—Partial or complete loss of consciousness caused by a temporary reduction in the supply of blood to the brain.

fallopian tubes—Oviducts; in the female, passageway for the ova (egg) from the ovary to uterus.

false imprisonment—Restraining an individual or restricting an individual's freedom.

fanfold—Folding in accordian pleats; done with bed linens.

fascia—Fibrous membrane covering, supporting, and separating muscles.

fasting blood sugar (FBS)—Blood test that measures blood serum levels of glucose (sugar) after a person has had nothing by mouth for a period of time.

fat—Also called a *lipid*; nutrient that provides the most concentrated form of energy; highest-calorie energy nutrient; overweight.

fat-restricted diet—Diet with limited amounts of fats, or lipids.

febrile—Pertaining to a fever, or elevated body temperature.

feces—Also called *stool*; waste material discharged from the bowel.

femur—Thigh bone of the leg; the longest and strongest bone in the body.

fertilization—Conception; impregnation of the ovum by the sperm.

fetus—Unborn infant from the end of the third month of pregnancy until birth.

fever—Elevated body temperature, usually above 101°F, or 38.3°C, rectally.

fibula—Outer and smaller bone of the lower leg.

filing—Arranging in order.

fire extinguisher—A device that can be used to put out fires.

first aid—Immediate care given to a victim of an injury or illness to minimize the effects of the injury or illness.

fixed expenses—Those items in a budget that are set and usually do not change (e.g., rent and car payments).

flatus—Air or gas in the intestines.

flexion—Decreasing the angle between two parts; bending a limb.

foramina—A passage or opening; a hole in a bone through which blood vessels or nerves pass.

Fowler's position—The patient lies on the back with the head elevated at one of several different angles.

fracture—A break (usually, a break in a bone or tooth).

frontal plane—Imaginary line that separates the body into a front section and a back section.

frostbite—Actual freezing of tissue fluid resulting in damage to the skin and underlying tissue.

full liquid diet—Diet consisting of liquids and foods that are liquid at body temperature.

fungi—Group of simple, plantlike animals that live on dead organic matter (e.g., yeast and molds).

gait—Method or manner of walking.

gallbladder—Small sac near the liver; concentrates and stores bile.

gastric—Pertaining to the stomach.

generic name—Chemical name of a drug; name not protected by a trademark.

genital—Pertaining to the organs of reproduction.

geriatrics, gerontology—The study of the aged or old age and treatment of related diseases and conditions.

gingiva—The gums (tissues surrounding the teeth).

glaucoma—Eye disease characterized by increased intraocular pressure.

glomerulus—Microscopic cluster of capillaries in Bowman's capsule of the nephron in the kidney.

glucometer—Instrument used to measure blood-glucose (blood-sugar) level.

glucose—The most common type of sugar in the body.

glycosuria—Presence of sugar in the urine.

Golgi apparatus—That structure in the cytoplasm of a cell that produces, stores, and packages secretions for discharge from the cell.

gonads—Sex glands, ovaries in the female and testes in the male.

Gram's stain—Technique of staining organisms to identify specific types of bacteria present.

graphic chart—Record used to record vital signs (e.g., temperature, pulse, and respirations) and other information.

groin—Area between the abdomen and upper inner thigh.

gross income—Amount of pay earned before deductions are taken out.

gynecology—The study of diseases of women, especially those affecting the reproductive organs.

halitosis—Bad breath.

hard copy—Computer term for a printed copy of information.

hard palate—Bony structure that forms the roof of the mouth.

hardware—Machine or physical components of a computer system (usually, the parts of the computer and the peripherals).

heading—That section of a letter containing the address of the person sending the letter and the date of writing.

heart attack—*See* **myocardial infarction**.

heat cramp—Muscle pain and spasm resulting from exposure to heat and inadequate fluid and salt intake.

heat exhaustion—Condition resulting from exposure to heat and excessive loss of fluid through sweating.

heat stroke—Medical emergency caused by prolonged exposure to heat, resulting in high body temperature and failure of sweat glands.

hemacytometer—Specially calibrated instrument with a measured and lined area for counting blood cells.

hematemesis—Vomiting of blood.

hematocrit—Blood test that measures the percentage of red blood cells per a given unit of blood.

hematology—The study of blood and blood diseases.

hematuria—Blood in the urine.

hemiplegia—Paralysis on one side of the body.

hemoglobin—The iron-containing pigment of the red blood cells; serves to carry oxygen from the lungs to the tissues.

hemolyze—Disintegration of red blood cells, causing cells to dissolve or go into solution.

hemoptysis—Spitting up blood; blood-stained sputum.

hemorrhage—Excessive loss of blood; bleeding.

hemorrhoids—Varicose veins of the anal canal or anus.

hemostat—Instrument used to compress (clamp) blood vessels to stop bleeding.

heparin—A substance formed in the liver to prevent the clotting of blood; an anticoagulant.

hepatitis—Inflammation of the liver.

high-fiber diet—Diet containing large amounts of fiber, or indigestible food.

high-protein diet—Diet containing large amounts of protein-rich foods.

high-velocity evacuator—Dental handpiece used to remove particles and large amounts of liquid from the oral cavity.

home health care—Any type of health care provided in a patient's home environment.

homeostasis—A constant state of natural balance within the body.

honesty—Truthfulness; integrity.

horizontal recumbent position—*See* **supine position**.

hormone—Chemical substance secreted by an organ or gland.

HOSA—Health Occupations Students of America, a national organization for students enrolled in health occupations programs.

hospice—Program designed to provide care for the terminally ill while allowing them to die with dignity.

hospital—Institution that provides medical or surgical care and treatment for the sick or injured.

humerus—Long bone of the upper arm.

hygiene—Principles for health preservation and disease prevention.

hyperglycemia—Presence of sugar in the blood; high blood sugar.

hyperopia—Farsightedness; defect in near vision.

hypertension—High blood pressure.

hyperthermia—Condition that occurs when body temperature exceeds 104°F, or 40°C, rectally.

hypoglycemia—Low blood sugar.

hypotension—Low blood pressure.

hypothalamus—That structure in the diencephalon of brain that regulates and controls many body functions.

hypothermia—Condition in which body temperature is below normal, usually below 95°F (35°C) and often in the range of 78° to 95°F (26° to 35°C).

hypoxia—Without oxygen.

ice bag/collar—Plastic or rubber device filled with ice to provide dry-cold application.

idiopathic—Without recognizable cause; self-originating.

ileostomy—A surgical opening connecting the ileum (small intestine) and the abdominal wall.

ileum—Final section of small intestine; connects the jejunum and large intestine.

immunity—Condition of being protected against a particular disease.

impaction—A large, hard mass of fecal material lodged in the intestine or rectum; a tooth that does not erupt into the mouth.

impression—Negative reproduction of a tooth or dental arch.

incisal surface—The cutting or biting surface of anterior teeth.

incision—Cut or wound of body tissue caused by a sharp object; a surgical cut.

incisors—Teeth located in the front and center of the mouth; used to cut food.

income—Total amount of money received in a given period (usually a year); salary is usually the main source.

incontinent—Unable to voluntarily control urination or defecation.

index—To put names in proper order for filing purposes.

infancy—Period of development from birth to 1 year of age.

infection—Invasion by organisms; contamination by disease-producing organisms, or pathogens.

inferior—Below; under.

inflammation—Tissue reaction to injury characterized by heat, redness, swelling, and pain.

informed consent—Permission granted voluntarily by a person who is of sound mind and aware of all factors involved.

inguinal—Pertaining to the region of body where the thighs join the trunk; the groin.

inhalation—Breathing in.

initiative—Ability to begin or follow through with a plan or task; determination.

input—Computer term for information that is entered into a computer.

inquiry—Search for information.

insertion—End or area of a muscle that moves when the muscle contracts.

inside address—That section of a letter that contains the name and address of the person or firm to whom the letter is being sent.

inspiration—Breathing in; taking air into the lungs.

insulin shock—Condition that occurs in diabetics when there is an excess amount of insulin and a low level of glucose (sugar) in the blood.

insurance form—A form used to apply for payment by an insurance company.

intake and output (I & O)—A record that notes all fluids taken in or eliminated by a person in a given period of time.

integumentary—Pertaining to the skin or a covering.

interactive video—The color, sound, and motion of video technology integrated with computer-assisted instruction to create a new technology.

intercostal—Pertaining to the space between the ribs (costae).

interproximal space—The area between two adjoining teeth.

intestine—That portion of the alimentary canal from the stomach to the rectum and anus.

intradermal—Inserted or put into the skin.

intramuscular—Injected or put into a muscle.

intravenous—Injected or put into a vein.

intubate—To insert a tube.

invasion of privacy—Revealing personal information about an individual without his or her consent.

invasive—Pertains to a test or procedure that involves penetrating or entering the body.

inversion—Turning a body part inward.

involuntary—Independent action not controlled by choice or desire.

iris—Colored portion of the eye; composed of muscular, or contractile, tissue that regulates the size of the pupil.

ischemia—Inadequate blood flow to the body tissues caused by an obstruction in circulation.

isolation—Method or technique of caring for persons who have communicable diseases.

jackknife position—The patient lies on the abdomen with both the head and legs inclined downward and the rectal area elevated.

jaundice—Yellow discoloration of the skin and eyes, frequently caused by liver or gallbladder disease.

jejunum—The middle section of the small intestine; connects the duodenum and ileum.

job interview—A face-to-face meeting or conversation between an employer and an applicant for a job.

joint—An articulation, or area where two bones meet or join.

kcal-controlled diet—Diet containing low-calorie foods; frequently prescribed for weight loss.

kidney—Bean-shaped organ that excretes urine; located high and in back of the abdominal cavity.

kilocalorie—Unit used to measure the energy value of food.

kilojoule—Metric unit used to measure the energy value of food.

knee-chest position—The patient rests his or her body weight on the knees and chest; used for sigmoidoscopic and rectal examinations.

labia majora—Two large folds of adipose tissue lying on each side of the vulva in the female; hairy outer lips.

labia minora—Two folds of membrane lying inside the labia majora; inner hairless lips.

labial surface—Crown surface of the anterior teeth that lies next to the lips; facial surface of the anterior teeth.

laboratory—A room or building where scientific tests, research, experiments, or learning takes place.

laceration—Wound or injury with jagged, irregular edges.

lacrimal—Pertaining to tears; glands that secrete and expel tears.

lactation—Process of secreting milk.

lancet—Sharp, pointed instrument used to pierce the skin to obtain blood.

laryngeal mirror—Instrument with a mirror, used to examine larynx.

larynx—Voice box, located between the pharynx and trachea.

late adulthood—Period of development beginning at 65 years of age and ending at death.

late childhood—Period of development from 6 to 12 years of age.

lateral—Pertaining to the side.

lead—An angle or view of the heart that is recorded in an electrocardiogram.

leadership—Ability to lead, guide, and direct others.

ledger card—A card or record that shows a financial account of money charged, received, or paid out.

left lateral position—*See* Sims's position.

legal—Authorized or based on law.

legal disability—A condition in which a person does not have legal capacity and is therefore unable to enter into a legal agreement (e.g., as is the case with a minor).

lens—Crystalline structure suspended behind the pupil of the eye; refracts or bends light rays onto the retina; also, the magnifying glass in a microscope.

lethargy—Abnormal drowsiness or sluggishness; state of indifference or stupor.

letterhead—Preprinted heading at the top of paper used for written correspondence.

leukocyte—White blood cell (WBC).

leukocyte count—Blood test that counts the total number of white blood cells (normally 5,000 to 10,000 cells per cubic millimeter of blood).

libel—False written statement that causes a person ridicule or contempt or causes damage to the person's reputation.

licensure—Process by which a government agency authorizes individuals to work in a given occupation.

life stages—Stages of growth and development experienced by an individual from birth to death.

ligament—Fibrous tissue that connects bone to bone.

light diet—Also called a *convalescent diet;* diet that contains easy-to-digest foods.

line angle—Area on crown surfaces of a tooth formed by a line drawn between two surfaces.

liner—Dental material that covers or lines exposed tooth tissue, usually in the form of a varnish.

lingual surface—The crown surface of teeth that is next to the tongue.

listen—To pay attention, make an effort to hear.

lithotomy position—The patient lies on the back with the feet in stirrups and knees flexed and separated.

liver—Largest gland in the body; located in the upper right quadrant of the abdomen; two of its main functions are excreting bile and storing glycogen.

living will—A legal document stating whether a person desires on what measures should or should not be taken to prolong life when his or her condition is terminal.

low-cholesterol diet—Diet that restricts foods high in saturated fat.

low-protein diet—Diet that limits foods high in protein.

low-residue diet—Diet that limits foods containing large amounts of residue, or indigestibles.

lung—Organ of respiration located in the thoracic cavity.

lymph—Fluid formed in body tissues and circulated in the lymphatic vessels.

lymph node—A round body of lymph tissue that filters lymph.

lymphatic duct—Short tube that drains purified lymph from the right sides of the head and neck and the right arm.

lymphatic vessels—Thin-walled vessels that carry lymph from tissues.

lysosomes—Those structures in the cytoplasm of a cell that contain digestive enzymes to digest and destroy old cells, bacteria, and foreign matter.

macule—A discolored but neither raised nor depressed spot or area on the skin.

magnetic resonance imaging (MRI)—Process that uses a computer and magnetic forces, instead of X rays, to visualize internal organs.

mainframe computer—Largest type of computer; many users can access this computer at the same time.

malignant—Harmful or dangerous; likely to spread and cause destruction and death (e.g., as can be the case with cancer).

malnutrition—Poor nutrition; without adequate food and nutrients.

malpractice—Providing improper or unprofessional treatment or care that results in injury to another person.

mammogram—X-ray examination of the breasts.

mandible—Horseshoe-shaped bone that forms the lower jaw; only movable bone of the skull.

master's degree—Degree awarded by a college or university after completion of 1 or more years of prescribed study beyond a bachelor's degree.

mastication—The process of chewing with the teeth.

maxilla—Upper jawbone; two bones fused or joined together.

meatus—External opening of a tube (e.g., the urinary meatus).

mechanical lift—Special device used to move or transfer patient.

medial—Pertaining to the middle or midline.

Medicaid—Government program that provides medical care for people whose incomes are below a certain level.

medical history—A record that shows all diseases, illness, and surgeries that a patient has had.

medical record—Also called a *patient chart;* written record of a patient's diagnosis, care, treatment, test results, and prognosis.

Medicare—Government program that provides medical care for elderly and/or disabled individuals.

medication—Drug used to treat a disease or condition.

medulla—Inner, or central, portion of an organ.

medulla oblongata—The lower part of the brain stem; controls vital processes such as respiration and heartbeat.

medullary canal—Inner, or central, portion of a long bone.

meiosis—The process of cell division that occurs in gametes, or sex cells (ovum and spermatozoa).

melanin—Brownish-black pigment found in the skin, hair, and eyes.

memorandum—A short, written statement or message.

meninge—Membrane that covers the brain and spinal cord.

menopause—Permanent cessation of menstruation.

mental—Pertaining to the mind.

mesial surface—The side surface of teeth that is toward the midline of the mouth.

metabolism—The use of food nutrients by the body to produce energy.

metacarpal—Bone of the hand between the wrist and each finger.

metastasis—The spread of tumor or cancer cells from the site of origin.

metatarsal—Bone of the foot between the instep and each toe.

microcomputer—Desktop or personal computer found in the home or office.

microorganism—Small, living plant or animal not visible to the naked eye.

microscope—Instrument used to magnify or enlarge objects for viewing.

micturate—Another word for *urinate;* to expel urine.

midbrain—That portion of the brain that connects the pons and cerebellum; relay center for impulses.

middle adulthood—Period of development from 40 to 65 years of age.

midsagittal—An imaginary line drawn down the midline of the body to divide the body into a right side and a left side.

midstream specimen—Urine specimen in which urination is begun before catching the specimen in the specimen cup.

minerals—Inorganic substances essential to life.

mitered corner—Special folding technique used to secure linen on a bed.

mitochondria—Those structures in a cell that provide energy and are involved in the metabolism of the cell.

mitosis—Process of asexual reproduction by which cells divide into two identical cells.

mitral valve—Flap or cusp between the left atrium and left ventricle in the heart.

model—Also called a *cast*; a positive reproduction of the dental arches or teeth in plaster or similar materials.

modified block—Letter-writing format in which all parts of the letter start at the left margin except the heading, complimentary close, signature, and title, which start at the center line.

moist cold—An application that provides cold temperature and is wet against the skin.

moist heat—An application that provides warm temperature and is wet against the skin.

molars—Teeth in the back of the mouth; largest and strongest teeth; used to grind food.

motivated—Stimulated into action; incentive to act.

mouth—Oral cavity; opening to the digestive tract, or alimentary canal.

muscle tissue—Body tissue composed of fibers that produce movement.

muscle tone—State of partial muscle contraction providing a state of readiness to act.

myocardial infarction—Heart attack; a reduction in the supply of blood to the heart resulting in damage to the muscle of the heart.

myocardium—Muscle layer of the heart.

myopia—Nearsightedness; defect in distant vision.

myth—A false belief; an established belief with no basis.

nasal cavity—Space between the cranium and the roof of the mouth.

nasal septum—Bony and cartilaginous partition that separates the nasal cavity into two sections.

nasogastric tube—A tube that is inserted through the nose and goes down the esophagus and into the stomach.

nausea—A feeling of discomfort in the region of the stomach accompanied by the tendency to vomit.

necrosis—Death of tissue.

need—Lack of something required or desired; urgent want or desire.

needle holder—Instrument used to hold or support a needle while sutures (stitches) are being inserted.

negligence—Failure to give care that is normally expected, resulting in injury to another person.

neonate—Newborn infant.

neoplasm—New growth or tumor.

nephron—Structural and functional unit of the kidney.

nerve—Group of nerve tissues that conducts impulses.

nerve tissue—Body tissue that conducts or transmits impulses throughout the body.

net income—Amount of pay received for hours worked after all deductions have been taken out; take-home pay.

neurology—The study of the nervous system.

neuron—Nerve cell.

nocturia—Excessive urination at night.

noninvasive—Pertaining to a test or procedure that does not require penetration or entrance into the body.

nonpathogen—A microorganism that is not capable of causing a disease.

nonverbal—Without words or speech.

nose—The projection in the center of the face; the organ for smelling and breathing.

nosocomial—Pertaining to or originating in a health care facility such as a hospital.

nucleolus—The spherical body in the nucleus of a cell that is important in reproduction of the cell.

nucleus—The structure in a cell that controls cell activities such as growth, metabolism, and reproduction.

nutrition—All body processes related to food; the body's use of food for growth, development, and health.

nutritional status—The state of one's nutrition.

observation—To look at, watch, perceive, or notice.

obstetrics—The branch of medicine dealing with pregnancy and childbirth.

occlusal surface—The chewing or biting surface of posterior teeth.

occult—Hidden, concealed, not visible (e.g., an internal [occult] hemorrhage).

occult blood—Blood that is hidden; also, a test done on stool to check for the presence of blood.

occupational therapy—Treatment directed at preparing a person requiring rehabilitation for a trade or for return to the activities of daily living.

occupied bed—A bed that is made while the patient is in bed.

olfactory—Pertaining to the sense of smell.

oliguria—Decreased or less-than-normal amounts of urine secretion.

ombudsman—Specially trained individual who acts as an advocate for others to improve care or conditions.

Omnibus Budget Reconciliation Act (OBRA)—Federal law that regulates the education and testing of nursing assistants.

oncology—The branch of medicine dealing with tumors or abnormal growths (e.g., cancer).

open bed—A bed with the top sheets fanfolded to the bottom.

ophthalmologist—A medical doctor who specializes in diseases of the eye.

ophthalmology—The study of the eye and diseases and disorders affecting the eye.

ophthalmoscope—An instrument used to examine the eye.

optician—An individual who makes or sells lenses, eyeglasses, and other optical supplies.

optometrist—A licensed, nonmedical practitioner who specializes in the diagnosis and treatment of vision defects.

oral cavity—The mouth.

oral hygiene—Care of the mouth and teeth.

oral-evacuation system—Special machine that uses water to form a suction or vacuum system to remove liquids and particles from the oral cavity.

organ—Body part made of tissues that have joined together to perform a special function.

organ of Corti—Structure in the cochlea of the ear; organ of hearing.

organelles—Structures in the cytoplasm of a cell, including the nucleus, mitochondria, ribosomes, lysosomes, and Golgi apparatus.

origin—End or area of a muscle that remains stationary when the muscle contracts.

originator—The person who writes a check to issue payment.

orthodontics—The branch of dentistry dealing with prevention and correction of irregularities of the alignment of teeth.

orthopedics—The branch of medicine/surgery dealing with the treatment of diseases and deformities of the bones, muscles, and joints.

orthotist—An individual skilled in straightening or correcting deformities by the use of orthopedic appliances (e.g., brace or special splints).

os coxae—The hipbone; formed by the union of the ilium, ischium, and pubis.

ossicles—Small bones, especially the three bones of the middle ear that amplify and transmit sound waves.

osteopathy—A field of medicine and treatment based on manipulation, especially of the bones, to treat disease.

osteoporosis—Condition in which bones become porous and brittle because of lack or loss of calcium, phosphorus, and other minerals.

ostomy—A surgically created opening into a body part.

otoscope—An instrument used to examine the ear.

output—Computer term for processed information, or the final product obtained from the computer; also, total amount of liquid expelled from the body.

ovary—Endocrine gland or gonad that produces hormones and the female sex cell, or ovum.

palate—Structure that separates the oral and nasal cavities; roof of the mouth.

pallor—Paleness; lack of color.

palpation—The act of using the hands to feel body parts during an examination.

pancreas—Gland that is dorsal to the stomach and that secretes insulin and digestive juices.

panoramic—Dental X ray that shows the entire dental arch, or all of the teeth and related structures, on one film.

Papanicolaou test—Also called a *pap test*; a test to classify abnormal cells obtained from the vagina or cervix.

papule—Solid, elevated spot or area on the skin.

paralysis—Loss or impairment of the ability to feel or move parts of the body.

paraplegia—Paralysis of the lower half of the body.

parasite—Organism that lives on or within another living organism.

parasympathetic—A division of the autonomic nervous system.

parathyroid—One of four small glands located on the thyroid gland; regulates calcium and phosphorus metabolism.

parenteral—Other than by mouth.

partial bath—Bath in which only certain body parts are bathed or in which the health care provider bathes those parts of the body that the patient is unable to bathe.

patella—The kneecap.

pathogen—Disease-producing organisms.

pathology—The study of the cause or nature of a disease.

patience—Ability to wait, persevere; capacity for calm endurance.

patients' rights—Factors of care that all patients can expect to receive.

patriotism—Love and devotion to one's country.

payee—Person receiving payment.

pediatrics—The branch of medicine dealing with care and treatment of diseases and disorders of children.

pedodontics—The branch of dentistry dealing with treatment of teeth and oral conditions of children.

pegboard system—Method of maintaining financial accounts and records in an office.

pelvic—Pertaining to the pelvis area below the abdominal region and near the sacrum and hip bones.

penis—External sex organ of the male.

percussion—Process of tapping various body parts during an examination.

percussion hammer—Instrument used to check reflexes.

periapical—Around the apex of a root of a tooth; dental X ray that shows the entire tooth and surrounding area.

pericardium—Membrane sac that covers the outside of the heart.

perineum—Region between the vagina and anus in the female and between the scrotum and anus in the male.

periodontics—The branch of dentistry dealing with the treatment of the gingiva (gum) and periodontium (supporting tissues) surrounding the teeth.

periodontium—Structures that surround and support the teeth.

periosteum—Fibrous membrane that covers the bones except at joint areas.

peripheral—That part of the nervous system apart from the brain and spinal cord; also, a device connected to a computer.

peristalsis—Rhythmic, wavelike motion of involuntary muscles.

peritoneal—Pertaining to the body cavity containing the liver, stomach, intestines, urinary bladder, and internal reproductive organs.

permanent teeth—*See* **secondary teeth**.

personal hygiene—Care of the body including bathing, hair and nail care, shaving, and oral hygiene.

perspiration—The secretion of sweat.

pH—A scale of 0 to 14 used to measure the degree of acidity or alkalinity of a substance, with 7 being neutral.

phalanges—Bones of the fingers and toes.

pharmacology—The study of drugs.

pharynx—The throat.

phlebitis—Inflammation of a vein.

phlebotomist—Also called a *venipuncture technician;* individual who collects blood and prepares it for tests.

physical—Of or pertaining to the body.

physical therapy—Treatment by physical means, such as heat, cold, water, massage, or electricity.

Physicians' Desk Reference **(PDR)**—Reference book that contains essential information on medications.

physiological needs—Basic physical or biological needs required by every human being to sustain life.

physiology—The study of the processes or functions of living organisms.

pineal—Glandlike structure in the brain.

pinna—Also called the *auricle;* external portion of the ear.

pituitary—Small, rounded endocrine gland at the base of the brain; regulates function of other endocrine glands and body processes.

placenta—Temporary endocrine gland created during pregnancy to provide nourishment for the fetus; the afterbirth.

plane—Flat or relatively smooth surface; an imaginary line drawn through the body at various parts to separate the body into sections.

plaque—Thin, tenacious, filmlike deposit that adheres (sticks) to the teeth and can lead to decay; made of protein and microorganisms.

plasma—Liquid portion of the blood.

platelet—*See* **thrombocyte**.

pleura—A serous membrane that covers the lungs and lines the thoracic cavity.

podiatrist—An individual who specializes in the diagnosis and treatment of diseases and disorders of the feet.

point angle—Area on the crown surface of a tooth that is formed when three surfaces meet.

poisoning—Condition that occurs when contact is made with any chemical substance that causes injury, illness, or death.

polycythemia—Excess number of red blood cells.

polydipsia—Excessive thirst.

polyuria—Increased production and discharge of urine; excessive urination.

pons—That portion of the brain stem that connects the medulla oblongata and cerebellum to the upper portions of the brain.

positron emission tomography (PET)—Computerized body scanning technique in which the computer detects a radioactive substance injected into a patient.

posterior—Toward the back; behind.

posterior teeth—Teeth toward the back of the oral cavity, including the bicuspids and molars.

postmortem care—Care given to the body immediately after death.

postoperative—After surgery.

postpartum—Following delivery of a baby.

Power of Attorney (POA)—A legal document authorizing a person to act as another person's legal representative or agent.

prefix—An affix attached to the beginning of a word.

preoperative—Before surgery.

primary teeth—*See* **deciduous teeth**.

privileged communications—All personal information given to health personnel by a patient; must be kept confidential.

proctoscope—Instrument used to examine the rectum.

prognosis—Prediction regarding the probable outcome of a disease.

projection—Defense mechanism in which an individual places the blame for his or her actions on someone else or circumstances.

pronation—Turning a body part downward; turning "palm down."

prone position—The patient lies on the abdomen, with the legs together and the face turned to the side.

prophylactic—Preventative; agent that prevents disease.

prophylaxis angle—Dental handpiece attachment that holds polishing cups, disks, and brushes used to clean the teeth or polish restorations.

prostate gland—In the male, gland near the urethra; contracts during ejaculation to prevent urine from leaving the bladder.

prosthesis—An artificial part that replaces a natural part (e.g., dentures or a limb).

prosthodontics—The branch of dentistry dealing with the construction of artificial appliances for the mouth.

protective isolation—*See* **reverse isolation**.

protein—One of six essential nutrients needed for growth and repair of tissues.

protoplasm—Thick, viscous substance that is the physical basis of all living things.

protozoa—Microscopic, one-celled animals often found in decayed materials and contaminated water.

proximal—Closest to the point of attachment or area of reference.

pruritus—Itching.

psychiatry—The branch of medicine dealing with the diagnosis, treatment, and prevention of mental illness.

psychology—The study of mental processes and their effects on behavior.

psychosomatic—Pertaining to the relationship between the mind or emotions and the body.

puberty—Period of growth and development during which secondary sexual characteristics begin to develop.

pulmonary—Pertaining to the lungs.

pulmonary valve—Flap or cusp between the right ventricle of the heart and the pulmonary artery.

pulp—Soft tissue in the innermost area of a tooth and made of nerves and blood vessels held in place by connective tissue.

pulse—Pressure of the blood felt against the wall of an artery as the heart contracts or beats.

pulse deficit—The difference between the rate of an apical pulse and the rate of a radial pulse.

puncture wound—Injury caused by a pointed object such as a needle or nail.

pupil—Opening or hole in the center of the iris of the eye; allows light to enter the eye.

pustule—Small, elevated, pus- or lymph-filled area of the skin.

pyrexia—Fever.

pyuria—Pus in the urine.

quadriplegia—Paralysis below the neck; paralysis of arms and legs.

radial deviation—Moving toward the thumb side of the hand.

radiology—The branch of medicine dealing with X rays and radioactive substances.

radiolucent—Transparent to X rays; permitting the passage of X rays or other forms of radiation.

radiopaque—Not transparent to X rays; not permitting the passage of X rays or other forms of radiation.

radius—Long bone of the forearm, between the wrist and elbow.

rale—Bubbling or noisy sound caused by fluid or mucus in the air passages.

random access memory (RAM)—Form of computer memory known as read/write memory because data can be stored or retrieved from it.

range of motion (ROM)—The full range of movement of a muscle or joint; exercises designed to move each joint and muscle through its full range of movement.

rate—Number per minute, as with pulse and respiration counts.

rationalization—Defense mechanism involving the use of a reasonable or acceptable excuse as explanation for behavior.

read only memory (ROM)—Nonerasable, permanent form of computer memory built into a computer to control many of the computer's internal operations.

reagent strip—Special test strip containing chemical substances that react to the presence of certain substances in the urine or blood.

reality orientation—Activities to help promote awareness of time, place, and person.

recall—To call back; letter or notice that reminds a patient to return for periodic treatment or examination.

receipt—Written record that money or goods has been received.

rectal, rectum—Pertaining to or the lower part of large intestine, the temporary storage area for indigestibles.

rectal tube—Tube inserted into the rectum to aid in the expulsion of flatus (gas).

red marrow—Soft tissue in the epiphyses of long bones.

reference initials—Initials placed at the bottom of a letter to indicate the writer and/or typist.

refractometer—An instrument used to measure the specific gravity of urine.

registration—Process whereby a regulatory body in a given health care area administers exams and/or maintains a list of qualified personnel.

rehabilitation—The restoration to useful life through therapy and education.

religion—Spiritual beliefs and practices of an individual.

repression—Defense mechanism involving the transfer of painful or unacceptable ideas, feelings, or thoughts into the subconscious.

resistant—Able to oppose; organisms that remain unaffected by harmful substances in the environment.

respiration—The process of taking in oxygen (inspiration) and expelling carbon dioxide (expiration) by way of the lungs and air passages.

responsibility—Being held accountable for actions or behaviors; willing to meet obligations.

restoration—Process of replacing a diseased portion of a tooth or a lost tooth by artificial means, including filling materials, crowns, bridges, or dentures.

restraints—Protective devices that limit or restrict movement.

resumé—A summary of a person's work history and experience, submitted when applying for a job.

retina—The sensory membrane that lines the eye and is the immediate instrument of vision.

retractor—Instrument used to hold or draw back the lips or sides of a wound or incision.

reverse isolation—Technique used to provide care to patients requiring protection from organisms in the environment.

rheostat—Foot control in dental units; used to operate handpieces.

rhythm—Referring to regularity; regular or irregular.

ribs—Also called *costae*; twelve pairs of narrow, curved bones that surround the thoracic cavity.

rickettsiae—Parasitic microorganisms that live on other living organisms.

root—The anatomic portion of a tooth that is below the gingiva (gums); helps hold the tooth in the mouth.

rotation—Movement around a central axis; a turning.

rubber base—Dental impression material that is elastic and rubbery in nature.

safety standards—Set of rules designed to protect both the patient and the health care worker.

saliva ejector—Handpiece in dental units that provides a constant, low-volume suction to remove saliva from the mouth.

salivary glands—Glands of the mouth that produce saliva, a digestive secretion.

salutation—A greeting; the greeting in a letter (e.g., "Dear").

satisfaction—Fulfillment or gratification of a desire or need.

scalpel—Instrument with a knife blade and used to incise (cut) skin and tissue.

scapula—Shoulder blade or bone.

sclera—White outer coat of the eye.

screen—To evaluate; to determine the purpose of telephone calls so they can be referred to the correct person.

scrotum—Double pouch containing the testes and epididymus in the male.

sebaceous gland—Oil-secreting gland of the skin.

secondary teeth—The thirty-two teeth that make up the second, or permanent, set of teeth.

secretion—Substance produced and expelled by a gland or other body part.

self-actualization—Achieving one's full potential.

self-esteem—Satisfaction with oneself.

semicircular canals—Structures of the inner ear that are involved in maintaining balance and equilibrium.

seminal vesicle—One of two saclike structures behind the bladder and connected to the vas deferens in the male; secretes thick, viscous fluid for semen.

senile lentigines—Dark-yellow or brown spots that develop on the skin as aging occurs.

senility—Feebleness of body or mind caused by aging.

sensitive—Susceptible to a substance; organisms that are affected by an antibiotic in a culture and sensitivity study.

septum—Membranous wall that divides two cavities.

serrated—Notched; toothed.

sharps container—A puncture-resistant container for disposal of needles, syringes, and other sharp objects contaminated by blood or body fluids.

shock—Clinical condition characterized by various symptoms and resulting in an inadequate supply of blood and oxygen to body organs, especially the brain and heart.

sigmoidoscope—Instrument used to examine the sigmoid, or S-shaped, section of the large intestine.

sign—Objective evidence of disease; something that is seen.

signature—A person's name written by that person.

Sims's position—The patient lies on his or her left side with the right leg bent up near the abdomen.

sinus—Cavity or air space in a bone.

sitz bath—Special bath given to apply moist heat to the genital or rectal area.

skeleton—The bony structure of the body.

skill—Expertness, dexterity; an art, trade, or technique.

skin puncture—A small puncture made in the skin to obtain capillary blood.

slander—Spoken comment that causes a person ridicule or contempt or damages the person's reputation.

small intestine—That section of the intestine that is between the stomach and large intestine; site of most absorption of nutrients.

smear—Material spread thinly on a slide for microscopic examination.

Snellen charts—Special charts that use letters or symbols in calibrated heights to check for vision defects.

social—Pertaining to relationships with others.

sodium-restricted diet—Special diet containing low or limited amounts of sodium (salt).

soft diet—Special diet containing only foods that are soft in texture.

soft palate—Tissue at the back of the roof of the mouth; separates the mouth from the nasopharynx.

software—Programs or instructions that allow computer hardware to function intelligently.

specific gravity—Weight or mass of a substance compared with an equal amount of another substance that is used as a standard.

speculum—Instrument used to dilate, or enlarge, an opening or passage in the body for examination purposes.

sphygmomanometer—Instrument calibrated for measuring blood pressure in millimeters of mercury (mm Hg).

spinal—Pertaining to the vertebral column or spinal cord.

spinal cord—A column of nervous tissue extending from the medulla oblongata of the brain to the second lumbar vertebra in vertebral column.

spleen—Ductless gland below the diaphragm and in the upper-left quadrant of the abdomen; serves to form, store, and filtrate blood.

sprain—Injury to a joint accompanied by stretching or tearing of the ligaments.

sputum—Substance coughed up from the bronchi; contains saliva and mucus.

statement-receipt—Financial form that shows charges, amounts paid, and balance due.

statistical data—Record containing basic facts about a patient, such as address, place of employment, insurance, and similar items.

sterile—Free of all organisms, including spores and viruses.

sterile field—An area that is set up for certain procedures and is free from all organisms.

sterilization—Process that results in total destruction of all microorganisms; also, surgical procedure that prevents conception of a child.

sternum—Breastbone.

stethoscope—Instrument used for listening to internal body sounds.

stomach—Enlarged section of the alimentary canal, between the esophagus and the small intestine; serves as an organ of digestion.

stool—Material evacuated from the bowels; feces.

strain—Injury caused by excessive stretching, overuse, or misuse of a muscle.

stroke—*See* cerebral vascular accident.

subcutaneous—Beneath the skin.

subcutaneous fascia—Layer of tissue that is under the skin and connects the skin to muscles and underlying tissues.

sublingual—Under the tongue.

sudoriferous gland—Sweat-secreting gland of the skin.

suffix—An affix attached to the end of a word.

suicide—Killing oneself.

superior—Above, on top of, or higher than.

supination—Turning a body part upward; turning "palm up."

supine position—The patient lies flat on the back, face upward.

suppository—Solid medication that has a base of cocoa butter or glycerine and is designed to melt after insertion into a body cavity (e.g., the rectum or vagina).

surgery—The branch of medicine dealing with operative procedures to correct deformities, repair injuries, or treat disease.

surgical hose—Elastic or support hose used to support leg veins and increase circulation.

surgical scissors—Special scissors used to cut tissue.

surgical shave—Removal of hair and cleansing of skin prior to an operation.

suture—Surgical stitch used to join the edges of an incision or wound; also, an area where bones join or fuse together.

suture-removal set—Set of instruments, including suture scissors and thumb forceps, used to remove stitches (sutures).

sympathetic—That division of the autonomic nervous system that allows the body to respond to emergencies and stress; also, to understand and attempt to solve the problems of another.

symptom—A subjective indication of disease that is felt by the patient.

syncope—Fainting; temporary period of unconsciousness.

system—A group of organs and other parts that work together to perform a certain function.

systole—Period of work, or contraction, of the heart.

systolic pressure—Measurement of blood pressure taken when the heart is contracting and forcing blood into the arteries.

tachycardia—Fast, or rapid, heart beat (usually more than 100 beats per minute in an adult).

tactful—Able to do or say the correct thing; thoughtful.

tarsal—One of seven bones that forms the instep of the foot.

tartar—*See* calculus.

technician—A level of proficiency usually requiring a 2-year associate's degree or 3 to 4 years of on-the-job training.

technologist—A class of expertise in a health career field, usually requiring at least 3 to 4 years of college plus work experience.

temperature—The measurement of the balance between heat lost and heat produced by the body.

temporary—Dental material used for restorative purposes for a short period of time until permanent restoration can be done.

tendon—Fibrous connective tissue that connects muscles to bones.

tension—Uncomfortable inner sensation, discomfort, strain, or stress that affects the mind.

terminal illness—An illness that will result in death.

testes—Gonads or endocrine glands that are located in the scrotum of the male and that produce sperm and male hormones.

thalamus—That structure in the diencephalon of the brain that acts as a relay center to direct sensory impulses to the cerebrum.

therapeutic diet—Diet used in the treatment of disease.

therapy—Remedial treatment of a disease or disorder.

thermometer—Instrument used to measure temperature.

thoracic—Pertaining to the chest or thorax.

thoracic duct—Main lymph duct of the body; drains lymph from the lymphatic vessels into the left subclavian vein.

thrombocyte—Also called a *platelet*; blood cell required for clotting of the blood.

thrombus—A blood clot.

thymus—Organ in the upper part of the chest, lymphatic tissue, and endocrine gland that atrophies at puberty.

thyroid—Endocrine gland that is located in the neck and regulates body metabolism.

tibia—Inner and larger bone of the lower leg, between the knee and ankle.

tissue—A group of similar cells that join together to perform a particular function.

tissue forcep—An instrument with one or more fine points (teeth) at the tips of blades; used to grasp tissue.

tongue—Muscular organ of the mouth; aids in speech, swallowing, and taste.

tonometer—An instrument used to measure intraocular (within the eye) pressure.

tonsil—Mass of lymphatic tissue found in the pharynx (throat) and mouth.

tort—A wrongful or illegal act of civil law not involving a contract.

tourniquet—Device used to compress the blood vessels.

trachea—Windpipe; air tube from the larynx to the bronchi.

transdermal—Through the skin.

transfusion—Transfer of blood from one person to another person; injection of blood or plasma.

transverse plane—Imaginary line drawn through the body to separate the body into a top half and a bottom half.

Trendelenburg position—The patient lies on the back with the head lower than the feet, or with both the head and feet inclined downward.

tricuspid valve—Flap or cusp between the right atrium and right ventricle in the heart.

tri-flow syringe—Handpiece in dental units that provides air, water, or a combination of air and water for various dental procedures.

trifurcated—Having three roots (as do some teeth).

tuning fork—An instrument that has two prongs and is used to test hearing acuity.

24-hour urine specimen—Special urine test in which all urine produced in a 24-hour period is collected in a special container.

tympanic membrane—The eardrum.

typing and crossmatch—A determination of blood types and antigens prior to a blood transfusion.

ulcer—An open lesion on the skin or mucous membrane.

ulna—Long bone in the forearm, between the wrist and elbow.

ulnar deviation—Moving toward the little finger side of the hand.

ultrasonic unit—Piece of equipment that cleans with sound waves.

ultrasonography—Noninvasive, computerized scanning technique that uses high-frequency sound waves to create pictures of body parts.

ultra-speed handpiece—High-speed handpiece used in dental units to cut and prepare a tooth during a dental procedure.

umbilicus—Naval; in slang, "belly button."

Universal Method—Abbreviated means of identifying the teeth.

universal precautions—Recommendations that must be followed to prevent transmission of pathogenic organisms by way of blood and body fluids.

Unopette—Disposable, self-filling, blood-diluting pipette unit used for blood cell counts.

uremia—Excessive amounts of urea (a waste product) in the blood.

ureter—Tube that carries urine from the kidney to the urinary bladder.

urethra—Tube that carries urine from the urinary bladder to outside the body.

urinalysis—Examination of urine by way of physical, chemical, or microscopic testing.

urinary-drainage unit—Special device used to collect urine and consisting of tubing and a collection container usually connected to a urinary catheter.

urinary meatus—External opening of the urethra.

urinary sediments—Solid materials suspended in urine.

urinate—To expel urine from the bladder.

urine—The fluid excreted by the kidney.

urinometer—Calibrated device used to measure the specific gravity of urine.

urology—The branch of medicine dealing with urine and diseases of the urinary tract.

uterus—Muscular, hollow organ that serves as the organ of menstruation and the area for development of the fetus in the female.

vaccine—Substance given to an individual to produce immunity to a disease.

vagina—Tube from the uterus to outside the body in a female.

vaginal irrigation—Also called *douche*; injection of fluid into the vagina.

variable expense—In a budget, an expense that can change or be adjusted (e.g., expenses for clothing and entertainment).

varicose—Pertaining to distended, swollen veins.

vas deferens—Also called the *ductus deferens*; the tube that carries sperm and semen from the epididymus to the ejaculatory duct in the male.

vasoconstriction—Constriction (decrease in diameter) of the blood vessels.

vasodilation—Dilation (increase in diameter) of the blood vessels.

vein—Blood vessel that carries blood back to the heart.

venipuncture—Surgical puncture of a vein; inserting a needle into a vein.

venous—Pertaining to the veins.

ventral—Pertaining to the front, or anterior, part of the body; in front of.

ventricle—One of two lower chambers of the heart; also, a cavity in the brain.

venule—The smallest type of vein; connect capillaries and veins.

vertebrae—Bones of the spinal column.

vertigo—Sensation of dizziness.

vesicle—Blister; a sac full of water or tissue fluid.

vestibule—Small space or cavity at the beginning of a canal.

veterinary—Pertaining to the medical treatment of animals.

VICA—Vocational Industrial Clubs of America, a student organization for students enrolled in trade and industrial vocational programs.

villi—Tiny projections from a surface; in the small intestine, projections that aid in the absorption of nutrients.

virus—One of a large group of very small microorganisms, many of which cause disease.

visceral—Pertaining to organs.

vital signs—Determinations that provide information about body conditions; include temperature, pulse, respirations, and blood pressure.

vitamins—Organic substances necessary for body processes and life.

vitreous humor—Jellylike mass that fills the cavity of the eyeball, behind the lens.

void—To empty the bladder; urinate.

volume—The degree of strength of a pulse (e.g., strong or weak).

voluntary—Under one's control; done by one's choice or desire.

vomit—To expel material from the stomach and/or intestine through the mouth and/or nose.

vulva—External female genitalia; includes the labia majora, labia minora, and clitoris.

walker—A device that has a metal framework and aids in walking.

warm-water bottle—Rubber or plastic device designed to hold warm water for dry-heat application.

wellness—State of being in good health; well.

word root—Main word or part of word to which prefixes and suffixes can be added.

Workers' Compensation—Payment and care provided to an individual who is injured on the job.

wound—An injury to tissues.

xiphoid process—The small, bony projection at the lower end of the sternum (breastbone).

yellow marrow—Soft tissue in the diaphyses of long bones.